PSYCHIATRIC CONTOURS

THEORY IN FORMS

Series Editors

Nancy Rose Hunt, Achille Mbembe, and Todd Meyers

NANCY ROSE HUNT
& HUBERTUS BÜSCHEL

Psychiatric Contours

New African Histories of Madness

DUKE UNIVERSITY PRESS
Durham and London
2024

Project Editor: Lisa Lawley
Typeset in Untitled Serif by Westchester Publishing Services

Library of Congress Cataloging-in-Publication Data
Names: Hunt, Nancy Rose, editor. | Büschel, Hubertus, editor.
Title: Psychiatric contours : new African histories of madness /
Nancy Rose Hunt and Hubertus Büschel.
Other titles: Theory in forms.
Description: Durham : Duke University Press, 2024. | Series:
Theory in forms | Includes bibliographical references and index.
Identifiers: LCCN 2023037216 (print)
LCCN 2023037217 (ebook)
ISBN 9781478030348 (paperback)
ISBN 9781478026112 (hardcover)
ISBN 9781478059325 (ebook)
Subjects: LCSH: Psychiatry—Africa—History. | Psychiatry—
Social aspects—Africa. | Psychiatry—Political aspects—Africa. |
Imperialism—Psychological aspects. | Africa—Colonial
influence—Psychological aspects. | BISAC: HISTORY / Africa /
General | MEDICAL / History
Classification: LCC RC451.A35 P79 2024 (print) | LCC RC451.A35
(ebook) | DDC 616.890096—dc23/eng/20231227
LC record available at https://lccn.loc.gov/2023037216
LC ebook record available at https://lccn.loc.gov/2023037217

Cover art: Photograph, 2007, by Nancy Rose Hunt.

CONTENTS

FIGURES

PREFACE

This volume began to materialize when Hubertus Büschel organized a conference on "Global Histories of Psychiatry" at the University of Groningen in 2018. He remains grateful to all conference participants for their papers and debates. Initial versions of several chapters here—those by Büschel, Matthew Heaton, Richard Hölzl, Richard Keller, Sloan Mahone, and Jonathan Sadowsky, as well as the keynote by Nancy Rose Hunt—were part of those proceedings. Nancy also organized a panel on madness for the 8th European Conference on African Studies in Edinburgh. This 2019 session, sponsored by the International Africa Institute, London, included early versions of the chapters by Romain Tiquet and Nana Quarshie.

Hubertus is most grateful to his German funders, notably the German Research Foundation, for the conference funding and much more, including our index. Here, we extend many thanks to Eric and Doreen Anderson and their colleagues at Arc Indexing for their meticulous and intellectual labor on the index. The thorough work of Finn Patrick Bourke and Manyakhalé Diawara, both of the University of Kassel, as well as Tancrede Pagés of the United Nations University Institute on Comparative Regional Integration Studies in Bruges, provided precious editorial assistance for this volume. As the English-language speaker of our editorial pair, Nancy took the lead in critique and editing, working with the chapter authors, and not only by our French- and German-language speakers. She also worked closely with Finn (a master's student of Irish origin), an outstanding assistant and proofreader whose painstaking copyediting and bibliographic work led to important improvements in legibility and quality. Enthusiastic,

Finn never lost patience with the countless tasks at hand. We thank him wholeheartedly.

We extend much gratitude to our anonymous readers, selected by Duke University Press, for their critical readings of this book in manuscript form. We are also grateful to Achille Mbembe for his immediate enthusiasm before our book proposal. Sincere thanks go too to our always astute editor at Duke, Elizabeth Ault, for her eagerness, dedication, and speed. The entire team at Duke has been enormously helpful, efficient, and skilled, and that includes Benjamin Kossak and Christopher Robinson, as well as John Donohue of Westchester Publishing Services, for their editorial and copyediting services.

Many other colleagues and friends helped along the way as readers and those who inspired. Nancy extends much gratitude to Steven Feierman, Jean Comaroff, Patricia Hayes, and Todd Meyers for their alert readings and advice. She also remembers fondly her 2018 weeks in Paris (before and after going to Agadez), where she was trying out her first ideas about Africa's psychiatric historiography and its "trauma zones" from the Great Lakes to the Sahel. Without Nicholas Henckes, to whom I am most grateful, none of this would have happened in the same beautiful, critical way. Lastly, we thank Professor Todd Meyers for that precarious deep-winter errand, camera in tow, into transcultural psychiatry archives at McGill University, which provided source documents for chapter 6.

Finally, we are grateful to each other, for the spirited intellectual camaraderie spanning months, with many Zoom sessions, and a convivial interlude over a home-cooked meal in Berlin. Resonant was our outing, arranged by Hubertus, into the Vienna Forest and the town of Maria Gugging, whose psychiatric history stretches back to the Maria Gugging Psychiatric Clinic, founded in 1889. There, in the 1950s, the Austrian psychiatrist and writer about schizophrenia and art, Leo Navratil (1921–2006), had his patients make "Zustandsgebundene Kunst": art created during acute clinical states of mental illness and later showed in art contexts. Most of all, wonderful were the critical readings we shared with each other about our own texts, as well as the generosity in time and money for serious engagement with so many theoretical ideas, historiographical approaches, and methods. More than once we had to grapple with a challenging text or passage. These occasions generated small bursts of intellectual and ethical co-thinking, and from there we moved on to our next tasks.

Nancy Rose Hunt

INTRODUCTION

Madness, the Psychopolitical, and the Vernacular

Rethinking Psychiatric Histories

This volume seeks to ignite debate and experimentation within a broad field: histories and anthropologies of psychiatry and madness. Let's ask: How are we able to discern madness in any history or archive? It is critical to widen the spectrum for what may count as madness, in keeping with history's many variations and also the fresh historiographical edge offered here.

Consider the *Oxford English Dictionary*. It defines madness capaciously, with telling quotations from 1384 through 1990, embracing imprudence, delusion, wild foolishness, exuberance, uncontrollable rage, insanity, psychosis, and mental impairment (*Oxford English Dictionary* 2023a). Michel Foucault ([1961] 2006), in his 1961 history of madness, extended his reach from social perceptions of madness to the experiences of the mad and transgressive. For Africa, the challenges of periodizing and characterizing madness and psychiatry are different. Foucault placed the key rupture in his European history of madness in the seventeenth century with the widespread arrival of custodial care and internment. Yet as Megan Vaughan (1983, 1991) has pointed out, in most of colonial Africa, asylums only appeared sparsely, and not until the late nineteenth century.

Still, something other than his focus on confinement and early psychiatric science is what makes Foucault's work scintillating and necessary reading—as generative as Frantz Fanon—for Africanists and others writing postcolonial histories today. Foucault stressed the creativities surrounding madness and its representations, and he longed to hear the speech and sounds of the mad. His yearnings linger afresh in the experimental lines of this book, with each chapter somehow digging for pleas, tones, and stories mined from an archive.

It would be wrong to strictly oppose madness to the psychiatric—a hollow, misguided binary that. Rather, it is precisely Africa's psychiatric spaces that offer up many of the vivid, patient-authored archival slices deciphered here. These fragments emit words, sounds, and deliria. They also enable the intensity in interpretation that is the hallmark of this volume. Madness veers from, or gets entangled with, the psychiatric and also the psychopolitical. This point is worth pursuing further by asking where else madness, its clatter, thresholds, and forms may be hiding.

This volume joins that emerging, still slender field: madness histories from the Global South. A highlight here is the many histories of Africa's long decolonization, though other epochs are present. This introduction signals key concepts and registers by which madness and psychiatry may be traced, since the volume is intended for scholars across geographic fields, including historians and anthropologists of Africa and of psychiatry, and for students in a wide diversity of classrooms.

Plying the archive is a basic technique here, with chapters hewing close to the perplexities of diverse fragments. The book aims to breathe fresh life into that long-standing problematic. It also engages textures, sensibilities, and silences, and technologies, politics, and forms (Foucault 1972; Farge 1989; Derrida 1995; Trouillot 1995; Steedman 2001; Hamilton 2002; Stoler 2002, 2009). The chapters demonstrate how lively unexpected archival bits may become as their authors unfasten slices and expose psychopolitical and mirroring effects. Amid such intricacies, intimate, official, and vernacular dimensions emerge. Subjectivities flicker in, in startling and generative ways.

Many chapters open new conceptual ground, working across institutional and intimate scales and attending to the perceptions of patients, kin, and clinicians, among other figures. Lurking are state, institutional, and clinical regimes, suggestive of the psychopolitics of state, policing, security, and persecutory platforms. Most terrains are Africa-based, but the implications extend across racialized worlds.

Most histories of madness, everywhere, draw near to the psychiatric (Eghigian 2017). A few follow that fervent literary tendency of the 1990s, when vast "waves of writing turned to 'madness' to signify everything" (Pietikäinen 2015, 3). Others combine the objective and the subjective, drawing on metaphorical, symbolic, or psychoanalytic registers. Complex textures, delinked from the clinical, unravel situations of madness.

Powerful histories, this book shows, join milieus, psychopathologies, and selves. Psychopathology often begins out of a toxic milieu (Canguilhem 2012; Hunt 2016). The poison or harm may stem from a family (Winnicott [1965] 2006), a racialized or colonial situation (Sadowsky 1996, 1999), or a camp—as defined by Giorgio Agamben (2000), a biopolitical space of exception.

Social exclusions and riots yield much about turbulence, madness, forms, and figurations. Such may be unmoored from psychiatry and its category work. Yet, for colonial worlds, racialized injury, stemming from violence, segregations, and exclusions, fueled agitation and insurgency (Hunt 2016). Still, vernacular healing and charms often intervened, in discreet, secretive, dramatic, or insurrectionary ways (Littlewood and Lipsedge 1982; Bhugra and Littlewood 2002; Mahone and Vaughan 2007).

The vernacular may embrace healing technologies, persons, and practices. It suggests a social category (healers), a spatiality (township or shrine), or a tonality (rage, ambivalence, or hankering). Small clues may be pressed to draw out objects, places, or frictions. And I argue here that, given the vexed nature of the word *vernacular*, it is rewarding to poise the vernacular in relation to the "residual," taking account of those elements in a present that were "effectively formed in the past," yet are "still active in the cultural process," "effective" in the present, as Raymond Williams (1977) luminously suggested. I return to this vexed word below.

Psychiatric Strands in Africa's Many Histories

Much can be gained by attending to singular episodes from African histories. Each discussed here suggests the continent's psychiatric contours of madness.

Psychopathologies associated with "difference" emerged in Africa's contact zones by the seventeenth century, and more powerfully from the nineteenth century, a time that Gilles Deleuze (2008, 16) glossed powerfully as "paranoid imperialist formations." Those who suffered or acted out had nightmares, heard voices, or sensed their special capacities for visionary seeing, divination, and spirit possession. Others developed skills in healing somatic, social, and psychic maladies. That affliction is a path for healing is an idea as old as the seventeenth century (Feierman 1979, 1981; Janzen 1982; Hunt 2013b), though likely much older (Schoenbrun 2007).

From the late nineteenth century, merchants, anthropologists, missionaries, and colonial officials brought European notions of madness to Africa, as they began to colonize the continent. The attentive among them noticed that Africans resorted to possession and trance, had diverse ways of organizing care, and used copious consecrated charms. Many epics (Biebuyck with Mateene 1969) and oral traditions from precolonial polities speak about trickster figures and deranged monarchs. Consider Shaka, the Zulu king gone mad (Eldredge 2014), rendered as insane in Thomas Mofolo's (1931) novel. Shaka's harshly autocratic reign (1816–28) blurred with perceptions of his madness and use of terror to govern (Hamilton 1998). Soon and nearby, a missionary was collecting Zulu traditions that told of vernacular nightmares, trembling, madness, and kind or vengeful ancestral interventions (Callaway [1885] 2019; Lee 2021).

In Johannes Fabian's (2000) study of nineteenth-century explorers in central Africa, madness manifested when some European men seemed "out of their minds." Their irrationalities went with quiet, cannabis-induced *ecstatis* within such early colonial scenes of scientific inquiry. Such madness could seem more lighthearted than pathological, while the "mad frenzies" (Hokkanen 2018) of early European colonialists in Malawi involved mental agony, imperial tensions, and the plentiful consumption of quinine.

Madness has long permeated colonial histories of crisis and alienation in Africa. The label *superstition* distorts maladies, therapeutics, and forms. Madness could erupt in a refuge, a religious gathering, or a rebellion, as in Simon Kimbangu's life (Martin 1975; Vellut 2005). Likewise, a Libreville man turned delirious after participating in Bwiti, a religion with rituals known for healing mental states, and one of Africa's finest ethnographies ever of mental images and the religious imagination (Fernandez 1982).

Maria N'koi emerged in 1915 as a disruptive, insurgent woman healer, a decade after a spate of suicides in a violent, derelict colony, King Leopold's

Congo. Madness lay not always with *reactive suicides* in this milieu. In poetic, analogical patterns, madness would appear through a strong idiom: trembling trees. Possessed, distraught women knotted themselves up in high branches and vines, as if cut asunder and quaking in the wind. In Maria N'koi's domain, women entered into months of ceremonial dancing, alternating between quaking and quiet (Hunt 2016).

Missionaries translated such afflictions as *neurasthenia* (Hunt 2016). This European psychiatric attribution had no clinical effect in this early colonial world with few doctors. Yet the language of nervous trembling, barrenness, and spirit-shaken trees was *residual* and thus *vernacular*, to use the vocabulary that I develop further below. Each disturbed woman also entered into a trancelike "crisis of presence" (Martino 2012): she was possessed. These healing methods from a Congolese *shrunken milieu*, shriveled by force and many disappointments, were part of a therapeutic pattern found across a wide region that morphed with nervous dances and insurgencies during this acute decade (Hunt 2016). Kenya's Taita context of the 1950s, explored in this volume by Mahone (chapter 7), also combined emergency and possession as crucial streams.

Megan Vaughan (1983) pointed out in her prized essay "Idioms of Madness" that only a tiny proportion of Nyasaland's mentally disturbed ever reached the notice of the colonial authorities. Yet diviners, healers, and the possessed were active, operating like psychotherapists. A different view of colonial madness emerges out of Albert Schweitzer's iconic hospital in rural Gabon, where the year 1927 saw a man named Njambi arriving in chains after murdering someone in a mad fit of rage. Schweitzer glossed etiology in pejorative and primitivist terms, aligning madness with superstition. Njambi was still present at Schweitzer's hospital three decades later. This special patient moved about aplenty, since the famous doctor's treatment was manual labor, except during his angry outbursts when confinement or pharmaceuticals were Schweitzer's remedies. Sometimes Schweitzer intervened by calming his patient with words or his mere presence. Njambi became an everyday element in this racialized clinical space. He perceived the hospital as home, a protector from menacing forces. Yet this patient was rare. This Gabonese hospital provided residential care for few *madmen* over the decades, even if it incorporated the special Njambi fervently (Zumthurm 2020).

Shula Marks (1988) worked from an amazing cache of letters and with special ethnographic sensibilities, and she portrayed a radically different web of colonial relations and spaces. With a strong epistolary strand, fraught words between a white British Fabian woman and Lily Moya, a lonely Black South African schoolgirl from the Transkei, come vividly alive. Marks tracked down the boarding school and the girl's kin relations, as well as the asylum where she landed. Similarly, Megan Vaughan (2005) sensed that a flurry of letters, written by a subaltern clerk in colonial Nyasaland through his relentless use of a typewriter, were an important trove, and she mined them for suggestions of lunacy and humiliation.

Who could write always matters. Asylum care—or harm—is a staple of Africa's psychiatric histories (Vaughan 1983; Deacon 1996; Marks 1999; Sadowsky 1999; Jackson 2005). The spaces have varied, with some more segregated and insidious than others. From the interwar years, it was not unusual to witness bursts of rage and categorize them as *acute mania*. Such was the case for Isaac O., a literate nineteen-year-old in colonial Nigeria. He began to act strangely and was seen nearly naked on a highway in 1932. Once arrested and interned, he contested his confinement in the Yaba Lunatic Asylum. A copious documentary trail followed, as did his release from a prison and asylum. Conflicts emerged between him and the authorities over a *juju* tree and a curse. Sadowsky (1996) contextualizes the patient's delusions in relation to colonial domination, and by 1945 Isaac O. was back in Yaba. To interject Raymond Williams's (1977) versatile language again, elaborated below, *residual*, *emergent*, and *dominant* colonial registers mingled in Isaac O.'s story. And they combined with *vernacular* elements—a curse and the juju tree. (These elements furthered Sadowsky's [1999, 48–52] subtle interpretations of patient writings found in case files.)

Wulf Sachs ([1937] 1996; Dubow 1993) is iconic. In 1928, this Jewish psychiatrist was working with Black schizophrenic patients at the Pretoria Mental Hospital. In 1929–30, Sachs underwent psychoanalysis in Berlin and came into contact with Sigmund Freud. Soon, Sachs was inviting an urban Rhodesian healer, John Chavafambira, onto his psychoanalytic couch in 1930s Johannesburg. This healer-entrepreneur, a fascinating human instance of the vernacular,[1] narrated to Sachs his autobiography and dreams. He harked back to his father and grandfather, healer figures, and was keen to find—through Sachs and their big city—modern forms of expression and success. Repertoires of vernacular healing a few generations deep unfold within Chavafambira's biography, enigmatically composed by Sachs. So did his current practice as a healer and diviner in the city. His aspirations were intense, and over time his ambivalence toward the white psychoanalyst grew. Sachs's affection, anger, and ambitions were fraught.

The discord that transpired within this strange colonial duet has enabled many significant reflections since (Dubow 1993).

Cold War historiography and traces (Geissler et al. 2016; Roschenthaler and Diawara 2016; Vaughan 2016; Herzog 2017) have become an important new edge in African history, including its histories of madness. Fine inquiries into ethnopsychiatry in colonial and fascist worlds as well as the figures who pushed forward transitions toward transcultural psychiatry and psychoanalysis are emerging (Deluz 1991; McCulloch 1995; Heaton 2013; Herzog 2017; Collignon 2018; Antic 2019; Kilroy-Marac 2019; Delille 2020), including some transformative Swiss ethnopsychoanalysts who visited Africa, like Paul Parin (Parin 1980; Reichmayr 2020; Conci 2023). Terror, torture, and madness have opened up the psychopolitics of postcolonial regimes, like those of Jean-Bedel Bokassa (Titley 1997; Shoumatoff 1988), Idi Amin (Pringle 2019; Leopold 2021), and Mobutu Sese Seko (Wrong 2000). Dictatorial ambitions mixed in Africa with psychopathology or that idiomatic word, madness.

Prophets, City Wanderers, and Global Mental Health

If we turn to everyday lives in African cities since the 1960s, the numbers of persons found wandering, ecstatic, or confused—often labeled with that vexed word, schizophrenic—deserve analysis, tallying, and phenomenological reflection (Corin 1998; Henckes 2019; cf. Bateson 1972). There is episodic data: some poetic (Yoka 1999; Tonda 2021), some individualized or intriguing. Some have gone far by studying the subjectivities and conditions of one striking and deranged figure in a setting of precarity (Biehl 2005). Others have theorized subjectivities and subjections around "postcolonial disorders" in diverse settings (Good et al. 2008).

Julien Bonhomme (2008) writes of one lunatic, André Ondo Mba of Libreville, seen with a colonial helmet and ever busy, wandering. This *schizophrenic*—the word is Bonhomme's—made graffiti all over Gabon's capital (among parallels, see Büschel, chapter 3). Using supernatural language, he wrote on city surfaces while "blending mystical, sexual, and political themes." Born in 1943, he fell mad during a 1980s Bwiti initiation, itself a foray into occult forces. His chronic psychotic condition, sometimes labeled paranoid, enabled creativity. Aligned with God, his life seemed a set of miracles. As he wrote his revelations down daily, thousands of pages on scrap paper and public walls mounted up. Obsessed with science and white people, he copied bureaucratic knowledge and listened to voices through a loudspeaker with supernatural shivers. While ridiculing the Gabonese state, his status as madman kept him from being arrested. His textuality in graffiti form, like his visibility as public wanderer, came to align the city with divination.

Hasty classifications will always be problematic. Prophetic deliria and other ascriptions of madness emerge out of all kinds of African settings, before moving into diverse scholarly reflections. A history of when and how the wandering of *les fous* (mad people) became so prominent in Africa's postcolonial cities is an important historical question. The answers will surely be multiple, related to precarity, chaos, and securitizing regimes. At the same time, the alignment of prophets with madness is very old in Africa and the Caribbean, where this conjuncture landed many insurgent and oracular rebels in hospitals, jails, asylums, and in everyday streets (Edgar and Sapire 2000; Palmié 2002; Brown 2003; Bilby and Handler 2004; Hunt 2016; Brown 2020).

Global Mental Health is a recent, partially scientific phenomenon. Unveiled in the 2000s, the powerful rubric has many ambitions and tentacles (Summerfield 2012; Lovell 2019a) and wide zones of activity: in poverty, clinical trials, NGOs. Mixed in are postwar trauma work, group therapy for paying middle classes, and community work in needy villages and refugee camps. Its reach extends to humanitarianism, evidence-based science, and technologies of securitization (Howell 2011). Global Mental Health beckons for sensitive ethnographic research on its "emergence" as well as accruing forms of "self-evidence" (Daston 2007, 808). Some criticize the imperial resonances and implications of Global Mental Health (Summerfield 2012; Ecks 2016; Rose 2018; Beneduce 2019). Yet its processes of translation and distortion are rarely studied with care. A critical analysis might take in a range of languages—psychoanalytic (Hall 2018), religious, pharmaceutical, carceral—or even draw on critical race theory (Du Bois 2007; Moodley, Mujtaba, and Kleiman 2018).

Relevant also is a "psycho-therapeutic turn" (De Vos 2011) within humanitarian aid. This strand began in the 1990s, when trauma eclipsed hunger as the most flagged issue by international aid agencies. Both streams—the psychiatric and the psychosocial—deserve sensitive attention to patient and expert experiences, textualities, and muteness. In central Africa, the word *madness* has long been on many lips. Yet the mental suffering of children and others in zones of war often knows waiting and unspeakability (Waugh et al. 2007; Goltermann 2010; Otake 2019;

Salisbury 2020), even if they have inspired theoretical and clinical innovation (Polat 2017).

In emergency zones of neoliberal Africa, *psy* discourses have been translating traumatic experience into new lexicons. New categories are conjoined with idioms, weighed down by the psychiatric yet shaped by vernacular elements speaking to residual traces from the past. These idioms may be adopted in speech, interiorized by those seeking care, or offer up confessional forms of exposure therapy. PTSD is a rich category and vein for investigation (Fassin and Rechtman 2009), just as Sadowsky (chapter 5) shows depression as a plentiful historical seam.

Most everywhere in Africa—chaotic city streets, PTSD zones, and carceral energies directed at migrants moving across borders—we find theaters of madness. Many are intermixed with healing churches, mosques, spirit possession, or the clinical kiosks of *tradi-practiciens,* healers often in a quasi-clinical, mimetic mode. Mixed into *psy* languages are vernacular words, linking pasts with a present. In our still neoliberal time, the psychiatric remains a dominant register, and only partly due to Global Mental Health (Lovell 2019a, 2019b). Yet many are the mediations of residual elements amid digital economies or the traumatic memories of a generation (Behrouzan 2020).

Niches and Category Work

How to categorize any mental illness is always refractory, while the distribution of care is an important matter to study. Which symptoms or maladies align with idiomatic words for "madness," with psychological disturbance, or specific categories? At the same time, Africa knows just a scattering of hospital psychiatrists.

Muted within this volume is the arrival into Africa of the psychotic medications that remade psychiatry globally from the 1950s, just as wards were emptying, restraint forms diminishing, and WHO pharmaceutical guidelines entering. Likewise, we still know too little about postcolonial psychiatry in Africa (yet see Akyeampong, Hill, and Kleinman 2015). The first African psychiatrists and psychiatric nurses are quietly suggested here, later generations not at all. A serious, sensitive, and well-trained African psychiatrist, who was working in a small Catholic psychiatric hospital in eastern Congo in 2019, now is working for a big international NGO in the Sahel. Money talks: he wants to support his family and keep up with school fees. In most of Congo, indeed across most of rural Africa, there are no or few psychiatrists and caseloads are immense.

Subaltern assistants in asylums and clinics have surely been important through their labor, care, transactions, and bricolage. "Middle figures" (Hunt 1999) would have reshaped vernacular fragments, lexemes, and claims. This is a rich area for which more research is needed for all periods. Little is known about how patient experiences align with vernacular or biomedical ideas, inside and outside of traumatized zones.

Clinical psychiatry, it should be remembered, hardly would have touched the lives of Africans across all epochs suggested here. Today, official discourse about mental health may suggest that 2–5 percent of the population are ill, while some 95 percent of Africans are still thinking and acting in terms of what I have generalized here as vernacular practice. Is the incoherent person walking through a countryside or city, with vines or collected debris trailing behind, and suffering from a relative's curse, bad or "mad" in emic eyes? It is helpful to embrace "techniques of nearness," to use Walter Benjamin's marvelous phrase (1999, 545; Hunt 2016) when unpacking local words and interpretations, as well as milieus. Africans arriving at war-zone clinics in some regions might be treated for one nonpsychological condition after another, while their afflictions stemmed from trauma. When is treatment strongly pharmacological in Africa, with what medications? In fact, relatives and neighbors deal with the vast majority of mental disturbance, at least in rural Africa. Many psychiatric cases coming into medical or carceral institutions arrive with violence: agitated, turbulent, they cannot be managed at home.

Category errors are difficult to avoid. Still, category work should begin with vernacular words and idioms, and also with psychiatric and medical words at play. The ambiguities and mixtures are legion. And, the researcher's evolving vocabulary—what is "mad," vernacular, emic, schizophrenic, and the like—needs to keep the uncertainties in mind while seeking out greater specificities about meanings and patterns of resort.

In *Mad Travelers* (1998), an important psychiatric history set in France, Ian Hacking narrated the emergence and decline of a diagnostic category in the nineteenth century. He argued for attending to *ecological niches* that enable new symptoms to swell. A new category goes with many persons presenting with the novel malady. A niche may be worked out through the nuanced factors that generated the new category. This European history resonates with several chapters here. A niche may explain the psychopathologies of slavery or colonial racism. Yet I still prefer Georges

Canguilhem's (2012) term *milieu*, which is in keeping with the way Georges Balandier (1951) signaled the magnitude of "social pathology" in the decolonizing of equatorial Africa of the 1950s. Many a milieu generated colonial psychopathologies, whether of a state, securitizing practices, nervous zones, or analogous registers and scales (Revel 1996; Hunt 2016).

Madness may be individualized, or it may take on collective forms. A person may ignite a mood or rebellion with implications for public order. Some psychoses erupt as violent madness, as Good and Good (2010) showed for the masses "running *amuk*" in 1997 Indonesia. Yolanda Pringle (2019) has investigated how Uganda's early postcolonial state confronted "mass hysteria" in the 1960s, when a "psychic epidemic" of unstoppable laughter mixed with violence and affliction. W. J. T. Mitchell found something similar in the "affective temporality of the Trump presidency" and American rallies of madness. He turned to a frequently quoted line of Friedrich Nietzsche: "Insanity in individuals is somewhat rare. But in groups, parties, nations, and epochs, it is the rule" (Mitchell 2018). These words are not unfitting for Africa or for most colonized worlds.

Just as *category work* is a growing thread of analysis, pulling in collective or individualized directions,[2] Delille and Crozier (2018), in their fine history of transcultural psychiatry since the 1950s, explain that *epistemic objects*—like *amok*, schizophrenia, and refugee suffering—may convert and standardize case histories and conditions. Such objects enabled transcultural psychiatry to emerge as semiautonomous in relation to psychiatry. Similarly, Henckes, Hess, and Reinholdt (2018, 2, 12) use psychopathological "fringes" to conceptualize "zones of vagueness" within psychiatric practice. Ranging from culture-bound syndromes to psychotic risk, some diagnoses may unsettle classifications or destabilize expert knowledge.

Working out such forms of doubt and hesitation in African zones may yield insights and nuance. Controversies over categorization may take place among some mixture of anthropologists, psychiatrists, psychoanalysts, "African moderns,"[3] or healers, whether in conversation or not, or provoke conflict or debate (Parle 2007). The interwar psychoanalyst Wulf Sachs ([1937] 1996) discussed diagnostic categories with the Rhodesian healer who he angled onto his psychoanalytic couch in 1930s Johannesburg. Similarly, in the 1960s, the Nigerian psychiatrist Thomas Adeoye Lambo overturned remnants of racism through reshaping colonial psychiatric categories (Heaton 2013). Moreover, from the 1940s, Kenya's too-powerful psychiatrist of that colony and of Mau Mau, J. C. Carothers, was busy honing diagnostics in demeaning, racist, and violent ways (Carothers 1947; McCulloch 1995).

In colonial or decolonizing situations, category work spills out everywhere, every day, well beyond conventional psychiatry of the day. Such a dispersal arises when mania, possession, insurgencies, and prophetic currents come into play. African patients, kin, and healers objectified illness beside colonial categories and suspicions. Tentative boundaries abound in fraught situations almost everywhere. The Italian anthropologist Ernesto de Martino (2012) clarified magic as a subaltern technique, one used to combat hate, poverty, and suffering before situations of humiliation and marginality. Spirit possession is liminal, its trance-like states situated between illness and healing, the visible and the invisible. In colonial Africa, missionaries, authorities, and medics were wont to translate spirit possession into coarse psychiatric categories. Yet Africans had their own diagnostic languages, drawing on "vampire stories" (White 2000) and other traces of accusation, resentment, and sorcery. The key actors were rarely psychiatrists. Yet sometimes, as Büschel, Mahone, and Keller (chapters 3, 7, and 8) tell in this volume, they would show up with reading suggestions, political sensibilities, or cameras, and work against dominant psychiatric strains.

Historians of psychiatry usually attend to experts—psychiatrists or others who published or left traces in institutional archives. Yet in situations saturated with racialized power, the categories of Europeans tended to be primitivist, while the category work of Africans unfolded in spaces of dominant, racialized control. Thus, it is important to ask: When and how did categories—African or European, "traditional" or modern—get reified or overlap? Psychiatric case notes may distort. Brittle clichés construe and condense the "primitive" (see Hölzl, chapter 2), while only some encounters with vernacular speech and practice involved seeking out knowledge and understanding (see Büschel, Heaton, and Keller, chapters 3, 6, and 8). At the same time, African knowledge about a colonial milieu as forceful, dangerous, or pathological circulated, often with rage. The ensuing friction could generate frenzy or "therapeutic insurgencies" (Hunt 2016).

Few colonial Africans, even self-identifying moderns, sought out cosmopolitan psychiatry. Nor was this clinical science much on offer. Yet the diagnostic grids of sensitive Europeans who listened and observed do suggest a broadening of categories through exchanges with patients and kin or grappling with ethnographic perplexities (Sachs [1937] 1996; Field 1960). As early as the 1850s, Lemba healing texts from the lower Congo (Janzen

1982) and Amazulu traditions from South Africa (Callaway [1885] 2019) told of derangement, deliria, uncontrollable hiccups, the vengeful anger of deceased ancestors, and wealth achieved through selling enslaved persons. Psychiatric experts, like Wulf Sachs in South Africa or Margaret Field in the Gold Coast (see Hunt, chapter 10), might condescend or stretch to understand emic terms and practices.

Whether enwrapped in the secular or religious, in the biomedical, carceral, or vernacular, category work in colonial psychiatric laboratories could either reproduce or unsettle conditions of power. Primitivist fancy could distort when facing clinical doubt (Henckes, Hess, and Reinholdt 2018) or when enmeshed in political entanglements. When historians find patient words or deeds, psychiatrists often seem to be nearby. Colonial psychiatry, dominant, battled with emergent vernacular scenes and spectacles. Such was the case with the frightful distortions of Mau Mau, shaped by Kenya's racist psychiatrist, J. C. Carothers, and the terrified British regime. Kenya's extraordinary *pipeline*, with many detention centers and work camps, was the way that the British moved rebels and detainees through a set of psychological spaces and stages. The idea was always to remake minds and separate out opponents (White 1990; McCulloch 1995).[4] Binary colonial juxtapositions—like the modern and the primitive (Cooper 1988)—assisted in generating ignorance and opacities during Mau Mau, and among them was the idea that the Mau Mau were madmen in need of psychiatrists like Carothers.

Seeking out the emergent in modern expressive forms may not undo such a contentious polarity. Yet the exercise can track effects, and even wander in new directions.

Sensing and Sensibilities

This book senses subjects from the eighteenth century forward—patients, kin, elites, the enslaved, experts—and it hears them in new kinds of ways. A common historiographic sensibility is suggested. Whether we use the words *connected* (Subrahmanyam 1997), *provincialized* (Chakrabarty 2007), or *decentered* (Davis 2006; Büschel 2020), global historians of madness aim to understand how psychiatric practice has metamorphosed over time.

Yet, the question is usually less about psychiatry's insistences than about what Africans did with such practices and experiments entering their lives. Many reworked the psychiatric through denial, refusal, or by upending figurations of the modern (cf. Chakrabarty 2007, 16, 22). Madness as the ordinary, as Mehdi and Tiquet (2020) importantly show, must be investigated in relation to spaces and epochs. Rather than applying strict chronologies, it is helpful to appreciate slow, uneven temporal shifts toward "modernity" (Koselleck 2018), concretely and within imaginaries.

Many of Africa's novelists have narrated madness alongside war, frightful regimes, and city streets. Treating novels as an archive yields a trove worth careful historical mining (Hunt 2007). Madness in Africa knows dazzling works by Wole Soyinka, Sony Labou Tansi, Bessie Head, Chinua Achebe, Alain Mabanckou, Antonio Antunes, David Diop, Bessie Head, and Biyi Bandele-Thomas. Their novels and short stories, whether suggesting magical realism or psychopolitics, probe madness beside the "borderlines of the body" (Veit-Wild 2006). All spark ideas for historical investigation. Consider Achebe's short story "The Madman" ([1972] 1991). Set in a seemingly timeless Nigerian village, his story turns on a series of confrontations between a naked madman and an eminent Igbo man who erred by ridiculing the mad one. When the iconic mad outcast spots the arrogant upstart bathing outdoors, he runs off with this big man's clothes. This parvenu, naked, flees in distress, tumbling into an occult and hazardous space where his madness is congealed. European and psychiatric places are absent. Rather, Achebe intertwines the costs of bombastic snickering with a vengeful lunatic within an ambiguous time suggesting the precolonial.

Three Key Concepts

Three concepts incite further reflection for histories of madness and psychiatry. Each may stir a heuristic or further theoretical debate, or together they may ignite historical and ethnographic imaginations before the many psychiatric contours found in African, indeed all subaltern worlds.

Concept 1. Madness

Madness is a word with many guises. Often slotted in as an alternative for psychosis, with neurosis lurking too, madness is a polysemic term that fell to the wayside within psychiatry as the classificatory dimensions to this science intensified. Yet the word *madness* retains value in histories of race and colonial processes, and well beyond forms of estrangement. The antagonisms of a racialized milieu breed bewilderment, paranoia, agitation, delusion, alienation, misrecognition, and melancholia. Madness as a heuristic is a way of reckoning with such dimensions and registers, taking in the eccentric (cf. Brecher 2013), the deranged, and the stigmatized.

Madness may blur with diagnostics: the classification of symptoms. Yet how did psychiatric categories meet other modes and materialities of a religious, literary, or vernacular nature, when sizing up the strange, the frenzied, or disturbed? Suicide often folds in, as it has in Africa's histories (Iliffe 2004; Vaughan 2012). Hokkanen (2018; cf. Schmidt 2008) offers good reasons to be careful before the capacious word *madness*, preferring crises of the mind in his history of white imperialists. Moving from imperial to vernacular dimensions can keep *madness* energetic, everyday, or metaphorical. The term often suggests the pathological, whether in a psychiatric sense, through colonial frictions, or due to an expanding range of figurations or decisive events.

Foucault's (1961, 195–97) words are important for those working on modern Africa. He distinguished the early modern as the epoch when madness was "present in the social horizon as an aesthetic and daily fact." Such a formulation—madness as an aesthetic horizon—is useful for thinking about derangements and crises in Africa across all epochs. It intimates the perceptible, the sensory, and the repugnant. Foucault is also useful since he yearned for voices of the mad while moving beyond social perceptions of them. He saw madness as integrally human, embracing insights unavailable to reason, like passionate deliria, unstructured paroxysms, and deviations from a norm. His chronology for Europe remains different than Africa's, since his key rupture fell in mid-seventeenth-century France or Europe when isolating the mad inside moralizing therapies and spaces of confinement was pivotal (Foucault 2006; Gutting 2019). Madness at that juncture, Foucault argued, became more silent and a realm of exclusion, aspects that remain quite rare in much of contemporary Africa.

Megan Vaughan (1983, 1991) pointed out long ago that Africa never knew a "great confinement," even if southern Africa's settler colonies knew many asylums, with more for European patients than Black (Swartz 2017). Foucault (1961, 197), importantly, also wrote that when psychiatry became dominant in Europe, "madness . . . in all its vivacity" faded away. This volume, implicitly and explicitly, draws attention to this word *vivacity*. Such exuberance goes well—in moods, tempo, and poetics—with African episodes and forms of madness, again for all periods. African imaginations—moral, religious, and therapeutic—have long combined human-caused misfortune (still often coined by Africans and scholars as *witchcraft*) with somatic and psychic maladies or with animate divine energies mediating between the visible and the invisible worlds. The visible leans toward the material, the observable, and the everyday. The invisible embraces the dead, the ancestors and spirits. In African histories, this divide is as ancient as farming societies, so often on the move.

Still, African histories are less marked by a singular rupture, in the transformative way imagined by Foucault for his European history of madness. Rather, many African healers, chiefs, and kings, especially in a precolonial time of long ago, passed through a phase of madness. Such liminality in initiation or possession, as a "psychic awakening," might entail insomnia, crying, and hearing voices. A Zulu healer became like a "house of dreams," demonstrating that a spell of madness may go with gaining "an appropriate frame of mind and sensitivity to the spirit world" (Lee 2021, 159; as found in the problematic yet valuable: Callaway [1885] 2019). Something similar happened when being initiated into Bwiti (Fernandez 1982; Bonhomme 2008), as we saw above, or with Zimbabwean children when handling the effects of postcolonial war (Reynolds 1996).

Foucault's word *vivacity*, I again insist, opens many registers of madness for African spaces, today or in various pasts. Animated, boisterous elements push interpretation in manifold directions, from a realm of fancy to therapeutic theaters of the occult (Achebe [1972] 1991). The performances of the deranged, like incessant motion of city wanderers, may frighten neighbors, strangers, and passersby. Or they may yield wonder, delight, even paranoia. Africa's streets continue to be a realm of vivacity, where the mad are visible, energetic, and frightful. It is worthwhile investigating vivacity further, during colonial conquest as well as some of Africa's diverse—labor, political, biopolitical—stabilizations. The stakes were often rough and gritty. Some went stark raving mad. Audacious mutinies landed rebels in jails, asylums, or unmarked graves (Martin 1975; Edgar and Sapire 2000). Africans still use effervescence to get by or insist no, with vivacious semblances of insanity in their uprisings, their streets, and their art forms.

Even if confinement in Africa's asylums tended to be relatively thin, historians are unrelenting when seeking out archives. Psychiatric historians have gravitated toward big and minor asylums for source material and, as this volume shows, some are unearthing new riches. Aesthetic attention has been slim, however, though we would do well to bring in this aspect more, in relation to smells, the sensory, the sartorial, nudity, or street graffiti (Collignon 1984; Bonhomme 2008; Akana 2013). If we deepen vernacular or hypermodern strands, Foucault's vocabulary of manifestation and revelation becomes relevant. Such is true for Africa's religious histories with prophets arising, speaking against state or missionary powers, before being sent to prisons or asylums, as was the case for Congo's Simon Kimbangu and South Africa's Nontetha Nkwenkwe (Edgar and Sapire 2000). Some quite educated patients manifested madness through their writing, revealing anger, illness, and the autobiographical (Marks 1988). Subtle approaches in history and anthropology suggest that the use of the word *madness* has been increasing and also mutating (Pinto 2020). The word's capaciousness remains precious for all imaginative histories of madness, and the chapters in this volume make important incisions into these fluid semantics.

Concept 2. Psychopolitics

I turn now to another protean term, *psychopolitics*, and its adjectival form, the psychopolitical. The meanings have shifted since Peter Sedgwick ([1982] 2015, 245) dared to critique the "politicization of mental illness" by radical antipsychiatrists during a British time of crisis over issues of mental health provision (Staub 2011; P. Thomas 2019; cf. Richert 2019). Psychopolitics returns us to Foucault on governmentalities (Burchell, Gordon, and Miller 1991; Prozorov 2021), as in the mental health policies of the World Health Organization (WHO) or of any national regime. More recently, the German-based philosopher Byung-Chul Han (2017) expressed neoliberal rage at totalitarian tendencies in mental health assistance: those that oblige the accepting of help. The term may also suggest "how to use psychology in politics," as the neuropsychiatrist Jean-Michel Oughourlian (2012, 4–5) declared in relation to scapegoating or violent rivalries among crowds and nations.

The *psychopolitical* may exude a political mood. Frenzy can bleed into insurgencies or mix with the euphoric, as in "a collective outbreak of madness" during some postcolonial Congolese lootings (Devisch 1995, 607). The mad have been aligned with kings, heads of state, and presidents in various histories on a global scale. When looking at monarchy- or state-based encounters with madness in Africa, taut scenes of fury and defiance surface across a *longue durée*. Moods, atmospheres, and spaces of experience are important, yet not all psychopolitics show up as aggression, diminution, or hospitalization. Nor were the so-called mad always subaltern.[5]

In an excellent discussion for European history, Freis (2019, 20) glosses the psychopolitical as "the encounter and entanglement of psychiatric and political thought," demonstrating intersections within psychiatry and mental hygiene in interwar Austria, Germany, and Switzerland. This fine way offers much but tends to leave out "patients," never mind emic interjections from a lower stratum. For Africa, interactions among the psychiatric and the political perhaps call for layers in relation to something unsettled, "braided" (Mukherji 2016), or a triggering milieu. The latter might be a slave ship (see chapter 10), a prison, a refugee camp, or tax rebellion.

Opposing madness and normality makes less sense in a situation where hostility was regular, racialized, and psychopathological. The psychopolitical also may go energetic or creative. It is important to question those discourses about mental illness that conceal "the creative, positive aspect of psychotic phenomena" or "discreet, everyday madness" (Leader 2011, 8, 329). How madness, vivacity, and humor become aligned depends on situation and genre. Within Africa's epics, stories, or psychiatric case files, some brimming with patient jottings, laughter may sound, erupt, or be heard.

If some forms of therapy aim to "create a safe place in which to live" (Leader 2011, 330), the hostilities and humiliations of a state of exception—whether the camp is colonial, racialized, or for the displaced as refugees—may render safety out of reach. Reading Frantz Fanon suggests "pressures of fantasy," and racialized dreams may work to constitute colonial cultures (Lebeau 1998, 113). His words about the persecutory effects of alienation remain very important. Following Jacques Lacan, Fanon knew language was key, with madness "lived within the register of meaning" with "every delusional phenomenon" ultimately "spoken" (Fanon in Khalfa and Young 2018, 171–72). Emily Apter (2018) pushes psychopolitics toward such racial experiences and affects, recalling Nietzsche's *ressentiments* and recuperating Fanon, alongside Achille Mbembe (2016) on everyday racism.

It is important to attend to practices of racialized hate that stigmatize, injure, and humiliate those made not to belong. Fanon sensed a "collective unconscious" to colonial racism and stratification, as well as rejected, subaltern layers of indignation and shame in colonial situations stretching from Martinique to Algeria and France (Fanon 1965; House 2005). He also witnessed subcultures vying for endurance amid the dominant "structuring values" of a colonial situation. Imposing psychiatric "methods from an 'outside' on an 'indigenous mentality'" should be avoided, Fanon thought, since "Algerian culture carried other values." He wanted Algerian aspects to "be taken on board" by his psychiatric staff treating colonized patients (Fanon in Khalfa and Young 2018, 190). Madness became entangled with psychiatry in this Algerian context of torture and a terrible war of decolonization, where Fanon witnessed "crumbling" and "dissolution" in clinical settings. His idea of madness, again following Lacan, resembled a limit or threshold. At stake was liberty, since madness was "one of the means by which we can lose our freedom." "Colonial dissolution" went with "a pathology of freedom." Likewise, psychiatry should act with a political edge (Khalfa and Young 2018, 201, 434, 184, 210, 190; cf. Keller 2007).

The psychopolitical offers detours away from diagnostic categories alone. Its very fusion shifts scales from rulers or regimes to micropolitics and the psychic in the ordinary and the everyday, with raw subjectivities included. In the process, the psychopolitical pries open important new political contours for all psychiatric histories while pointing to forms of imbrication among the psychiatric, the political, and often the vernacular in Africa and beyond.

Concept 3. The Vernacular

It is time to return to the vernacular. The word seems on the rise in and beyond African studies, where Johannes Fabian (1990) long wielded it with panache. In medical and psychiatric histories, the term seems risky, as if an easy substitute for vexed terms like traditional, primitive, or Other, which too often keep alive a "savage slot" (Trouillot 2021). The vernacular surely may avoid the *traditional*, of course, with its suggestions of continuity, as has long troubled canny historians (White, Miescher, and Cohen 2001; Hobsbawm and Ranger 2012). Vernacular is also distinct from the *popular*, a term used to rethink healing (Feierman 1985) and cultural production as dynamic in African worlds (Barber 1987; Fabian 1998).

Etymologically, *vernacular* has long meant ordinary, domestic, native, or indigenous, and pertained to a language, idiom, or style (*Oxford English Dictionary* 2023b). A connotation of lowborn can creep in, as in that rare usage of a *vernacular slave* or one homeborn on a master's estate. Such reductions are in keeping with racialized diminutions and pejorative affronts. It is clear: vernacular will never be a perfect word (Orsini 2020) for Africa, a continent long distorted through troublesome culturalist glosses. The hazard of this admittedly problematic word lies in its easy purifications and its suggestions of a continuous and static realm, tradition.

The word *vernacular* is best kept unresolved, while observing how it becomes latticed in relation to zones or moments of power. By glimpsing it in speech, outbursts, materialities, and practices, historians may untangle symptoms, signs, or affinities, and across spaces. In other words, the vernacular may be made and kept plastic, with room for wealth and skill in healing knowledge as well in the objects—charms—used and surely much else in African histories.

Raymond Williams has not exactly been a leading light among those writing histories of Africa; he is mentioned in only a few book reviews since 1996 in the *Journal of African History*, the field's leading journal. Still, I make a case here for reading and rereading him, as this cultural critic and theorist offers an enormous amount when we are wrestling with refractory issues of time, duration, and practices, the vernacular and the most vexed binaries. Williams gives us a way to entangle the vernacular (a word he does not use) with his salient words: the *residual*, the *emergent,* and the *dominant*. He seeks out the materialist and the contingent within dynamic, interrelated forces shaping cultural forms.

To avoid, say, a contentious binary (for example, a colonial psychiatrist pitted against a healer or a charm), Williams's triadic formulation urges for embracing emergent categories and forms as well as energies and dreams. In the process, it strongly widens a social spectrum. Williams was against fixities. Residual elements, he cautioned, knew not any one past. The residual, he also wrote, is "effectively formed in the past" and it is "still active in the cultural process, not only and often not at all as an element of the past" (1977, 122). The emergent, he emphasized, "depends crucially on finding new forms." A healer may be busy seeking modern trappings, just as a trained medical assistant laboring in a modern clinic may mix in—or refuse—vernacular substances or methods (Hunt 1999; Langwick 2008, 2011). Williams spoke to distances between residual and dominant cultures, with the residual—and perhaps the emergent—incorporated into or excluded from dominant culture, even opposing it.

In the history of psychiatry most everywhere, the dominant culture lies in psychiatric practice, backed by state, carceral, and pharmaceutical powers. The vernacular may be many things, but for Africa often stems from religious practices, healing forms, and subaltern energies. The vernacular in Africa surely dates back to pre-European pasts, yet it involves no unbroken temporality. Instead, an eruptive, discontinuous tempo surely punctuated life and time. The vernacular can also just show up, as if in a flash, in a hasty appearance suggesting social visibility or a few archival lines, before receding again almost as swiftly.

Forms of madness preexisted conquest and the arrival of Europeans in Africa. The shift to colonial power was often abrupt and it had extractive, custodial, and psychiatric dimensions. The question, therefore, is less whether psychiatry imposed Eurocentric modalities, but rather how Africans remade colonial experiments, and when and how vernacular modes or idioms—whether leaning to the residual or emergent—came into play. In histories of madness, such elements get mixed up with persons, catastrophes, deliria, and that important idiom of Ernesto de Martino (2012): "crises of presence."

Williams (1977, 121–22) wrote that experiences and meanings, those "lived and practiced on the basis of the residue" and apart from previous formations, may entail "an idealization or fantasy" or express "an exotic," all from the perspective of dominant culture. With his words, we enter afresh into that long, vexed history of Africa's charms or *fetishes*, long construed by outsiders as outlandish, dreadful, and profoundly aesthetic. Yet these vernacular objects aligned with healing were part of contentious encounters of theft and exchange from the sixteenth century (Pietz 1987), just as they were increasingly snatched up as gorgeous or curious *fetish* objects late in the nineteenth century and increasingly as assets and aesthetic objects for European museums, galleries, and private collections, in keeping with *art nègre* (Black art) and Parisian and Belgian avant-garde tastes.

If we jump forward in time, to that epoch following most national decolonizations in Africa (1957–64), we see that vernacular healing was often incorporated as part of official "authenticity" movements (Bibeau 1976). The rituals and meanings of these could go strangely awry (Roberts 1994). Yet African healing has never been only kind and beneficent but also directed at harming enemies through curses and witchcraft (Hunt 2013b), and some of Africa's dictators became specialists at such cursing and also iconic of madness in Africa (Shoumatoff 1988). Common within psychiatric consultations, witchcraft is easily distorted as superstitious or backward. Still, sorcery remains active as politics and the everyday in postcolonial Africa (Geschiere 1997).

Murray Last's (1981) ideas about medical systems and "non-systems" are invaluable. Biomedicine and Islamic medicine were confident, visible forms of codified knowledge in late twentieth-century northern Nigeria. Spirit possession appeared as fractured, hidden, sometimes chaotic, and regardless as a noncodified form of knowledge. In this Islamic zone of Africa, such vernacular healing comprises a nonsystem (while Islamic elements might be construed as vernacular, too). Last's formulation is a vast enhancement on therapeutic pluralism (Janzen 1978), where the emphasis has been on tracking patterns of resort by subjects and kin in relation to therapeutic modes. Still, we can debate when—if ever—psychiatry became dominant within colonial and postcolonial fields. Residual elements may seem in tatters, mixed with secrecy or shame. Yet nonsystems may be utterly alive, with elements like the occult, magic, or charm objects suggesting pasts, even if largely operating underground.

The chapters circle around vernacular practice, even if obliquely. Many challenge the hegemony of psychiatric expertise. Most suggest new strata, forms of expression, and sources while innovating through historical narratives. Madness often comes down to suffering: whether of patients, kin, the deranged, or collectives, enmeshed in translation. The vernacular gains from being kept suspect. It also offers up slender strands to be "sutured in" (Hunt 2013a).

Ego-documents (Wilbraham 2014; Fumanti 2018, 2020) suggest gray zones, claims, deliria, and resentments, as can other archival traces. In keeping our evidentiary strategies complex and attending to all possible elements, including those suggesting a vernacular, we can arrive at nuanced interpretations, stories about psychiatry and madness that have gone unheard in African histories. Many chapters suggest the class aspirations of colonial subjects seeking to be part of a dominant, mixed, or emergent culture, seen through their writing, schooling, and other forms of striving and dreaming about upward mobility and whiteness. Tiquet (chapter 9) shows something contrary: how many Senegalese in 1960s Dakar sought to unload their agitated, insane kin in mental health institutions. Deliria, depression, and psychopathology appear, unequally, across the contributions.

Less obvious are the attempts to connect with a valorized or disdained past. Yet such endeavors are present in these chapters: with vernacular bits contained in delirious speech or writing (see chapters 1 and 3), in the vicious mishandling of therapeutic dancing on slave ships (chapter 10), in highly investigated forms of spirit possession in 1950s Taita (chapter 7), in commercialized healing shrines that mushroomed in the Gold Coast from the 1930s (chapter 10), and in countercultural psychiatric practice during Frantz Fanon's time in Algeria (chapter 8). Transcultural psychiatry (Collignon 2018) always had to account for vernaculars and residuals, even if in racist ways. Keller renders such a reckoning among a few brave, defiant, antiracist psychiatrists working against dominant psychiatric culture during Algeria's terrible colonial war.

The Chapters

The book is divided into four parts, with some chapters bleeding across these themes.

Part I, "Writing, Biography, and the Psychopolitics of Decolonization," opens narratives that have gone largely unnoticed in both African and psychiatric histories. By unwrapping new histories of decolonization, the chapters move between archival traces and colonial and postcolonial tensions. The writings of psychiatric patients and other subaltern subjects disclose the psychopolitics to decolonization. These texts draw on case files, autobiographical texts, biographies, and research remains, most of it generated by patients. It is the oblique approaches to hospital and institutional spaces that surprise here. These chapters also mine subjective interactions and intimate texts with sometimes the writings of patients or one slandered as mad. They move toward "worldmaking" in Ghana (chapter 1), pernicious racialized diminution on a Catholic mission (chapter 2), and the epistemic production of schizophrenia as a West African and global object (chapter 3). Each investigates diverse frames—spatial, political, nervous, or scientific— while thickly tracking peculiarities to their themes and subjects.

The Accra Psychiatric Hospital (1969–76) is the site for Nana Quarshie's (chapter 1) psychopolitical analysis of delusional patient speech. Figures like Kwame Nkrumah and a money-doubling prophet are lurking. This postcolonial history stems from one patient's long petition to authorities in Ghana, itself a paranoid regime with terror. Richard Hölzl (chapter 2) rethinks method while mining the biography of an African Catholic priest in Tanzania. A 1947 syphilis diagnosis within a Benedictine mission morphed into madness allegations during times of Africanization, when an African priest dared to question racial inequalities. Letters reveal this segregationist mission as violent and uncanny: a place of breakdowns, exclusions, damning psychiatric labels, and late colonial psychopathologies. Finally, Hubertus Büschel (chapter 3) interweaves autobiography and global psychiatric research with decolonizing processes. Central are the copious writing of a Cameroonian clerk who heard voices in 1968 and traveled to a WHO-affiliated schizophrenia clinic in Ibadan, Nigeria, where his German doctor, Alexander Boroffka, encouraged him to write and also read Daniel Schreber's memoir of nervous illness. Critical here are mirroring currents between patient textualities with dreams and global technoscience.

Part II, "Patient Words Meet Diagnostic Categories," foregrounds African words of patients and research subjects. These chapters consider diagnostic categories, research experimentalities, and mental derangement. Psychological, infrastructural, and situational dimensions come to the fore, as do colonial breakdowns, depression, and a "psychic stress disorder." Four interned Malagasy from the 1920s are Raphaël Gallien's subject (chapter 4), and he reads their case files for trajectories and horizons. These patients longed to move up in rank, materially or symbolically, within colonial or monarchical hierarchies. The way each fell apart when promotions proved out of reach underlines the psychic harm—of feeling socially blocked—in this French colonial situation. Jonathan Sadowsky (chapter 5) considers depression's categorization in relation to somatization, guilt, and the incommensurability of knowledge, in relation to the work of leading research figures in colonial Africa's psychiatric history: Frantz Fanon, Margaret Field, Raymond Prince, and J. C. Carothers. Whether as a disease of civilization or as capacities within colonial ideology, psychiatric research developed within both global and African spaces and scales. Complicated imaginaries emerging from the Nigerian survey work of Raymond Prince are investigated by Matthew Heaton (chapter 6). Prince's research concerned "psychic stress disorder." Student responses to his questionnaires suggest the intense pressures of the work of studying. The surveys disclose nervous words, puzzled reactions, and the fears of these youth of Nigeria's elite boarding schools, especially when confronted by this research intervention.

Part III, "Practices and Long Durations," examines colonial ideologies emerging beside practice and time. Psychiatric tensions and ambivalent mixtures were common to colonial situations. These chapters turn to colonial moments of urgency and violence, and also to unusual research formations, psychiatric approaches, and fraught locations. Remarkably different scenes from colonial Kenya and colonial Algeria suggest vernacular symptoms and theaters, sometimes still mediated in postcolonial metropoles. The wide range of sources suggests that psychiatric historiography is beginning afresh from the unforeseen and the bewildering, though often from the canonical sources of experts. Sloan Mahone (chapter 7) tells of a perplexing, psychiatric urgency in a late colonial situation. Amid psychiatric, anthropological, and governmental layers as well as the fixations and camerawork of a Canadian psychiatrist, stress and "possession hysteria" drew much attention during violent state outbursts in Kenya's isolated Taita Hills. Competing claims about colonial tensions and modernity speak to perceptions of madness during decolonization. Resistance among two exceptional psychiatrists in colonial Algeria is Richard Keller's subject (chapter 8). He also considers vexed colonial legacies lingering still in contemporary France. Considering not only Frantz Fanon but also Suzanne Taïeb, Keller shows how these sensitive clinicians attended to suffering under such fraught conditions, reframing dominant French narratives in the process, and also politicizing care before French Algeria's racist psychiatry.

Many chapters derive from curious archives, disclosing patient words or collective suffering. Subjectivities are not the point of all the chapters. Rather, several other analytics and methods surface: painting in a colonial scene, unpacking a research enterprise, or grappling with the psychopathologies of a situation. Some chapters track moods, selves, or collective dimensions, and they do so through patient case files, biography, autobiography, or microhistorical techniques. From "illness narratives" (Kleinman 1988) to banalities, the chapters realign African histories of psychiatry through that long-standing stance of Africanist historiography: locating unexpected archives and seeking unconventional shapes and genres.

These impulses are alive in Part IV, "Unexpected Archives and Ethnographic Investigations," where often thin yet unusual archives or ethnographic notes are mined in innovative ways. Revisited is a timeworn idea from Africa's important field, health and healing studies, that kin are key in African situations of health, healing, and care (Janzen 1978; Feierman 1981; Hunt 2013b). Anthropology and mobility as revelatory themes in African history also find fresh treatments here as part of psychiatric histories of Africa. Other themes are present: hospitalization and its arrangements, decolonization's slowness, and the historical depth to psychopathologies and racialized enclosures.

A thin yet granular archive is stretched far, and beautifully so, by Romain Tiquet (chapter 9), who studies letters written by kin seeking to intern mentally ill relatives in Dakar. Family disquiet unfolded before sick relatives who became objects of 1960s state processes, just as Senegalese authorities prioritized order and security. The final chapter, authored by me, juxtaposes two West African scenes and discusses matters of milieu, mobility, and racialized harm. From 1950s velocities in the Gold Coast to late eighteenth-century slow-moving slave ships, transport contrivances unveil radically different experiences and nightmares. Easy notions of the vernacular are troubled by these unlike worlds with dreams of modern lorries, ship suicides, and coerced dancing.

Final Words

Three concepts arise here, we have seen: madness, psychopolitics, and the vernacular. Madness remains a capacious term, while psychopolitics—rich and important—will surely flourish analytically in the years to come. For a continent where witchcraft remains an everyday word, it is crucial to grapple with the vernacular. However fraught this word, it takes us to vital strands, signs, and practices: overt or lying in shadows.

Madness persists as a refractory domain. Through their diverse modes of exposition, inquiry, and theorization, these chapters are quite unlike each other, yet together they provide a broad view amid serious stories. Many expose modes of doing and suffering. They combine patient narratives, diagnostic categories, harmful milieus, and mirroring effects, related to quite different colonialisms and also to innovations in method. Everyday forms of dissent burst forth in some. Several investigate a scene or figuration from Africa's decolonizing years, or quite a different era as well. The work of decoding utterances and idioms yields a diversity of interpretations of social rankings and spaces.

Key is to preclude the vernacular as something fixed. Vernacular bits regularly arrive in clinical settings. Patients and kin carry them in with their words, objects, and expectations. Conceptually, the vernacular urges for discerning, not the authentic, but mixed idioms and materials, for pairing an element with another trace of some kind.

Finally, let us also touch on two matters that remain slight or absent here. Gender and women are present, though usually tacitly. Enslaved women figure on eighteenth-century slave ships (chapter 10) and reveal how these inhuman enclosures generated death, suicide, and feisty forms of female refusal. Men dominate in this volume as patients, clinicians, and experts. A diversity of female *psy* specialists—Margaret Field (chapter 10), Grace Harris (chapter 7), and Suzanne Taïeb (chapter 8)—bring to the fore the labor and convictions of these experts. Pioneers in transcultural psychiatry remained on the margins of dominant practice in Africa. The visibility and accomplishments of these few women are an important counterpoint to the masculinist nature of psychiatric practice in Africa. Some of these women confronted the charged situations of the decolonizing years with courage and audacity.

The second matter is ethics, a theme usually broached in relation to the findings in a clinical archive or a hospital field site (Kilroy-Marac 2019). Ethics need concerted and canny attention, and chapters 1–3 grapple with them. Ethics also need a special underlining for Africa, given its many unregulated clinical spaces with vulnerable yet serendipitous archives. Since the archival may embrace clinic-based or patient-authored information, telling of delusions, dreams, and diagnoses, it is vital to grapple with matters of confidentiality, consent, and discretion. Secrecy and disguise may obfuscate much in field situations, with researchers speaking with living subjects. Asking a person construed as mentally ill to speak aloud or to seek to "capture" their minor voice suggests an unsettling naïveté about subaltern historiography and ethics. Within this wide moral realm, gritty and granular alike, matters of stigmatization, shame, and disclosure are at stake, as are the rights, wishes, and the need for informed consent of patients and kin.

Most of Africa's histories of psychiatry end by the 1980s. Often missing, therefore, are the way that "trauma zones" (Hunt 2021) came to prevail, roughly from the neoliberal 1990s, along with psychiatric practices and suffering within Africa's humanitarian, migratory, and confessional zones. If we were to only include Rwanda's 1994 genocide and South Africa's Truth and Reconciliation Commission here, we would miss many other traumatic zones (Brachet 2009; Beneduce 2019; Veronese et al. 2020; yet see Jones 2012). Some therapeutic modalities in these zones date from at least the eighteenth century, quite likely earlier (Janzen 1982; Hunt 2013b; Lee 2021). Their healing practices may be read as strongly residual, though an emergent, entrepreneurial energy may be present as they vacillate between pasts and futures while creating new forms. Such ways of healing and being modern were common in Africa from the interwar years (Feierman 1979, 1985; Iliffe 1998; Hunt 1999; Langwick 2011). Africa's new *tradi-practiciens* have been working in the same social spaces as doctors, pastors, humanitiarian workers, PTSD-psychologists, and psychiatrists: within precarious trauma zones. And, the new energies of these entrepreneurial healers are reminiscent of the mushrooming in commercial healing shrines that Margaret

Field documented for southern Gold Coast from the 1930s. In each, one finds much swaying into a residual vernacular as well as a moving forward into emergent and animated forms.

It is time to close. These chapters abound with crises, symptoms, and psychopathologies from racialized and decolonizing worlds, with much speech and penned textualities by suffering patients (Porter 1985). Present are intimacies and claims, with African subjects straining to realize unfettered, modern, and novel selves. Psychic suffering surfaces here alongside tears, impudence, and dreams. There are copious affective traces with phantasms and deliria. So it seems fitting to close with two big stars, theorists, in the history of psychiatry and psychoanalysis. Perhaps their words should become pivotal in the aspirations and labors of psychiatric historians, and at a time when the field—history itself—turns strongly toward sound, the unconscious, and the uncanny. I refer to Gilles Deleuze and Félix Guattari (1972, 106), who declared: "Every delirium has strong historical, geographical, political, and racial content." May their words instruct and inspire.

Indeed, in this volume, it is as if we see the labor of a new generation of talented, imaginative historians, winding this profound and versatile dictum with very specific layers around a chosen African milieu and its archival traces. Expansively they do so, almost as if twirling round and round, as they spawn a lattice of insights and a novel intellectual constellation.

Acknowledgments

My thanks to Steven Feierman for his decisive critique of an earlier version of this introduction, to Patricia Hayes for her important insights, and to Hubertus Büschel for his generous reading and for insisting on many fine, critical points.

Notes

1   Pushing between the residual and the emergent, as in Williams (1977).

2   I first wrote these lines on category work as a conference abstract for Nicholas Henckes, and later expanded them during a 2018 stay that he generously assembled for me in Paris, before and after my fascinating few research weeks

spent in Agadez and Niamey, Niger. I remain very grateful to him for his splendid organization, his kindness, and his superb critical suggestions.

3   An "African modern" suggests an aspiring "middle figure" (Hunt 1999) as drawn out brilliantly by Lynn Thomas (Cole and Thomas 2009; L. Thomas 2020) in relation to Africa's "modern girl" subjects, figurations, identifications, posturing, and bodily remaking, like the modernity-aspiring Nigerian students described by Heaton in chapter 6 of this volume.

4   See the impressive digital archive of the Museum of British Colonialism, https://museumofbritishcolonialism.org/2018-9-28-the-pipeline-dpzc5/#, accessed August 23, 2023.

5   It is worth wondering why parallel vocabulary, the *psychosocial*, has been bursting out of Budapest (Auestad and Kabesh 2017; Borgos, Gyimesi, and Erős 2019). Compare the 2015 international conference in Budapest, "Psycho Politics: The Cross Sections of Science and Ideology in the History of Psy Sciences," https://cognitivescience.ceu.edu/events/2015-10-30/psycho-politics-cross-sections-science-and-ideology-history-psy-sciences, accessed April 25, 2023.

Sources

Achebe, Chinua. (1972) 1991. "The Madman." In *Girls at War and Other Stories*, n.p. Reprint, New York: Anchor Books.

Agamben, Giorgio. 2000. *Means without End: Notes on Politics*. Minneapolis: University of Minnesota Press.

Akana, Parfait D. 2013. "Note sur la dénudation publique du corps au Cameroun: À propos d'une explication médiatique." *L'Autre, Cliniques, Cultures, Sociétés* 14, no. 2: 236–43.

Akyeampong, Emmanuel Kwaku, Allan G. Hill, and Arthur Kleinman, eds. 2015. *The Culture of Mental Illness and Psychiatric Practice in Africa*. Bloomington: Indiana University Press, 2015.

Antic, Ana. 2019. "Imagining Africa in Eastern Europe: Transcultural Psychiatry and Psychoanalysis in Cold War Yugoslavia." *Contemporary European History* 28:234–51.

Apter, Emily S. 2018. *Unexceptional Politics: On Obstruction, Impasse, and the Impolitic*. Brooklyn, NY: Verso.

Auestad, Lene, and Amal Treacher Kabesh, eds. 2017. *Traces of Violence and Freedom of Thought*. London: Palgrave Macmillan.

Balandier, Georges. 1951. "La situation coloniale: Approche théorique." *Cahiers Internationaux de Sociologie* 11:44–79.

Barber, Karin. 1987. "The Popular Arts in Africa." *African Studies Review* 30:1–78.

Bateson, Gregory. 1972. *Steps to an Ecology of Mind: Collected Essays in Anthropology, Psychiatry, Evolution, and Epistemology*. San Francisco: Chandler.

Behrouzan, Orkideh. 2020. *Prozak Diaries: Psychiatry and Generational Memory in Iran*. Stanford, CA: Stanford University Press.

Beneduce, Roberto. 2019. "'Madness and Despair Are a Force': Global Mental Health, and How People and Cultures Challenge the Hegemony of Western Psychiatry." *Culture, Medicine, and Psychiatry* 43:710–23.

Benjamin, Walter. 1999. *The Arcades Project*. Translated by Howard Eiland and Kevin McLaughlin; prepared on the basis of the German volume edited by Rolf Tiedemann. Cambridge, MA: Belknap Press of Harvard University Press.

Bhugra, Dinesh, and Roland Littlewood, eds. 2002. *Colonialism and Psychiatry*. New Delhi: Oxford University Press.

Bibeau, Gilles. 1976. "Mbindo Lala: Un hôpital en forme de village." *Médecine traditionnelle au Zaïre et en Afrique* 1:57–69.

Biebuyck, Daniel P., with Kahombo C. Mateene. 1969. *The Mwindo Epic from the Banyanga*. Berkeley: University of California Press.

Biehl, João Guilherme. 2005. *Vita: Life in a Zone of Social Abandonment*. Berkeley: University of California Press.

Bilby, Kenneth M., and Jerome S. Handler. 2004. "Obeah: Healing and Protection in West Indian Slave Life." *Journal of Caribbean History* 38, no. 2: 153–83.

Bonhomme, Julien. 2008. "God's Graffiti: Prophetic Agency and the Pragmatics of Writing in Postcolonial Gabon." In *Anthropologies*, edited by Richard Baxstrom and Todd Meyers, 31–55. Baltimore, MD: Creative Capitalism.

Borgos, Anna, Júlia Gyimesi, and Ferenc Erős, eds. 2019. *Psychology and Politics: Intersections of Science and Ideology in the History of Psy-Sciences*. Budapest: Central European University Press.

Brachet, Julien. 2009. *Migrations transsahariennes: Vers un désert cosmopolite et morcelé, Niger*. Bellecombe-en-Bauges, France: Croquant.

Brecher, W. Puck. 2013. *The Aesthetics of Strangeness: Eccentricity and Madness in Early Modern Japan*. Honolulu: University of Hawai'i Press.

Brown, Vincent. 2003. "Spiritual Terror and Sacred Authority in Jamaican Slave Society." *Slavery and Abolition* 24, no. 1: 24–53.

Brown, Vincent. 2020. *Tacky's Revolt: The Story of an Atlantic Slave War*. Cambridge, MA: Harvard University Press.

Burchell, Graham, Colin Gordon, and Peter Miller. 1991. *The Foucault Effect: Studies in Governmentality with Two Lectures by and an Interview with Michel Foucault*. Chicago: University of Chicago Press.

Büschel, Hubertus. 2020. "Beyond the Colonial Shadow? Delinking, Border Thinking, and Theoretical Futures of Cultural History." In *Futures of the Study of Culture:*

Interdisciplinary Perspectives, Global Challenges, edited by Doris Bachmann-Medick, Jens Kugele, and Ansgar Nünning, 123–38. Berlin: De Gruyter.

Callaway, Henry. (1885) 2019. *The Religious System of the Amazulu, Izinyanga Zo-kubula, or: Divination, as Existing among the Amazulu, in Their Own Words*. Natal: J. A. Blair. Reprint, Cambridge, MA: MIT Press.

Canguilhem, Georges. 2012. *Writings on Medicine*. New York: Fordham University Press.

Carothers, J. C. 1947. "A Study of Mental Derangement in Africans, and an Attempt to Explain Its Peculiarities, More Especially in Relation to the African Attitude to Life." *Journal of Mental Science* 93, no. 392: 548–97.

Chakrabarty, Dipesh. 2007. *Provincializing Europe: Postcolonial Thought and Historical Difference*. Princeton, NJ: Princeton University Press.

Cole, Jennifer, and Lynn M. Thomas, eds. 2009. *Love in Africa*. Chicago: University of Chicago Press.

Collignon, René. 1984. "La lutte des pouvoirs publics contre les 'encombrements humains' à Dakar." *Canadian Journal of African Studies* 18, no. 3: 573–82.

Collignon, René. 2018. "Henri Collomb and the Emergence of a Psychiatry Open to Otherness through Interdisciplinary Dialogue in Post-Independence Dakar." *History of Psychiatry* 29, no. 3: 350–62.

Conci, Marco. 2023. "Psychoanalytic Ego Psychology: A European Perspective." *International Forum of Psychoanalysis* 32, no. 1: 4–22.

Cooper, Frederick. 1988. "Mau Mau and the Discourses of Decolonization." *Journal of African History* 29, no. 2: 313–20.

Corin, Ellen. 1998. "The Thickness of Being: Intentional Worlds, Strategies of Identity, and Experience among Schizophrenics." *Psychiatry* 61, no. 2: 133–46.

Daston, Lorraine. 2007. "The History of Emergences." *Isis* 98, no. 4: 801–8.

Davis, Natalie. 2006. *Trickster Travels: A Sixteenth-Century Muslim between Worlds*. New York: Hill and Wang.

Deacon, Harriett J. 1996. "Madness, Race and Moral Treatment: Robben Island Lunatic Asylum, 1846–1890." *History of Psychiatry* 7, no. 26: 287–97.

Deleuze, Gilles. 2008. *Two Regimes of Madness: Texts and Interviews, 1975–1995*, edited by David Lapoujade. Cambridge, MA: MIT Press.

Deleuze, Gilles, and Félix Guattari. 1972. *L'anti-Œdipe*. Paris: Minuit.

Delille, Emmanuel, ed. 2020. *Ethnopsychiatry*. Montreal: McGill–Queen's University Press.

Delille, Emmanuel, and Ivan Crozier. 2018. "Historicizing Transcultural Psychiatry: People, Epistemic Objects, Networks, and Practices." *History of Psychiatry* 29, no. 3: 257–62.

Deluz, Ariane. 1991. "Ethnopsychiatrie." In *Dictionnaire de l'ethnologie et de l'anthropologie*, edited by Pierre Bonte and Michel Izard, 251–52. Paris: PUF.

Derrida, Jacques. 1995. *Mal d'archive: Une impression freudienne*. Paris: Galilée.

Devisch, René. 1995. "Frenzy, Violence, and Ethical Renewal in Kinshasa." *Public Culture* 7, no. 3: 593–629.

De Vos, Jan. 2011. "The Psychologization of Humanitarian Aid: Skimming the Battlefield and the Disaster Zone." *History of the Human Sciences* 24, no. 3: 103–22.

Du Bois, W. E. B. 2007. *The Souls of Black Folk*. Oxford: Oxford University Press.

Dubow, Saul. 1993. "Wulf Sach's *Black Hamlet*: A Case of 'Psychic Vivisection'?" *African Affairs* 92, no. 369 (October): 519–56.

Ecks, Stefan. 2016. "Commentary: Ethnographic Critiques of Global Mental Health." *Transcultural Psychiatry* 53, no. 6: 804–8.

Edgar, Robert, and Hilary Sapire. 2000. *African Apocalypse: The Story of Nontetha Nkwenkwe, a Twentieth-Century South African Prophet*. Athens: Ohio University, Center for International Studies.

Eghigian, Greg, ed. 2017. "Introduction to the History of Madness and Mental Health." In *The Routledge History of Madness and Mental Health*, 1–15. London: Routledge.

Eldredge, Elizabeth A. 2014. *The Creation of the Zulu Kingdom, 1815–1828: War, Shaka, and the Consolidation of Power*. Cambridge: Cambridge University Press.

Fabian, Johannes, ed. and trans., with Kalundi Mango and W. Schicho. 1990. *History from Below: The "Vocabulary of Elisabethville" by André Yav. Text, Translations and Interpretive Essay*. Amsterdam: John Benjamins.

Fabian, Johannes. 1998. *Moments of Freedom: Anthropology and Popular Culture*. Charlottesville: University Press of Virginia.

Fabian, Johannes. 2000. *Out of Our Minds: Reason and Madness in the Exploration of Central Africa*. Berkeley: University of California Press.

Fanon, Frantz. 1965. "Medicine and Colonialism." In *A Dying Colonialism*, translated by Haakon Chevalier, 121–146. New York: Grove Press.

Farge, Arlette. 1989. *Le goût de l'archive*. Paris: Éditions du Seuil.

Fassin, Didier, and Richard Rechtman. 2009. *The Empire of Trauma: An Inquiry into the Condition of Victimhood*. Princeton, NJ: Princeton University Press.

Feierman, Steven. 1979. "Change in African Therapeutic Systems." *Social Science and Medicine. Part B, Medical Anthropology* 13, no. 4: 277–84.

Feierman, Steven. 1981. "Therapy as a System-in-Action in Northeastern Tanzania." *Social Science and Medicine. Part B, Medical Anthropology* 15, no. 3: 353–60.

Feierman, Steven. 1985. "Struggles for Control: The Social Roots of Health and Healing in Modern Africa." *African Studies Review* 28, no. 2–3: 73–147.

Fernandez, James W. 1982. *Bwiti: An Ethnography of the Religious Imagination in Africa*. Princeton, NJ: Princeton University Press.

Field, Margaret Joyce. 1960. *Search for Security: An Ethno-Psychiatric Study of Rural Ghana*. Evanston, IL: Northwestern University Press.

Foucault, Michel. (1961) 2006. *History of Madness*. London: Routledge.

Foucault, Michel. 1961. "La folie n'existe pas que dans une société." In *Dits et écrits I: 1954–1975*, 195–97. Paris: Editions Gallimard.

Foucault, Michel. 1972. *The Archaeology of Knowledge*. New York: Pantheon Books.

Freis, David. 2019. *Psycho-Politics between the World Wars: Psychiatry and Society in Germany, Austria, and Switzerland*. Cham, Switzerland: Springer.

Fumanti, Mattia. 2018. "Conjuring Madness: Self/Non Self and Mental Illness in Post-Apartheid Namibia." *Somatosphere*, April 6. http://somatosphere.net/2018/04/conjuring-madness.html.

Fumanti, Mattia. 2020. "'A German Whore and No Money at That': Insanity and the Moral and Political Economies of German South West Africa." *Culture, Medicine and Psychiatry* 44, no. 3: 382–402.

Geissler, Paul Wenzel, Guillaume Lachenal, John Manton, and Noémi Tousignant. 2016. *Traces of the Future: An Archaeology of Medical Science in Africa*. Chicago: University of Chicago Press.

Geschiere, Peter. 1997. *The Modernity of Witchcraft: Politics and the Occult in Post-colonial Africa*. Charlottesville: University Press of Virginia.

Goltermann, Svenja. 2010. "On Silence, Madness, and Lassitude: Negotiating the Past in Post-war West Germany." In *Shadows of War: A Social History of Silence in the Twentieth Century*, edited by Efrat Ben-Ze'ev, Ruth Ginio, and Jay Winter, 91–112. Cambridge: Cambridge University Press.

Good, Byron J., and Mary-Jo DelVecchio Good. 2010. "Amuk in Java: Madness and Violence in Indonesian Politics." In *A Reader in Medical Anthropology: Theoretical Trajectories, Emergent Realities*, edited by Byron J. Good, Michael M. J. Fischer, Sarah S. Willen, and Mary-Jo DelVecchio Good, 473–80. Hoboken, NJ: Wiley-Blackwell.

Good, Mary-Jo DelVecchio, Byron Good, Sandra Hyde, and Sarah Pinto, eds. 2008. *Postcolonial Disorders*. Berkeley: University of California Press.

Gutting, Gary. 2019. *Foucault: A Very Short Introduction*. 2nd ed. Oxford: Oxford University Press.

Hacking, Ian. 1998. *Mad Travelers: Reflections on the Reality of Transient Mental Illnesses*. Charlottesville: University Press of Virginia.

Hall, Stuart. 2018. "Psychoanalysis and Cultural Studies." *Cultural Studies* 32:889–96.

Hamilton, Carolyn. 1998. *Terrific Majesty: The Powers of Shaka Zulu and the Limits of Historical Invention*. Cambridge, MA: Harvard University Press.

Hamilton, Carolyn, ed. 2002. *Refiguring the Archive*. Cape Town, South Africa: David Philip.

Han, Byung-Chul. 2017. *Psychopolitics: Neoliberalism and New Technologies of Power*. London: Verso.

Heaton, Matthew M. 2013. *Black Skin, White Coats: Nigerian Psychiatrists, Decolonization, and the Globalization of Psychiatry*. Athens: Ohio University Press.

Henckes, Nicholas. 2019. "Schizophrenia Infrastructures: Local and Global Dynamics of Transformation in Psychiatric Diagnosis-Making in the Twentieth and Twenty-First Centuries." *Culture, Medicine and Psychiatry* 43, no. 4: 548–73.

Henckes, Nicolas, Volker Hess, and Marie Reinholdt. 2018. "Exploring the Fringes of Psychopathology: Boundary Entities, Category Work and Other Borderline Phenomena in the History of 20th Century Psychopathology." *History of the Human Sciences* 31, no. 2: 3–21.

Herzog, Dagmar. 2017. *Cold War Freud: Psychoanalysis in an Age of Catastrophes*. Cambridge: Cambridge University Press.

Hobsbawm, Eric, and Terence Ranger. 2012. *The Invention of Tradition*. New York: Cambridge University Press.

Hokkanen, Markku. 2018. "'Madness', Emotions and Loss of Control in a Colonial Frontier: Methodological Challenges of Crises of Mind." In *Encountering Crises of the Mind*, edited by Tuomas Laine-Frigren, Jari Eilola, and Markku Hokkanen, 277–95. Leiden: Brill.

House, Jim. 2005. "Colonial Racisms in the 'Métropole': Reading *Peau noire, masques blancs* in Context." In *Frantz Fanon's Black Skin, White Masks: New Interdisciplinary Essays*, edited by Max Silverman, 46–73. Manchester: Manchester University Press.

Howell, Alison. 2011. *Madness in International Relations: Psychology, Security, and the Global Governance of Mental Health*. London: Routledge.

Hunt, Nancy Rose. 1999. *A Colonial Lexicon: Of Birth Ritual, Medicalization, and Mobility in the Congo*. Durham, NC: Duke University Press.

Hunt, Nancy Rose. 2007. "Between Fiction and History: Modes of Writing Abortion." *Cahiers d'études africaines* 47, no. 186: 277–312.

Hunt, Nancy Rose. 2013a. *Suturing New Medical Histories of Africa*. Berlin: LIT Verlag.

Hunt, Nancy Rose. 2013b. "Health and Healing." In *Oxford Handbook of Modern African History*, edited by John Parker and Richard Reid, 378–95. Oxford: Oxford University Press.

Hunt, Nancy Rose. 2016. *A Nervous State: Violence, Remedies, and Reverie in Colonial Congo*. Durham, NC: Duke University Press.

Hunt, Nancy Rose. 2021. "Beyond Trauma? Notes on a Word, a Frame, and a Diagnostic Category." In *Historical Trauma and Memory: Living with the Haunting Power of the Past*, edited by Pumla Gobodo-Madikizela, Eric Ndushabandi, and Kopano Ratele, 17–30. Stellenbosch, South Africa: Sun Media.

Iliffe, John. 1998. *East African Doctors: A History of the Modern Profession*. Cambridge: Cambridge University Press.

Iliffe, John. 2004. *Honour in African History*. New York: Cambridge University Press.

Jackson, Lynette. 2005. *Surfacing Up: Psychiatry and Social Order in Colonial Zimbabwe, 1908–1968*. Ithaca, NY: Cornell University Press.

Janzen, John M. 1978. *The Quest for Therapy in Lower Zaire*. Berkeley: University of California Press.

Janzen, John M. 1982. *Lemba, 1650–1930: A Drum of Affliction in Africa and the New World*. New York: Garland.

Jones, Tiffany Fawn. 2012. *Psychiatry, Mental Institutions, and the Mad in Apartheid South Africa*. London: Routledge.

Keller, Richard C. 2007. *Colonial Madness: Psychiatry in French North Africa*. Chicago: University of Chicago Press.

Khalfa, Jean, and Robert J. C. Young. 2018. *Frantz Fanon: Alienation and Freedom*. London: Bloomsbury Academic.

Kilroy-Marac, Katie. 2019. *An Impossible Inheritance: Postcolonial Psychiatry and the Work of Memory in a West African Clinic*. Berkeley: University of California Press.

Kleinman, Arthur. 1988. *The Illness Narratives: Suffering, Healing, and the Human Condition*. New York: Basic Books.

Koselleck, Reinhart. 2018. *Sediments of Time: On Possible Histories*. Stanford, CA: Stanford University Press.

Langwick, Stacey. 2008. "Articulate(d) Bodies: Traditional Medicine in a Tanzanian Hospital." *American Ethnologist* 35, no. 3: 428–39.

Langwick, Stacey. 2011. *Bodies, Politics, and African Healing: The Matter of Maladies in Tanzania*. Bloomington: Indiana University Press.

Last, Murray. 1981. "The Importance of Knowing about Not Knowing." *Social Science and Medicine. Part B, Medical Anthropology* 15, no. 3: 387–92.

Leader, Darian. 2011. *What Is Madness?* London: Hamish Hamilton.

Lebeau, Vicky. 1998. "Psychopolitics: Frantz Fanon's *Black Skin, White Masks*." In *Psycho-Politics and Cultural Desires*, edited by Jan Campbell and Janet Harbord, 107–17. London: UCL Press.

Lee, Rebekah. 2021. *Health, Healing and Illness in African History*. London: Bloomsbury Academic.

Leopold, Mark. 2021. *Idi Amin: The Story of Africa's Icon of Evil*. New Haven, CT: Yale University Press.

Littlewood, Roland, and Maurice Lipsedge. 1982. *Aliens and Alienists: Ethnic Minorities and Psychiatry*. Harmondsworth, UK: Penguin.

Lovell, Anne M. 2019a. "Genealogies and Anthropologies of Global Mental Health." *Culture, Medicine and Psychiatry* 43, no. 4: 519–47.

Lovell, Anne M. 2019b. "Falling, Dying Sheep, and the Divine: Notes on Thick Therapeutics in Peri-Urban Senegal." *Culture, Medicine and Psychiatry* 43, no. 4: 663–85.

Mahone, Sloan, and Megan Vaughan. 2007. *Psychiatry and Empire*. London: Palgrave Macmillan.

Marks, Shula. 1988. *Not Either an Experimental Doll: The Separate Worlds of Three South African Women*. Bloomingdale: Indiana University Press.

Marks, Shula. 1999. "'Every Facility That Modern Science and Enlightened Humanity Have Devised': Race and Progress in a Colonial Hospital, Valkenberg, Cape Colony, 1894–1910." In *Insanity, Institutions and Society, 1800–1914: A Social History of Madness in Comparative Perspective*, edited by Joseph Melling and Bill Forsythe, 268–91. London: Routledge.

Martin, Marie-Louise. 1975. *Kimbangu: An African Prophet and His Church*. Grand Rapids, MI: Wm. B. Eerdmans.

Martino, Ernesto de. 2012. "Crisis of Presence and Religious Reintegration." *HAU: Journal of Ethnographic Theory* 2, no. 2: 434–50.

Mbembe, Achille. 2016. *Politiques de l'inimitié*. Paris: La Découverte.

McCulloch, Jock. 1995. *Colonial Psychiatry and "the African Mind."* Cambridge: Cambridge University Press.

Mehdi, Gina Aït, and Romain Tiquet. 2020. "Introduction au theme: Penser la folie au quotidien." *Politique africaine*, no. 157: 17–38.

Mitchell, William John Thomas. 2018. "Present Tense: Time, Madness, and Democracy around 6 November 2018." *In the Moment*, website of *Critical Inquiry*. Accessed September 12, 2021. https://critinq.wordpress.com/2018/10/30/present-tense-time-madness-and-democracy-around-6-november-2018/.

Mofolo, Thomas. 1931. *Chaka: An Historical Romance*. London: International Institute of African Languages and Cultures, Oxford University Press.

Moodley, Roy, Falak Mujtaba, and Sela Kleiman. 2018. "Critical Race Theory and Mental Health." In *Routledge International Handbook of Critical Mental Health*, edited by Bruce M. Z. Cohen, 79–88. Abingdon, UK: Routledge.

Mukherji, Projit Bihari. 2016. *Doctoring Tradition: Ayurveda, Small Technologies and Braided Sciences*. Chicago: University of Chicago Press.

Orsini, Francesca. 2020. "Vernacular: Flawed but Necessary?" *South Asian Review* 41, no. 2: 204–6.

Otake, Yuko. 2019. "Suffering of Silenced People in Northern Rwanda." *Social Science and Medicine* 222:171–79.

Oughourlian, Jean-Michel. 2012. *Psychopolitics: Conversations with Trevor Cribben Merrill*. East Lansing: Michigan State University Press.

Oxford English Dictionary. 2023a. s.v. "madness, n." https://doi.org/10.1093/OED/1122797550.

Oxford English Dictionary. 2023b. s.v. "vernacular, adj. and n." https://doi.org/10.1093/OED/1309095969.

Palmié, Stephan. 2002. *Wizards and Scientists: Explorations in Afro-Cuban Modernity and Tradition*. Durham, NC: Duke University Press.

Parin, Paul. 1980. *Fear Thy Neighbor as Thyself: Psychoanalysis and Society among the Anyi of West Africa*. Chicago: University of Chicago Press.

Parle, Julie. 2007. *States of Mind: Mental Illness and the Quest for Mental Health in Natal and Zululand, 1868–1918*. Pietermaritzburg, South Africa: University of KwaZulu-Natal Press.

Pietikäinen, Petteri. 2015. *Madness: A History*. New York: Routledge.

Pietz, William. 1987. "The Problem of the Fetish: The Origin of the Fetish." *Res*, no. 13: 23–45.

Pinto, Sarah. 2020. "Madness: Recursive Ethnography and the Critical Uses of Psychopathology." *Annual Review of Anthropology* 49:299–316.

Polat, Bican. 2017. "Before Attachment Theory: Separation Research at the Tavistock Clinic, 1948–1956." *Journal of the History of the Behavioral Sciences* 53, no. 1: 48–70.

Porter, Roy. 1985. "The Patient's View: Doing Medical History from Below." *Theory and Society* 14, no. 2: 175–98.

Pringle, Yolanda. 2019. *Psychiatry and Decolonisation in Uganda*. London: Palgrave Macmillan.

Prozorov, Sergei. 2021. "Foucault and the Birth of Psychopolitics: Towards a Genealogy of Crisis Governance." *Security Dialogue* 52, no. 5: 436–51.

Reichmayr, Michael, ed. 2020. *Zurück aus Afrika: Die ethnopsychoanalytische Erweiterung der Psychoanalyse, Schriften 1975–1982*. Vol. 7 of *Werkausgabe Paul Parin*, edited by Johannes and Michael Reichmayr. Vienna: Mandelbaum Verlag.

Revel, Jacques. 1996. *Jeux d'échelles: La micro-analyse à l'expérience*. Paris: Gallimard.

Reynolds, Pamela. 1996. *Traditional Healers and Childhood in Zimbabwe*. Athens: Ohio University Press.

Richert, Lucas. 2019. *Break on Through: Radical Psychiatry and the American Counterculture*. Cambridge, MA: MIT Press.

Roberts, Allen F. 1994. "'Authenticity' and Ritual Gone Awry in Mobutu's Zaire: Looking beyond Turnerian Models." *Journal of Religion in Africa* 24, no. 2: 134–59.

Roschenthaler, Ute, and Mamadou Diawara, eds. 2016. *Copyright Africa: How Intellectual Property, Media and Markets Transform Immaterial Cultural Goods*. Canon Pyon, UK: Sean Kingston.

Rose, Nikolas. 2018. *Our Psychiatric Future*. Cambridge, UK: Polity.

Sachs, Wulf. (1937) 1996. *Black Hamlet*. Reprint, Baltimore, MD: Johns Hopkins University Press.

Sadowsky, Jonathan. 1996. "The Confinements of Isaac O.: A Case of 'Acute Mania' in Colonial Nigeria." *History of Psychiatry* 7, no. 25: 91–112.

Sadowsky, Jonathan. 1999. *Imperial Bedlam: Institutions of Madness in Colonial Southwest Nigeria*. Berkeley: University of California Press.

Salisbury, Laura. 2020. "Between-Time Stories: Waiting, War and the Temporalities of Care." *Medical Humanities* 46, no. 2: 96–106.

Schmidt, Heike. 2008. "Colonial Intimacy: The Rechenberg Scandal and Homosexuality in German East Africa." *Journal of the History of Sexuality* 17, no. 1: 25–59.

Schoenbrun, David. 2007. "Conjuring the Modern in Africa: Durability and Rupture in Histories of Public Healing between the Great Lakes of East Africa." *American Historical Review* 111:1403–39.

Sedgwick, Peter. (1982) 2015. *Psycho Politics*. Reprint, London: Pluto Press.

Shoumatoff, Alex. 1988. *African Madness*. New York: Alfred A. Knopf.

Staub, Michael E. 2011. *Madness Is Civilization: When the Diagnosis Was Social, 1948–1980*. Chicago: University of Chicago Press.

Steedman, Carolyn. 2001. *Dust: The Archive and Cultural History*. New Brunswick, NJ: Rutgers University Press.

Stoler, Ann. 2002. "Colonial Archives and the Arts of Governance." *Archival Science* 2:87–109.

Stoler, Ann. 2009. *Along the Archival Grain: Epistemic Anxieties and Colonial Common Sense*. Princeton, NJ: Princeton University Press.

Subrahmanyam, Sanjay. 1997. "Connected Histories: Notes towards a Reconfiguration of Early Modern Eurasia." *Modern Asian Studies* 31, no. 3: 735–62.

Summerfield, Derek. 2012. "Afterword: Against 'Global Mental Health.'" *Transcultural Psychiatry* 49, no. 3–4: 519–30.

Swartz, Sally. 2017. "Mad Africa." In *The Routledge History of Madness and Mental Health*, edited by Greg Eghigian, 229–44. London: Routledge.

Thomas, Lynn M. 2020. *Beneath the Surface: A Transnational History of Skin Lighteners*. Durham, NC: Duke University Press.

Thomas, Philip. 2019. "Neoliberal Governmentality, Austerity, and Psycho-Politics." In *Psychology and Politics: Intersections of Science and Ideology in the History of Psy-Sciences*, edited by Anna Borgos, Júlia Gyimesi, and Ferenc Erős, 321–28. Budapest: Central European University Press.

Titley, Brian. 1997. *Dark Age: The Political Odyssey of Emperor Bokassa*. Montreal: McGill–Queen's University Press.

Tonda, Joseph. 2021. *Afrodystopie: La vie dans le rêve d'autrui*. Paris: Éditions Karthala.

Trouillot, Michel-Rolph. 1995. *Silencing the Past: Power and the Production of History*. Boston: Beacon Press.

Trouillot, Michel-Rolph. 2021. "Anthropology and the Savage Slot: The Poetics and Politics of Otherness." In *Trouillot Remixed: The Michel-Rolph Trouillot Reader*, edited by Yarimar Bonilla, Greg Beckett, and Mayanthi L. Fernando, 53–84. Durham, NC: Duke University Press.

Vaughan, Megan. 1983. "Idioms of Madness: Zomba Lunatic Asylum, Nyasaland, in the Colonial Period." *Journal of Southern African Studies* 9, no. 2: 218–38.

Vaughan, Megan. 1991. *Curing Their Ills: Colonial Power and African Illness*. Cambridge, UK: Polity.

Vaughan, Megan. 2005. "Mr Mdala Writes to the Governor: Negotiating Colonial Rule in Nyasaland." *History Workshop Journal* 60, no. 1: 171–88.

Vaughan, Megan. 2012. "The Discovery of Suicide in Eastern and Southern Africa." *African Studies* 71, no. 2: 234–50.

Vaughan, Megan. 2016. "Changing the Subject? Psychological Counseling in Eastern Africa." *Public Culture* 28, no. 3: 499–517.

Veit-Wild, Flora. 2006. *Writing Madness: Borderlines of the Body in African Literature*. Oxford, UK: James Currey.

Vellut, Jean-Luc. 2005. *Simon Kimbangu, 1921, de la prédication à la déportation: Les sources*. Brussels: Académie royale des sciences d'outre-mer.

Veronese, Guido, Alessandro Pepe, Loredana Addimando, Giovanni Sala, and Marzia Vigliaroni. 2020. "'It's Paradise There, I Saw It on TV': Psychological Wellbeing, Migratory Motivators, and Expectations of Return among West African Migrants." *Nordic Psychology* 72, no. 1: 33–50.

Waugh, Melinda J., Ian Robbins, Stephen Davies, and Janet Feigenbaum. 2007. "The Long-Term Impact of War Experiences and Evacuation on People Who Were Children during World War Two." *Aging and Mental Health* 11, no. 2: 168–74.

White, Luise. 1990. "Separating the Men from the Boys: Constructions of Gender, Sexuality, and Terrorism in Central Kenya, 1939–1959." *International Journal of African Historical Studies* 23:1–25.

White, Luise. 2000. *Speaking with Vampires: Rumor and History in Colonial Africa*. Berkeley: University of California Press.

White, Luise, Stephan Miescher, and David William Cohen. 2001. *African Words, African Voices: Critical Practices in Oral History*. Bloomington: Indiana University Press.

Wilbraham, Lindy. 2014. "Reconstructing Harry: A Genealogical Study of a Colonial Family 'Inside' and 'Outside' the Grahamstown Asylum, 1888–1918." *Medical History* 58, no. 2: 166–87.

Williams, Raymond. 1977. "Dominant, Residual and Emergent." In *Marxism and Literature*, 121–27. Oxford: Oxford University Press.

Winnicott, Derek W. (1965) 2006. *The Family and Individual Development*. Reprint, London: Routledge.

Wrong, Michela. 2000. *In the Footsteps of Mr Kurtz: Living on the Brink of Disaster in the Congo*. London: Fourth Estate.

Yoka, Lye. 1999. *Kinshasa, signes de vie*. Paris: Harmattan.

Zumthurm, Tizian. 2020. *Practicing Biomedicine at the Albert Schweitzer Hospital 1913–1965: Ideas and Improvisations*. Leiden: Brill.

PART I

WRITING, BIOGRAPHY, AND THE PSYCHOPOLITICS OF DECOLONIZATION

Nana Osei Quarshie

1

Archives of False Prophets

Inventing the Future in
a West African Psychiatric Hospital

You cannot carry out fundamental change without a certain amount of madness. In this case, it comes from nonconformity, the courage to turn your back on the old formulas, the courage to invent the future. It took the madmen of yesterday for us to be able to act with extreme clarity today. I want to be one of those madmen. *We must dare to invent the future.*

Thomas Sankara, first president of Burkina Faso, 1983–1987

To regain my good health permanently, all foes depriving me of Girls, Money, Spiritual and Political GODLY Powers whilst they attack me with germs, drugs, and privacy invading MENTAL TRANSISTORS must be executed or jailed for life by the Ghana Government for me, right now, as demanded and directed by DIVINE VENGEANCE.

Akla-Osu, SUPERLANDLORD of Ghana

To his psychiatrists, Akla-Osu was a false prophet.[1] Admitted to the Accra Psychiatric Hospital on January 6, 1969, he was a recidivist inpatient until 1976. During this seven-year period, he was confined four times. Discharged a final time on September 16, 1976, Akla-Osu's dialogue with the psychiatric hospital continued, off and on, for a total of nine years. In 1978, he traveled hundreds of miles from his family's home in the Volta Region of Ghana to the coastal city of Accra, Ghana's capital, where he presented hospital authorities with a four-page handwritten petition for financial relief. Akla-Osu was, by then, a lapsed architecture student and unemployed boarding school instructor. He audaciously signed his petition as "GHANA's SUPERLANDLORD, the GOOD GOLDMANGOD."[2] Medical authorities at the Accra Psychiatric Hospital were unmoved by the petition. Psychiatrists had previously diagnosed Akla-Osu as suffering from schizophrenia, featuring delusions of grandeur and persecution.[3] From the doctors' clinical standpoint, the claims made in the petition were products of his delusions. They evaluated his statements as false and socially unsubstantiated, as symptoms of schizophrenia.

Akla-Osu's petition is drawn from the large depository of delusional utterances preserved in the Accra Psychiatric Hospital's patient files. But its length and detail offer unusually rich documentation of the personal and political worldview of a psychiatric patient in postcolonial Africa. In this chapter, I argue that Akla-Osu's petition, and the depositories in which utterances such as his reside on the African continent, constitute the *archives of false prophets*. They are historical repositories of the unrealized "callings" that haunt African colonial asylums and postcolonial psychiatric hospitals (Kilroy-Marac 2019). These archives lay bare, but are also built on, the inherent discursive alterity that slots the African mind as simultaneously "savage" and "mad" in the colonial library (Abraham 1962; Mudimbe 1988; Trouillot 1991; Vaughan 1991; McCulloch 1995). They signal the world of alternative claims to authority, and to imagining the political future, that competed on a crowded stage of political programs and rivalries in the early decades of independence in much of Africa (Cooper 2014; Wilder 2015; Getachew 2019).

African and expatriate psychiatrists working in postcolonial Africa, as well as scholars of psychiatry, have long theorized that delusions are medical symptoms, but ones uniquely shaped by political and social circumstances (Forster 1958; Collignon 1983). As early as the 1960s, psychiatric and psychoanalytically informed anthropologists working in West Africa explored the political implications of the delusional utterances of people seeking care for mental distress (Jahoda 1957, 1961; Field 1960; Fortes and Mayer 1966; Ortigues and Ortigues 1966). They aimed to distinguish delusions from hallucinations and shared cultural persecutory beliefs (Zempleni and Collomb 1968; Collignon 2015). Though historical examinations of the problem remain few and bound to the colonial period (du Plessis 2019, 2), historians, like anthropologists, have been concerned with the "epistemic standing" of delusional representations (Srinivasan 2019). They seek to understand how politics shape psychopathology; how sociopolitical contexts inform the content of delusions (Swartz 2008). Acknowledging the criticism that it may be naive to compare psychiatric patients to prophets, Jonathan Sadowsky (1999, 71) reads the delusions of colonial-era Nigerian patients as akin to the revelatory insight of the unfiltered ramblings of the inebriated. Lynette Jackson (2018, 90–98) suggests that some forms of speech identified as delusional in Zimbabwe's colonial asylum might have reflected a form of ideological rebellion against white supremacy. Rory du Plessis (2019) uncovers the political biases of colonial psychiatrists by exploring how certain delusions expressed by Black patients were silenced and censored in psychiatric publications in colonial South Africa.

Discussions of the political significance of delusional speech are more common in histories of psychiatry in Europe and North America than in Africa (Wright 2004; Murat 2014; du Plessis 2019). This is perhaps because historians of psychiatry in Africa have more to offer than studies figuring the delusions of psychiatric patients as reflective of sociopolitical circumstances. We must also interrogate the potential that delusional utterances hold for engendering future-oriented theories alongside reimaginings of historical conditions of possibility, particularly during periods of political transition (Sass 1994; Metzl 2010; Gerrans 2014; Bortolotti 2018). Akla-Osu did not simply reflect the world. Rather, I argue, he attempted to reinvent it, to mold future actions, by injecting the revisionist claims in his petition into his relationships with his psychiatric caregivers. Understood in this light, delusional utterances actualize a geography of patient "gnosis" (Fabian 1969; Mudimbe 1988, 9), contesting the knowledge claims of allopathic medicine, and the medical opinions of physicians and therapists. Delusions reveal how the putatively "insane," the mentally distressed, perform the transition from functional objects or beings-in-themselves, mere mirrors of the social world, to freedom-thinking subjects or beings-for-themselves. They are a starting point for what Valentin-Yves Mudimbe frames as an "absolute discourse":

sources for intellectual—as much as medical or political—histories of colonial and postcolonial Africa.

By placing Akla-Osu's petition within broader archives of false prophets, this chapter proposes a new method for conducting histories of postcolonial African psychiatry. Ironically, the tentative engagement of the history of psychiatry in Africa with delusional utterances places the subfield at odds with broader trends in African history, which has sustained a rich conversation on the use of unconventional oral genres as historical evidence. Such genres include oracles, accusations of witchcraft, vampire stories, and dreams—utterances that are categorizable as delusional in some clinical or political circumstances. In the 1960s, Africa's historians were burdened by proving the evidentiary base of oral sources and narratives (Vansina 1965). But the 1970s and 1980s brought new examinations of the positivism of oral traditions research, a turn away from nationalist to populist historical accounts, and concerns about memory, gender, and political struggle. Life history research, a feminist methodological innovation of this era (Geiger 1990; Hofmeyr 1993), offered an alternative to the earlier structuralist emphasis on the universal and symbolic aspects of African oral traditions. But, as noted by Luise White (2000) and David William Cohen and E. S. Atieno Odhiambo (2004), life history risked overvalorizing unmediated individual voices, ignoring the ways in which oral testimonies operate as social performances of speech genres.

Anthropologists of psychiatry in postcolonial Africa have built on insights derived from life history research and its critics to fruitful ends (Davis 2012; Nakamura 2013; Pinto 2014; Luhrmann and Marrow 2016; Pandolfo 2018). Julien Bonhomme (2009), in his examination of Ondo Mba—a schizophrenic graffiti prophet of Libreville, Gabon—tacks between the individual voice and the social genre at play. Bonhomme asks how delusional utterances construct and perform agency. For the ethnographer, who lives in the time of the patient, the pitfalls of overprivileging voices can be avoided by placing delusional speech in its sociopolitical context and in conversation with contemporaneous genres of speech. Historians, who may be more temporally distanced from their subjects (Lévi-Strauss 1963; Fabian 1983), must situate such utterances within historically specific genres of speech. If not, historians risk turning delusional utterances into voices without selves: "voices," in the words of White (2000, 68), in which no "embodiments, interests, and powers strive to be reinvented and reinterpreted as they speak."

This chapter models a new interpretive approach to delusional utterances that takes cues from life-history-informed anthropology and microhistorical approaches in African history, which triangulate the scanty archival traces produced by minor events and little-known individuals with political forces and conjunctures in order to uncover larger but unexplored social worlds (Hunt 1999; McCaskie 2000). This approach calls for both a temporal and a methodological shift. We are only just beginning to write the postcolonial history of psychiatry due to uneven access to archives for this era, and a shift in taste toward the postcolonial. In part, the paucity of historical work on delusional utterances of psychiatric patients in Africa is materially determined. The archival sources that give direct access to patients' voices, whether as reported speech in court or hospital records, or reflections written in their own hand, are often difficult to access. But Ghana's National Archives, and those of the Accra Psychiatric Hospital's Biostatistics Department, are littered with petitions regarding the cases of mentally distressed individuals. The petitions are often situated within correspondence from medical authorities, the police, and other government officials. The letters located in the Ghanaian National Archives are mainly written by the family members of patients between the 1920s and the 1950s. Conversely, the archive of the Accra Psychiatric Hospital's Biostatistics Department holds letters from the postindependence era. Some family-written letters in the colonial library strategically frame confined patients as passive persons in need of rescue from the mental asylum. By contrast, letters written by postcolonial patients reveal their active engagement in debates regarding confinement and treatment (Porter 1985; Risse and Warner 1992).

Postcolonial letters are windows into the political worldviews that frame patient experiences with psychiatric care. But public knowledge about lived experiences with psychiatric care and confinement often leads to the sociopolitical exclusion of distressed individuals and their families. In much of the world, this stigma accounts for why most psychiatric patient files are under a century-long moratorium. At the Accra Psychiatric Hospital, however, practical limitations to individual patient privacy have long impacted ideological frameworks and policies concerning researchers' access to postcolonial patient files. Dr. Edward Francis Bani Forster, who arrived from Gambia in 1951 as the first African with a medical degree in psychiatry, instituted the rule, still in place today, that patients must be accompanied by kin, or a member of their therapy management group, during outpatient clinic consultations. This policy limits the patient's privacy in the hope of collecting more accurate case notes and patient histories so as to facilitate better treatment practices. Privacy is also impacted by spatial limitations. With two doctors to an office during outpatient clinics, patients easily overhear other cases, and the confidentiality of the content of patient files is relatively ambiguous. A social scientist with multidisciplinary interests, Forster recognized this ambiguity when he established the patient file archive of the Accra Psychiatric Hospital. In his first decade in Accra, he selectively granted anthropologists and social psychologists access to the archive for anonymized research. In his own writing, Forster interpreted anonymized letters from Ghana's psychiatric archives to help explain the psychological impacts of independence-era political change. Building on Forster's method, this chapter turns to the postcolonial archive to bring into vision the delusional utterances in Akla-Osu's long and richly textured handwritten petition—a veritable political manifesto. This manifesto calls attention to the methodological question that undergirds my interpretive orientation: How do the delusional strive to remake and reinvent their sociopolitical context as they speak?

The chapter is divided into three sections. The first examines Akla-Osu's personal and medical history, covering his early life from 1949 to 1968 and his diagnosis as mentally ill between 1968 and 1969, and it concludes with Akla-Osu's interactions with the Accra Psychiatric Hospital from 1969 to 1978, the year he delivered his petition to hospital authorities. The other two sections explore the intellectual content of Akla-Osu's petition in the context of postcolonial West Africa. My reading of Akla-Osu's statements inverts the common historiographical emphasis on how political contexts shaped delusions in Africa. Instead, I center how Akla-Osu dared to invent the future—to use the words of Thomas Sankara—by reframing his psychiatric treatment as a set of ideologically consequential impending acts destined to justify his political and spiritual authority across time. Attention to the creative political work of Akla-Osu's speech highlights efforts of psychiatric patients to transform social perceptions by shaping people's future actions through the manifestation of novel forms of sociopolitical belonging and the foreclosure of others. This approach is a starting point for placing Akla-Osu's provocative and delusional conceptual arguments in dialogue with the ideas of politicians and intellectual thinkers of his day, who sit at the center of most political histories of this period.

Akla-Osu

Akla-Osu's multiple stints in the mental hospital for schizophrenia between 1969 and 1976, and his self-appointment in 1977 as Ghana's president-elect and SUPERLANDLORD, unfolded within the political and psychiatric history of early postcolonial Ghana. Akla-Osu's paternal family was Ewe, an ethnic group and language variety straddling the border of contemporary Ghana and Togo. The second of seven children, Akla-Osu was born in Ho, British Togoland, in July 1949. This was the year that Kwame Nkrumah, the future president of independent Ghana, founded the Convention People's Party (CPP). A precocious and intelligent child, Akla-Osu graduated from primary school in Dzalele, British Togoland in 1955.[4] During this period, he lived in the home of his uncle, a popular priest for an Ewe spirit in the town of Ave-Dzalele.[5] Akla-Osu likely served after school as a priest's assistant and runner: delivering messages and goods for his uncle, and gaining intimate knowledge of the practice (Field 1937). Between 1956 and 1959, Akla-Osu studied at a middle school in Nsawam, a town forty miles northwest of Accra in Ghana's Eastern Region. His first two years of middle school were tracked with Ghana's move toward independence and the consolidation of its national borders. In 1956, citizens of British Togoland voted in a plebiscite to decide whether to remain a British-administered United Nations mandate or to join a nascent Ghana, which became the first independent nation in sub-Saharan Africa in 1957. Many Ewe ethnic nationalists argued that British Togoland should temporarily remain a British mandate in order to establish a union with French Togoland (contemporary Togo), which would reconstitute the former borders of German Togoland. Integration with Ghana won the day, however, with 58 percent of the vote.[6] British Togoland became the Volta Region of independent Ghana. In Akla-Osu's second year of middle school, Ghana gained independence, with Nkrumah and the CPP leading the first government.

During middle school, Akla-Osu lived in his parents' home in a cosmopolitan and multiethnic neighborhood surrounded by a mix of Ga, Ewe, and Twi speakers. Added to this milieu were his American teachers, members of the first-ever cohort of Peace Corps volunteers.[7] His father was an employee of the Ghana State Farms Corporation in Nsawam.[8] Like many Ewe-speaking people, Akla-Osu's kin transgressed the British and French colonial mandate borders dividing the formerly unified German Togoland. Colonial administrators in the Gold Coast had long desired to recruit labor from French West Africa. Nkrumah similarly encouraged the movement of people, like Akla-Osu's father, from French Togoland into the Gold Coast. Nkrumah promoted a united Togoland—albeit under the Ghanaian flag—as part of his "United States of Africa." But after the plebiscite, the Ghanaian state conducted violent attacks on Togolese reunification activists that encouraged, between 1958 and 1961, over 5,700 refugees to flee the Volta Region for French Togoland (Skinner 2015, 170). Akla-Osu's youth was marked by Ghanaian state reprisals against Ewe migrants from French Togoland, such as his father.

We do not have much information on Akla-Osu's mother, who died when he was ten years old. But his petition suggests she may have been Ga, from Osu, Accra.[9] Early dissatisfaction with the promises of independence emanated not only from the Ewe-speaking Volta Region, but also from the CPP's stronghold of Accra, where the Ga Shifimokpee, a political organization representing ethnic Ga people, was formed. Ga activists, many of whom were descendants of Accra's long-standing political authorities, claimed the CPP was complicit in taking their land. At rallies, they chanted such slogans as, "Ga lands are for Ga people," "People of Ga descent, arise," and "We are being despoiled by strangers" (Quarcoopome 1992). In November 1958, a bomb exploded near Flagstaff House, Nkrumah's official residence. The prime minister decried it as an assassination attempt and had forty-three members of the Ga Shifimokpee arrested. Nkrumah plunged into a prolonged state of paranoia, triggering a cycle of state terror and counterterror between 1958 and 1966 that created political and personal insecurity for many Ghanaian citizens, and ultimately led to Nkrumah's overthrow.

Between 1959 and 1964, Akla-Osu attended a secondary school in Akropong in the Eastern Region. He graduated with high standing and was admitted to the preliminary architecture program at the University of Science and Technology in Kumasi. Akla-Osu entered university during the moment in Ghanaian history referred to as "the period of crisis" (1961–66) by Dr. Edward Francis Bani Forster, the nation's first psychiatrist. A Gambian-born doctor who had worked in Ghana since 1951, Forster (1972, 383) used the rate of first admissions from 1951 to 1971 at the Accra Psychiatric Hospital as a metric for gauging the level of social disintegration in Ghana. This was, in his words, "an attempt to correlate the effects of political, economic, and social pressures on a people and to see whether these forces in their varying intensities, produced any adverse effects, identifiable from the vantage point of psychiatric observation." From 1961 to 1966, Forster found that the Accra

Psychiatric Hospital encountered more outpatients, more first admissions, and more psychiatric symptoms than during any other period in Ghana's first twenty years of popular rule. During the crisis period, Forster noted that suspicions grew between husbands and wives, and between parents and children, who were trained to inform the state of their parents' suspicious activities (Forster 1972; Ahlman 2017). By January of 1966, the state's balance of payments deficit was in shambles, and the citizenry responded to CPP-sponsored state terror with their own anti-CPP acts of terrorism. Within the month, Nkrumah was overthrown in a military coup, leading to the establishment of the National Liberation Council (1966–69).

In early November 1968, Akla-Osu, now a twenty-one-year-old architecture student, delivered a petition letter to the inspector in charge of the police post at the University of Science and Technology. Mirroring the antagonisms between parent and child that Forster witnessed in the Nkrumah era, Akla-Osu wrote, "I have reasons to believe that my father has sold me to either the Ghana Government or to a group of scientists such that I could be used anyhow for experimental purposes."[10] He concluded the letter with three concerns that justified his broader claims. First, that he was injected with "the virus of Chronic Bronchitis" in October 1962. Second, that he was the owner of 40.8 British pounds' million worth of premium bonds that the Nkrumah regime bought in 1964. In a curious statement marking a conflation of his person with financial capital, he noted "my father might have been duped to sell me because of my wealth." Third, that an "organized group of people," including some close friends and colleagues, had "been using a variety of incriminatory tactics to show me to the public as (1) a liar, (2) a block-head, (3) a womanizer, (4) a drunkard, (5) a smoker, (6) a drug addict and (7) an insane person!" Pleading desperately for help from the police, Akla-Osu pledged to "re-act on my own" if they did not save him.[11]

Within a month of delivering this note to police, Akla-Osu threatened the vice-chancellor of the university.[12] He was subsequently placed under the care and observation of Dr. Emmanuel William Quartey Bannerman, the resident medical officer at the university's hospital. Writing to the medical officer in charge of the Accra Psychiatric Hospital on December 21, 1968, Bannerman suggested that Akla-Osu was suffering from persecutory and grandiose delusions.[13] As evidence, the doctor pointed to the patient's belief that his senior tutor, also the leader of the university's Christian Fellowship Group, had stolen his lottery winnings from 1965, and that the Roman Catholic chaplain supported this theft. When he finally sent Akla-Osu to the psychiatric hospital on January 5, 1969, Bannerman noted the patient was "known to have drawn a knife on two occasions."[14] Akla-Osu was a danger to society.

Between 1969 and 1974, Akla-Osu was admitted four separate times to inpatient treatment at the Accra Psychiatric Hospital: twice under certificates of urgency (under police escort), and twice as a voluntary patient (brought in by his family). His first two periods of confinement in the hospital came after referrals from Bannerman. The first took place from January to early May 1969, when he was granted a two-week trial leave. Instead of returning from leave, Akla-Osu made his way back to Kumasi to continue his studies.[15] Five months later, Bannerman filed another certificate of urgency to have Akla-Osu reexamined at the Accra Psychiatric Hospital. He arrived on October 8, 1969, and was released just short of two months later. After his second confinement, Akla-Osu found work as a teacher at an elite girls' secondary school in the Ashanti Region.[16] But the headmaster accused Akla-Osu of erratic behavior and fired him shortly thereafter. Akla-Osu's brother took him to the mental hospital, where he stayed as a voluntary patient from November 23, 1970, to December 21, 1971. Four years later, Akla-Osu endured a final extended voluntary stay at the Accra Psychiatric Hospital, arriving on December 3, 1975, and leaving on September 16, 1976. He returned to the Accra Psychiatric Hospital on February 1, 1978, sixteen months after his final date of discharge. Doctors took a brief note regarding the visit. These were the final words written in his patient file: "Says people are using mental transistors to damage him.[17] These people persistently annoy him and make him lose any job he gets. He also hears these people's [sic] voices talking to him. He is dressed in a very bizarre fashion."[18] The doctor's note emphasized Akla-Osu's concerns about his job prospects and the persistence of his auditory hallucinations. But it neither discussed Akla-Osu's proposed solutions to his employment woes nor the content of his hallucinations. To access that information, we now turn to the petition Akla-Osu delivered to authorities at the Accra Psychiatric Hospital in 1978.

The GOOD GOLDMANGOD

Doctors must have found Akla-Osu's voluminous petition remarkable. He framed it as his application for a certificate of fitness: a letter from the hospital authorities affirming a recovering patient's readiness to obtain employment. But such letters were usually brief, not three-thousand-word political exegeses. The first page of the petition began with the following salutation: "N. B. = Nota Bene (THOUGH I AM GHANA'S SUPERLANDLORD, OWNER OF THE LAND OF GHANA, YET I AM THE MOST HUMBLE 'PATIENT.' GOOD BUT NOT PROUD.)"[19] The heading of the second page stated, "THOUGH I NEED MORE THAN ONE MILLION CEDIS (¢1,000,000) ANNUAL INCOME, I AM NOT YET RECEIVING EVEN A CEDI."[20] If Akla-Osu's goal was to convince medical authorities of the validity of his concerns, these headings likely had the opposite effect. Doctors at the Accra Psychiatric Hospital would have interpreted these bold-faced statements as classic manifestations of delusions of grandeur.

Two thematic threads drive the petition's central requests. The first is Akla-Osu's status as the GOLDMANGOD, the avatar of a deity that he believed had won him riches and glory through "lucky chance games"—a euphemism for the lottery. Despite his alleged winnings, Akla-Osu wrote to the hospital authorities: "I AM ASHAMED OF MY POVERTY. I AM SOCIALLY ISOLATED AND SEXUALLY STARVED, IN DIRE NEED OF SEX WITH GOOD GIRLS (SWEETHEARTS), JUST AS I NEED MY SUBSISTENCE MONEY MYSELF TO BUY RADIO CASSETTE RECORDER, SOME NEW CLOTHES, FURNITURE AND OTHER THINGS (AMENITIES) TO MEET THE DEMANDS OF THE INFLATION AND HIGH COST OF LIVING." Akla-Osu insisted that nefarious enemies—including his father, American Peace Corps teachers from his childhood, the police, and hospital staff—conspired to steal money from him. Writing "I am the GOLDMANGOD; and Money is God in manifestation to me as freedom from want (poverty) and limitation for me and my true lovers,"[21] Akla-Osu slotted his God into the category of what were known as "money-doubling spirits" in independence-era Ghana. Money-doubling (*atsrɛlɛ* in Ga, Akla-Osu's maternal language) was a historical form of ritual intercession, in which a supplicant offered a shrine priest money on the promise that it would be increased by an interceding spirit and then returned to the client (McCaskie 1995, 122). Gustav Jahoda, a psychiatric anthropologist working in Ghana in the 1950s, noted that the term itself was a misnomer, as supplicants were often promised far more than double the profits (Jahoda 1957, 271). Money-doubling spirits bore a resemblance to evangelical prosperity gospel, popular in the United States during the first half of the twentieth century. In 1937, the anthropologist Margaret Field noted a changing tide in the landscape of healing in Accra, whereby "private medicine men" were being replaced by a new class of healer that she characterized as "the American type of superstitious or villain-ous quack" (Field 1937, 133). Field was referring to scientific herbalists—innovators within Ghana's healing landscape who combined historical ritual and herbal healing techniques with the semiotics and sartorial practices of Euro-American allopathic medicine (Osseo-Asare 2016). In Field's estima-tion, semiliterate and literate Africans made up most of the gullible victims of these con men because "they believe every word of the patent medicine advertisements that they read and freely spend their money on such things as 'Brain and Memory Pills' and subscriptions to correspondence 'colleges' selling courses of instruction in Ancient Egyptian mysteries of the Soul" (Field 1937, 133). On the one hand, Field's analysis of scientific herbalists minimized the long-standing Euro-American influences on the Ga healing repertoires she studied (Roberts 2015, 207–10). On the other hand, there seems to have been some truth to her observations that "scientific herbal-ists" deceived their clientele. By the late 1950s, the Criminal Investigation Division of the Accra Police were investigating numerous cases of the notori-ous practice of "money-doubling," by then officially considered a confidence game, a scam, by the Ghanaian government (Jahoda 1957).

While it is easy to see money-doubling as fraud, its roots suggest a far more complex history, one starting in the early colonial era, a moment when the historical imperative to accumulate cash intersected intensely with con-cerns around belief in the financial potency of spirits (ɔbosom in Twi) in the former Asante Territories (McCaskie 1995, 122). Money-doubling be-came widespread in the Asante forest region following the Fourth Anglo-Asante War (1900–1901), after which the British exiled the Asantehene to the Seychelles and annexed Asante. After the war, the Asante state became increasingly enrolled in the British colonial economy, which was based on the use of a new, singular form of currency: the British pound. But most Asante citizens had limited access to cash. Many men and women migrated to work on cocoa farms and in gold mines to meet British head tax demands, which could only be paid in pounds. Traveling shrine priests went from village to village offering to intercede with spirits that could ritually increase one's cash. Among the Asante, it was conjecturally understood that the sharpness of a spirit's powers was linked to their ability to accumulate acolytes and of-ferings (McCaskie 1995, 123).[22] At the same time, a spirit's power was seen as inherently ambiguous, as spirits could abscond with the money given to them for doubling. This fate was familiar to Akla-Osu. Only an extremely generous supplicant could ensure financial reward rather than harm. Despite the inherent risks entailed, avarice took hold because of desperation for access to cash. Many people willingly ceded their money to the shrine priests of doubling spirits. Their chances of success were likely as good as Akla-Osu's prospects with the "lucky chance games."

In the mid-1950s, Jahoda (1957, 270–71) noted that the avatars of money-doubling spirits in Ghana were often young men who were allegedly educated enough to have ambitious desires, but not enough to actually receive a lucrative position. Like Akla-Osu, most avatars were literate, but of "illiterate parentage," and were newcomers to the city from the countryside. These individuals were upwardly mobile but encountered a glass ceiling early in their careers. Field's literate Africans of the early 1930s were fooled by fake correspondence degrees in the quest to better their lot. Jahoda's intermediate literates eschewed correspondence courses for "short cuts and hit upon an easy way of exploiting the greed and gullibility of their luckier fellows" (Jahoda 1957, 270). Similar to Akla-Osu, who lived with his uncle—a famous Ewe spirit priest—during his primary school years, doublers often worked as, or with, ritual herbalists. Jahoda differentiated between "magical" and "technological" money-doublers, although the two modes overlapped at times. The magical variety operated through the power of spirits, much like their counterparts in early colonial Asante. A client would go to a field of invocation, often a sacred grove, where a shrine priest gave them instructions. The client would return to the meeting place with an offering (a set quantity of cash) and be instructed to return a day later for their blessings. If the offering was pleasing to the spirit, the client's money would be doubled. The client would then inform other people they knew about the doubler, who might patronize the doubler's services. When this new mass of clients returned for their increase, however, they often found that the doubler was nowhere to be seen, and their money had been "eaten" by the spirit (McCaskie 1995, 122). Meanwhile, technological money-doublers sold machines, often toasters adorned with bells and buzzers, that allegedly produced banknotes. According to Jahoda (1957, 271), technological doublers relied on "the high prestige of Western technology, together with the widespread ignorance of its most elementary principles." The doubler would demonstrate that the machine worked in his shop and offer it for free, charging clients for the medicine, an herb or a liquid, which they would take home and feed into the machine to make it function.

Akla-Osu was an unsuccessful avatar for his money-doubling spirit. One might say his only real success in capital accumulation was allegedly obtaining a 200-cedi monthly welfare payment for subsistence from the government. In his words: "I deserve this my little monthly allowance of only two hundred cedis (₵200) more than any other handicapped Ghanaian because I am the only person under MENTAL TRANSISTOR TORTURE and the only GOLDMANGOD, Avatar of God."[23] If Akla-Osu was the "GOLDMANGOD, Avatar of God," a money-doubling prophet, as he claimed, then he should have benefited from the spirit's accumulative will. But his lot as a pauper, recidivist psychiatric patient, architectural student dropout, and sacked high school teacher, was more akin to the clients than to the prophets of money-doubling spirits. It was as if the spirit for which he was the avatar lacked clients. Needing tributes in order to survive, the spirit dispossessed its own prophet. Akla-Osu's petition suggests he was bankrupt. And yet, like many victims of money-doubling scams, he still believed his blessings were yet to come.

Ghana's SUPERLANDLORD

Another significant thematic thread in Akla-Osu's petition was his claim to be Ghana's "SUPERLANDLORD, OWNER OF THE LAND OF GHANA." As we saw above, his uncle, a famous Ewe spirit priest in Ave-Dzalele, was a model of spiritual authority for the young Akla-Osu. Likewise, Nkrumah, who rose to fame in the year of his birth, was a distant but prominent model of political sovereignty. The popularity of money-doubling in the late 1950s presaged an increasingly popular critique of Nkrumah's regime by the mid-1960s. As noted in a letter written to Marxist humanist scholar Raya Dunyaveskaya by a young Ghanaian interlocutor named Kofi, "SIKADICIOUS is a word which has been coined by Ghanaians to describe Nkrumaists, because they love money, women, wine and luxurious things more than the people."[24] Akla-Osu's stated desires for "SEX WITH GOOD GIRLS," money, new clothes, and furniture,[25] suggests that he also suffered from "sikadiciousness," a money-eating disorder; the term coming from the Twi word for "gold/money" (*sika*), and the verb "to eat" (*di*). The term came into widespread usage in the early 1960s as a lay critique of Nkrumaist politicians who enriched themselves while lay citizens and soldiers were subjected to austerity measures (Nugent 2019, 442). Although Nkrumah and his CPP fashioned themselves as scientific herbalists healing the nation, many citizens saw them more like money-doublers, who fed shrine spirits the cash of their clients, harming acolytes to heal themselves (Quarshie 2020). Sikadiciousness was a popular sociopsychological diagnosis of a form of economic, political, and sexual pica, marking the lay concerns about the alleged growth of the Nkrumah regime at the expense of the people.

By the late 1970s, Akla-Osu presented himself as the legitimate political sovereign of Ghana, a pretender to the throne relinquished by Nkrumah in the 1966 coup.

> My Ewe foster relatives often call me AKLAOSU, named after my hometown of ACCRA-OSU, that area in the ACCRA CITY where the seat of the Government of Ghana is. Due to the strong undercurrent of tribalism in our Ghana, my Ewe foster relatives also hate good me, envy me and LOVE BEING CRUEL TO ME because of my being a Ga youngster with money and future greatness as the one and only God destined Life-President of Ghana just as the Akans who wrongly believed I was a Togolese-Ewe also envied me and hated me for my God-given money and God-destined future Presidency.[26]

It is in this statement, at the intersection of his sikadiciousness and xenophobic claims to political authority, that we see the future-oriented potential of Akla-Osu's delusions. Akla-Osu was not the only prophet figure in the history of modern Ghana to claim political authority as the manifestation of a historic political leader. In fact, he shared the Accra Psychiatric Hospital with two Jesus Christs,[27] a king,[28] Julius Caesar,[29] Kwame Nkrumah,[30] his friend Kojo Botsio,[31] former Ghanaian prime minister K. A. Busia,[32] former Asantehene Nana Prempeh II,[33] and many others. Consider, for example, the Domankama cult of late precolonial Asante and its founding priest, who claimed to be the rebirth of Asantehene Osei Tutu I, the political founder of the Asante Empire. Historian Tom McCaskie (1981) notes the important role played by such appeals to historic greatness, "to a basic and indispensable ur-law," in shoring up ritual authority.

Akla-Osu's declaration, in contrast, calls for a slightly different reading, because he relied on an alleged Ga heritage to back his claim to political authority. Again, in his words: "Since I am a Ga by tribe and a true Ghanaian by citizenship, I have a strong desire to return home, ACCRA-OSU, right now, to really develop, become more civilized and better oriented in the city into the swing of life for the Presidency, so important to my country Ghana."[34] Akla-Osu equated civilizational attainment with his neighborhood, Osu, in his home city of Accra, which he also noted as the location of the "seat of the Government of Ghana." In so doing, Akla-Osu underscored the importance of his Ga heritage for his claim to political authority over the nation. The Ga are not an obvious choice for such a claim, as their authority in Accra had been in decline long before Akla-Osu's birth. By the early twentieth century, British consolidation of rule in the Gold Coast fissured the political authority of Ga elites over coastal cities, including Accra, setting into motion succession disputes, the removal and reassignment of stools from chiefs, and conflicts over landownership. Long before Nkrumah's rise to political power, Ga authorities were losing control over coastal cities to demographic shift, colonial occupation, and British empowerment of Asante elites (Quarcoopome 1993; Sackeyfio-Lenoch 2014).

Akla-Osu's Ga-centered justifications of his status as Ghana's SUPER-LANDLORD cannot be read as a conservative invocation of a popularly recognized historic greatness. Such a reading would be plausible, for example, if he drew on a real or imagined connection to Asante royalty, who achieved significant economic gains during the colonial period despite major political losses. By contrast, Akla-Osu's appeal to his Ga heritage was a mode of revisionism akin to people from enslaved backgrounds reinventing their heritage by tracking descent back to an alleged ancestor who was not enslaved. Such revisionism facilitated claims to political belonging, generating access to land and future resources, and influencing the treatment of the descendants of the formerly enslaved by people outside of their immediate kin group (Klein 1981). In this case, Akla-Osu called on a Ga heritage in Osu, Accra, that, although real, was unlikely a significant factor in his upbringing in the Eastern and Volta regions.[35] He did so to claim political power to restructure the future actions of his doctors according to his desires. The same declarations made about his Ga heritage, to substantiate his authority as Ghana's SUPERLANDLORD, appear in one other place—his demands about his future psychiatric care:

> I still don't want to be re-admitted into the hospital . . . I hate being
> a patient . . . I HAVE A STRONG DESIRE TO RETURN HOME. Accra
> is my homecity. True. Accra-Osu Cantonments is my home. This is
> very true. But the Accra Psychiatric Hospital at Asylum Down is NOT
> my home. For those who find happiness in that stinking old delapi-
> dated [sic] hospital it can be a permanent home and a mentally sick
> one at that. I hate the indelible stigma of public abhorrence (that

"HE IS A MAD MAN") often stamped on mental patients in this country Ghana and I am trying to erase mine by avoiding further RE-ADMISSIONS.[36]

On the one hand, it was against "the Akans who wrongly believed [he] was a Togolese-Ewe" and against his allegedly "primitive" Ewe foster relatives, the "envious greedy brutes" that took him in 1976 after his final discharge and nicknamed him Akla-Osu, that he appealed to his Ga heritage.[37] But by taking on the persona of a political sovereign of Ga descent, Akla-Osu also signaled a reorientation of the relevant political distinctions that governed the domains of social belonging and psychological security in Ghana at the time. If in the aftermath of Nkrumah's downfall Ghanaian citizens felt renewed hope for their nation's prospects, that moment was short lived. The consequences of years of economic instability and austerity soon became apparent. Politicians scapegoated immigrants, playing on popular fears of economic competition with "foreigners." Unable to improve on the economic inheritances of the CPP regime, the new National Liberation Council military government released "statistics" claiming the negative impact of West African immigrants, who allegedly made up 70 percent of the beggars, on the national economy (Peil 1971, 223). The National Liberation Council passed new and enforced old "Ghanaianization" laws to exclude immigrants from various sectors. The crescendo of this process came with the return to democratic rule and the establishment of Ghana's Second Republic under Prime Minister Kofi Abrefa Busia. On November 18, 1969, Busia's government published the Aliens Compliance Order, requiring all foreigners without residence permits to vacate the country within two weeks. Within a year of the mass expulsion order, it is estimated that over 140,000 people fled Ghana (Adida 2014).

Whether doctors provided him the certificate of fitness he requested, confined him, or ignored him, Akla-Osu's delusions of grandeur and paranoia manifested in the petition in such a way that all three responses played into his genealogical game, validating his authority claims. Akla-Osu, who saw himself as a victim of "Busia authorized criminals," was cognizant of the political ramifications of mass expulsion.[38] His father's family, Ewe speakers living along the Ghana–Togo border, would have been targets of mass expulsion. But he took his mother's Ga heritage—supposedly the cause of the mistreatment he faced from his "xenophobic" Ewe relatives, and the factor ignored by the Akan speakers who framed him as Togolese Ewe—transformed it into a hegemony-authorizing genealogy, and inserted that claim into his demands of his doctors. In doing so, Akla-Osu drew attention to the family resemblance between expulsion from the nation, the family, and the public. His petition was a blueprint for reconceptualizing Ghanaian political and psychic worlds along novel contours of enmity and conviviality. This was no conservative appeal to authority of the Nkrumaist era. If anything, it was a cry for that era's openness to the radical transformation of political life. Akla-Osu insisted on an alternate political reality: one that was not only a work of historical revisionism, not only an ideology of the past, but also a simultaneous inventing of potential political futures.

False Prophets

Delusional utterances in African psychiatric hospitals constitute the *archives of false prophets*: troves of hauntings, unrealized callings, failed and unintelligible representations. They also offer starting points for intellectual, as well as medical and political, histories of Africa. Historians have read the delusional utterances of African psychiatric patients for what they reveal about contemporaneous social, racial, and political tensions. But these readings, rooted in studies of colonial psychiatry, leave unexamined the creative political work intended by Akla-Osu and other psychiatric patients who lived through the tumultuous decades of early independence on the continent. Delusional utterances offer historians more than filters through which a "real world" is refracted. Postcolonial delusions of grandeur that draw on a historic leader are more than conservative appeals to the colonial or precolonial past, shoring up claims to authority. Delusional utterances are vectors of gnosis with a potential to invent the future. Like Akla-Osu's petition, they may entail proactive accounts that revise history and demand systematic political theorization. Such delusional utterances literally spill out of the boxes in the archives of psychiatric hospitals in Africa.[39] They should be examined for their epistemic standing and their sociopolitical justifications, but also for how they invent the future: to identify "the power of the future inscribed within the present" (Mbembe 2010; Radin 2019; Donovan 2020).

Akla-Osu was not just a sponge, nor a social mirror, casting back at the world the truths it would rather conveniently ignore. Rather, he interjected revisionist personal and political historical claims into his relationships with psychiatric caregivers. In this frame, he was similar to those Amia Srinivasan (2019, 150) describes as "successful worldmakers, who often appear to be people—we might call them moral prophets—who simply see the world as no one else yet sees it. Such people are truth-makers who speak and act as truth-tellers: who speak and act as if they are genealogically lucky." Akla-Osu was one such truth-maker, who spoke and acted as a truth-teller. He framed the possibility of his readmission to inpatient care as a justification for his claims to political and ritual authority in the past, present, and future. But successful worldmaking also requires social uptake. Others must accept your representational transformations, or you appear as a deluded charlatan. Akla-Osu was a false prophet, not because his delusions revealed him to be the unsuccessful avatar of a money-doubling spirit, but because he failed to convert others to his version of the future. He was deemed insane, his words evidence of his delusions of grandeur. That Akla-Osu was mentally distressed is clear. However, his words also signal a heretofore untold intellectual history of postcolonial Ghana, one suggestive of the consequences of Burkinabe president Thomas Sankara's call for Africa's postindependence politicians to dare to invent the future like the madmen of yesterday: a world of alternative claims to authority that competed for uptake on a crowded stage of political programs and rivalries that characterized the early decades of independence in much of Africa (Quarshie 2020). At the very least, Akla-Osu's words demand a new methodological approach to the history of psychiatry in postcolonial Africa: one that engages the creative conceptual work of patients.

Notes

Epigraphs: Thomas Sankara (interview with J. P. Rapp, 1985, cited in Prairie 2007); Akla-Osu (Petition—Application for My Certificate of Fitness, October 17, 1977).

1   From 2016 to 2017 I conducted anonymized research in the patient file archives of the Accra Psychiatric Hospital with permission from the Ghana Mental Health Authority. As was the case with this patient, it is often logistically impossible to trace the families of former patients in the archive. But as a sign of respect to their engagement with their mentally distressed kin, I refer to the patient by his family-given pseudonym as reported in the petition: Akla-Osu. I have chosen to maintain, as much as possible, Akla-Osu's orthographic choices in his petition to give the reader a sense of his writing style and intensity.

2 "Letter of Application for Certificate of Fitness [The Petition]," October 17, 1977, Accra Psychiatric Hospital Biostatistics Department Archives (henceforth APHBDA), Box 7A, Unit 340.

3 Certificate of Urgency, January 5, 1969, APHBDA, Box 7A, Unit 340.

4 History from Patient, January 6, 1969, APHBDA, Box 7A, Unit 340.

5 Letter from Social Welfare Officer to Fetish Priest M. A. in Ave-Dzalele, November 21, 1975, APHBDA, Box 7A, Unit 340.

6 Notably, separation from the Gold Coast won by 55 percent in the predominantly Ewe-speaking southern regions of British Togoland.

7 "Letter of Application."

8 Letter from University Registrar to Mr. A. S. at Ghana State Farms Corporation, September 17, 1969, APHBDA, Box 7A, Unit 340.

9 "Letter of Application."

10 "Undated Petition Asking Police to Investigate Father," APHBDA, Box 7A, Unit 340.

11 "Undated Petition."

12 Petition to Vice Chancellor, November 24, 1968, APHBDA, Box 7A, Unit 340.

13 Letter from Dr. Bannerman to Dr. Adomakoh, December 21, 1968, APHBDA, Box 7A, Unit 340.

14 Certificate of Urgency.

15 Letter from Dr. Bannerman to Dr. Adomakoh, May 2, 1969, APHBDA, Box 7A, Unit 340.

16 Letter from Boarding School Principal to Dr. Adomakoh, date unknown, APHBDA, Box 7A, Unit 340.

17 Likely a reference to electroconvulsive therapy, which he previously refused at the hospital.

18 Entry dated February 1, 1978, APHBDA, Box 7A, Unit 340.

19 "Letter of Application."

20 "Letter of Application." Cedi is the name of Ghana's currency.

21 "Letter of Application."

22 This was likely an outgrowth of the incorporation of "foreign" spirits and persons at the "fetish shrines" of Atlantic-era West Africa (Maier 1983; Pietz 1987).

23 "Letter of Application."

24 This letter was later published as "Exclusive Report from a Ghanaian: 'Nkrumah Rules by Terror, Intimidation, and Bribery.'" *The Worker's Journal* (August–September 1963): 7.

25 In a notorious case, Krobo Edusei, one of Nkrumah's cabinet ministers, became the target of a national scandal when it became known that his wife purchased a gold-plated bed in London.

26 "Letter of Application." Life-president was the title held by Nkrumah until the 1966 coup that ousted him.

27 APHBDA, Box 12/13, Unit 788; APHBDA, Box 190, Unit 11085.

28 APHBDA, Box 217, Unit 139.

29 APHBDA, Box 2, Unit 87.

30 APHBDA, Box 217, Unit 12503.

31 APHBDA, Box 14A, Unit 843.

32 APHBDA, Box 11B, Unit 681.

33 APHBDA, Box 2, Unit 87.

34 "Letter of Application."

35 While communities of Ga speakers have long resided in British Togoland (Nugent 2019), there is no suggestion that Akla-Osu was linked to these communities in the various intake interviews and medical histories conducted with him and his family by doctors at the Accra Psychiatric Hospital.

36 "Letter of Application."

37 "Letter of Application."

38 "Letter of Application."

39 More work must be done to confirm the ubiquity of these archives in lusophone Africa, but the scholarship of historians of psychiatry working in anglophone and francophone Africa is suggestive (du Plessis 2019; Kilroy-Marac 2019).

Sources

Archival Material

Accra Psychiatric Hospital Biostatistics Department Archives (APHBDA).

Literature

Abraham, Willie E. 1962. *The Mind of Africa*. London: Weidenfeld and Nicolson.

Adida, Claire L. 2014. *Immigrant Exclusion and Insecurity in Africa*. Cambridge: Cambridge University Press.

Ahlman, Jeffrey S. 2017. *Living with Nkrumahism: Nation, State, and Pan-Africanism in Ghana*. Athens: Ohio University Press.

Bonhomme, Julien. 2009. "Dieu par décret: Les écritures d'un prophète africain." *Annales: Histoires, sciences sociales* 64, no. 4: 887–924.

Bortolotti, Lisa. 2018. "Delusions and Three Myths of Irrational Belief." In *Delusions in Context*, edited by Lisa Bortolotti, 97–116. Cham, Switzerland: Springer.

Cohen, David William, and E. S. Atieno Odhiambo. 2004. *The Risks of Knowledge: Investigations into the Death of the Hon. Minister John Robert Ouko in Kenya, 1990*. Athens: Ohio University Press.

Collignon, René. 1983. "À propos de psychiatrie communautaire en Afrique noire: Les dispositifs villageois d'assistance. Éléments pour un dossier." *Psychopathologie africaine* 19, no. 3: 287–328.

Collignon, René. 2015. "Some Aspects of Mental Illness in French-Speaking West Africa." In *The Culture of Mental Illness and Psychiatric Practice in Africa*, edited by Emmanuel Akyeampong, Alan G. Hill, and Arthur Kleinman, 163–85. Bloomington: Indiana University Press.

Cooper, Frederick. 2014. *Citizenship between Empire and Nation*. Princeton, NJ: Princeton University Press.

Davis, Elizabeth Anne. 2012. *Bad Souls: Madness and Responsibility in Modern Greece*. Durham, NC: Duke University Press.

Donovan, Kevin P. 2020. "Colonizing the Future." *Boston Review*, September 28. https://bostonreview.net/articles/kevin-p-donovan-tk/.

Du Plessis, Rory. 2019. "A Hermeneutic Analysis of Delusion Content from the Casebooks of the Grahamstown Lunatic Asylum, 1890–1907." *South African Journal of Psychiatry* 25, no. 1: 1–7.

Fabian, Johannes. 1969. "An African Gnosis—for a Reconsideration of an Authoritative Definition." *History of Religions* 9, no. 1: 42–58.

Fabian, Johannes. 1983. *Time and the Other: How Anthropology Makes Its Object*. New York: Columbia University Press.

Field, Margaret J. 1937. *Religion and Medicine of the Ga People*. Oxford: Oxford University Press.

Field, Margaret J. 1960. *Search for Security: An Ethno-Psychiatric Study of Rural Ghana*. London: Faber and Faber.

Forster, Edward Francis Bani. 1958. "A Short Psychiatric Review from Ghana." In *Health, Mental Disorders and Mental Health in Africa South of the Sahara: CCTA/CSA-WFMH-WHO Meeting of Specialists on Mental Health*, 37–41. Bukavu, Democratic Republic of Congo: Commission for Technical Co-operation South of the Sahara.

Forster, Edward Francis Bani. 1972. "Mental Health and Political Change in Ghana 1951–1971." *Psychopathologie africaine* 8, no. 3: 383–417.

Fortes, Meyer, and Doris Y. Mayer. 1966. "Psychosis and Social Change among the Tallensi of Northern Ghana." *Cahiers d'études africaines* 6, no. 21: 5–40.

Geiger, Susan. 1990. "What's So Feminist about Women's Oral History?" *Journal of Women's History* 2, no. 1: 169–82.

Gerrans, Philip. 2014. *The Measure of Madness: Philosophy of Mind, Cognitive Neuroscience, and Delusional Thought*. Cambridge, MA: MIT Press.

Getachew, Adom. 2019. *Worldmaking after Empire: The Rise and Fall of Self-Determination*. Princeton, NJ: Princeton University Press.

Hofmeyr, Isabel. 1993. *"We Spend Our Years as a Tale That Is Told": Oral Historical Narrative in a South African Chiefdom*. Portsmouth, NH: Heinemann.

Hunt, Nancy Rose. 1999. *A Colonial Lexicon: Of Birth Ritual, Medicalization, and Mobility in the Congo*. Durham, NC: Duke University Press.

Jackson, Lynette A. 2018. *Surfacing Up: Psychiatry and Social Order in Colonial Zimbabwe, 1908–1968*. Ithaca, NY: Cornell University Press.

Jahoda, Gustav. 1957. "'Money-Doubling in the Gold Coast': With Some Cross-Cultural Comparisons." *British Journal of Delinquency* 8, no. 4: 266–76.

Jahoda, Gustav. 1961. "Traditional Healers and Other Institutions Concerned with Mental Illness in Ghana." *International Journal of Social Psychiatry* 7, no. 4: 245–68.

Kilroy-Marac, Katie. 2019. *An Impossible Inheritance: Postcolonial Psychiatry and the Work of Memory in a West African Clinic*. Berkeley: University of California Press.

Klein, Alexandre Norman. 1981. "The Two Asantes: Competing Interpretation of 'Slavery' in Akan-Asante Culture and Society." In *Ideology of Slavery in Africa*, edited by Paul Lovejoy, 149–67. Beverly Hills, CA: Sage.

Lévi-Strauss, Claude. 1963. *Structural Anthropology*. New York: Basic Books.

Luhrmann, Tanya Marie, and Jocelyn Marrow. 2016. *Our Most Troubling Madness: Case Studies in Schizophrenia across Cultures*. Berkeley: University of California Press.

Maier, Donna J. 1983. *Priests and Power: The Case of the Dente Shrine in Nineteenth-Century Ghana*. Bloomington: Indiana University Press.

Mbembe, Achille. 2010. "Faut-il provincialiser la France?" *Politique africaine* 3:159–88.

McCaskie, Tom C. 1981. "Anti-Witchcraft Cults in Asante: An Essay in the Social History of an African People." *History in Africa* 8:125–54.

McCaskie, Tom C. 1995. *State and Society in Pre-Colonial Asante*. Cambridge: Cambridge University Press.

McCaskie, Tom C. 2000. *Asante Identities: History and Modernity in an African Village, 1850–1950*. Bloomington: Indiana University Press.

McCulloch, Jock. 1995. *Colonial Psychiatry and "the African Mind."* Cambridge: Cambridge University Press.

Metzl, Jonathan. 2010. *The Protest Psychosis: How Schizophrenia Became a Black Disease*. Boston: Beacon Press.

Mudimbe, Valentin-Yves. 1988. *The Invention of Africa: Gnosis, Philosophy, and the Order of Knowledge*. Bloomington: Indiana University Press.

Murat, Laure. 2014. *The Man Who Thought He Was Napoleon: Toward a Political History of Madness*. Chicago: University of Chicago Press.

Nakamura, Karen. 2013. *A Disability of the Soul: An Ethnography of Schizophrenia and Mental Illness in Contemporary Japan*. Ithaca, NY: Cornell University Press.

Nugent, Paul. 2019. *Boundaries, Communities and State-Making in West Africa: The Centrality of the Margins*. Cambridge: Cambridge University Press.

Ortigues, Marie-Cécilie, and Edmund Ortigues. 1966. *Oedipe africain*. Paris: Plon.

Osseo-Asare, Abena Dove. 2016. "Writing Medical Authority: The Rise of Literate Healers in Ghana, 1930–70." *Journal of African History* 57, no. 1: 69–91.

Pandolfo, Stefania. 2018. *Knot of the Soul: Madness, Psychoanalysis, Islam*. Chicago: University of Chicago Press.

Peil, Margaret. 1971. "The Expulsion of West African Aliens." *Journal of Modern African Studies* 9, no. 2: 205–29.

Pietz, William. 1987. "The Problem of the Fetish, II: The Origin of the Fetish." *Anthropology and Aesthetics* 13, no. 1: 23–45.

Pinto, Sarah. 2014. *Daughters of Parvati: Women and Madness in Contemporary India*. Philadelphia: University of Pennsylvania Press.

Porter, Roy. 1985. "The Patient's View." *Theory and Society* 14, no. 2: 175–98.

Prairie, Michel. 2007. *Thomas Sankara Speaks: The Burkina Faso Revolution, 1983–1987*. London: Pathfinder Press.

Quarcoopome, Samuel Sackey. 1992. "Urbanisation, Land Alienation and Politics in Accra." *Research Review* 8, no. 1–2: 40–54.

Quarcoopome, Samuel Sackey. 1993. "The Impact of Urbanisation on the Socio-Political History of the Ga Mashie People of Accra: 1877–1957." PhD diss., University of Ghana.

Quarshie, Nana Osei. 2020. "Bounding 'Alien Lunatics' in Modern Ghana." PhD diss., University of Michigan.

Radin, Joanna. 2019. "The Speculative Present: How Michael Crichton Colonized the Future of Science and Technology." *Osiris* 34, no. 1: 297–315.

Risse, Guenter B., and John Harley Warner. 1992. "Reconstructing Clinical Activities: Patient Records in Medical History." *Social History of Medicine* 5, no. 2: 183–205.

Roberts, Jonathan. 2015. "Sharing the Burden of Sickness: A History of Healing in Accra, Gold Coast, 1677 to 1957." PhD diss., Dalhousie University.

Sackeyfio-Lenoch, Naaborko. 2014. *The Politics of Chieftaincy: Authority and Property in Colonial Ghana, 1920–1950*. Rochester, NY: University of Rochester Press.

Sadowsky, Jonathan. 1999. *Imperial Bedlam: Institutions of Madness in Colonial Southwest Nigeria*. Berkeley: University of California Press.

Sass, Louis A. 1994. "'My So-Called Delusions': Solipsism, Madness, and the Schreber Case." *Journal of Phenomenological Psychology* 25, no. 1: 70–103.

Skinner, Kate. 2015. *The Fruits of Freedom in British Togoland: Literacy, Politics and Nationalism, 1914–2014*. Cambridge: Cambridge University Press.

Srinivasan, Amia. 2019. "VII: Genealogy, Epistemology and Worldmaking." *Proceedings of the Aristotelian Society* 119, no. 2: 127–56.

Swartz, Sally. 2008. "Colonial Lunatic Asylum Archives: Challenges to Historiography." *Kronos* 34, no. 1: 285–302.

Trouillot, Michel-Rolph. 1991. "Anthropology and the Savage Slot: The Poetics and Politics of Otherness." In *Recapturing Anthropology: Working in the Present*, edited by Richard G. Fox, 17–45. Santa Fe, NM: School of American Research Press.

Vansina, Jan. 1965. *Oral Tradition*. Translated by H. M. Wright. London: Routledge.

Vaughan, Megan. 1991. *Curing Their Ills: Colonial Power and African Illness*. Cambridge, UK: Polity.

White, Luise. 2000. *Speaking with Vampires: Rumor and History in Colonial Africa*. Berkeley: University of California Press.

Wilder, Gary. 2015. *Freedom Time: Negritude, Decolonization, and the Future of the World*. Durham, NC: Duke University Press.

Wright, David. 2004. "Delusions of Gender? Lay Identification and Clinical Diagnosis of Insanity in Victorian England." In *Sex and Seclusion, Class and Custody: Perspectives on Gender and Class in the History of British and Irish Psychiatry*, edited by Anne Digby, 149–76. Leiden: Brill.

Zempleni, Andras, and Henri Collomb. 1968. "Sur la position médiatrice et le domaine propre de la psychologie sociale dans l'Afrique actuelle." *Journal of Social Issues* 24, no. 2: 57–67.

Richard Hölzl

2

Missionary Anxieties, Psychopathology, and Decolonization

A Biographical Approach

There is something uncanny about religious missions. At a superficial level of scrutiny, their task is straightforward. Spread the word (the gospel, holy scripture, rules, or a set of religious practices) and see who is listening and who is willing to follow. But missions—and their missionaries—have strong urges. They wish to feel at home in a new territory. Fulfilling this impulse is difficult, since missionaries are alien to the colonies, countries, and people among whom they proselytize. Even more troublesome, most missionaries realized almost from the very beginning of their work that "spreading the word" is not a simple transaction. Religious messages are not handed over like a well-sealed parcel from giving hands to receiving ones. Traveling missionaries rely on experienced cultural brokers and local experts, whose services are necessary for all kinds of tasks: finding pathways, shelter, sustenance, and protection, for mutual introduction during cultural encounters, and for translation in literal and cultural senses. Moreover, once missionaries have arrived in a mission field, settled, established a perimeter, contacted the locals, and gathered a small community of believers, their chosen task becomes neither easier nor less uncanny.

Why this is the case and what the effects of this configuration were for East African Christians will be the subject of this chapter. It will discuss colonial mission work and its decolonization by taking a close look at the biography of Father John (name altered by me; lived, 1911–99). He was an African priest who was baptized at the Benedictine mission of Peramiho in southwest Tanzania and served in the Archdiocese of Songea for more than fifty-five years, from his ordination in 1943 until the end of his life. He is named with a pseudonym here because his biography contains the story of an alleged psychiatric illness.[1]

In this chapter, I engage with the discussion regarding the "psychopathologies of colonialism." As Megan Vaughan and Dane Kennedy have argued, medical and psychiatric discourses reflect political and social conditions beyond the immediate medical field (Vaughan 1993; Kennedy 2016). One may add that they also impacted on political and social discourses beyond their immediate fields of practice and knowledge. Reading an interplay of subjective experiences, with individuals gaining subjectivity within a colonial framework, and entire colonial cultures of anxiety that bound together Africans and Europeans, I ask: How did the decolonization of church and state affect these subjective and political relations? Father John's biography serves as a "looking glass," mirroring the violent practices and anxieties of missionary colonialism and decolonization. Moreover, it provides a unique vantage point for understanding an individual's subjective negotiations within and against this painful process.

The preceding paragraph to some extent paraphrases the beginning of Ranajit Guha's "Not at Home in Empire" (1997). Guha portrays the "empire" as seen from the perspective of the colonizers as "uncanny."[2] My intention is to draw attention to similarities and differences between colonizers and missionaries. Guha sets out to describe the colonizers as beset by "anxiety" about something existential, limitless—something that they cannot name, but which is out there in the vast territory of the colony, beyond the circumscribed, fortified locales of white colonial rule. With reference to Kierkegaard and Heidegger, Guha contrasts anxiety with fear. Fear faces an actual or imagined but nevertheless direct threat, nothing that could not "be dealt with" by the practices of colonial rule. On the contrary, anxiety, according to Guha, is rooted in the profound isolation of the colonizer from the colonized.

More than a few missionaries of the colonial age will have shared this experience of colonial anxiety. However, there is a more characteristic form of anxiety connected to the insecurities particular to the missionary situation, which I refer to as "missionary anxiety." It is important to note the role of missions as independent and distinctive agents of colonialism here, with a focus on colonial education, public health systems, religious organization, and intellectual history. Understanding these peculiar anxieties is of great importance to the larger enterprise of a history of colonialism.

Let us for a moment follow Guha's distinction between fear and anxiety. Missionary anxiety is related to several fears, which directly concern the moment of conversion. As Heather Sharkey notes, "missionaries, their ostensible converts, and local communities were often uncertain about what 'conversion' meant (or should mean) in practice, and how it affected (or should affect) earlier loyalties and traditions" (Sharkey 2013, 2).[3] From this uncertainty, questions arise: How does one determine or prove whether conversion is sincere or complete? How does one prevent "conversion light" and a relapse into allegedly heathen ways? How does one avoid dilutions and subversions of the religious message? And, how does one keep the core values and convictions of the faith pure, while also accommodating the cultural specificities of the converted? Missions of various creeds set up procedures and practices to counter these insecurities. Potential converts underwent instruction, took oaths, and performed rituals, and their peers and religious experts monitored them. Yet, as in the case of colonial rule, these practices and regulations operated on the surface of a vast space which, in the case of missions, was mostly cultural. Like a child with a magnifying glass, the closer we stare, the more we discover that the space of the cultural is infinitely deep and complex. Seemingly fixed lines and boundaries begin to blur for anyone but staunch pragmatists. It is from this vastness and abysmal depth of culture that missionary anxiety took root.

The German Benedictine missionary Benno Heckel wrote in 1922: "Thirty years of preaching to the heathens *without* knowing the people. . . . Yes, we preached at the people, but they did not take it to heart, because it did not come from the heart, a heart that is truly comprehending, empathetic, living and thinking with the people. How might we have preached from the heart without knowing the culture of those we addressed. . . . We tried our best and sacrificed all, even lives. But still it was not delivered in the language of the heart necessary to convert our matrilineal people."[4] Acknowledging failure and insecurities is something not often found in the public transcripts of missions, but is instead buried in archives. At the time, Heckel's mission in southeast Tanzania lay in disarray. Not only had World War I disrupted missionary efforts, but the local population, independent of their creed, adhered to initiation processes that the missions had incriminated as sexually deviant and counter to the beliefs and morality of Christianity. Missionaries acted in a state of moral panic, trying to end initiations by attempting to steer the German and later English colonial administrations toward prohibition, violently disrupting rituals, sequestering children from parents, and excluding allegedly lapsed Christians from the parishes (on colonial moral panic, see Fischer-Tiné and White 2016, 8–10). By the late 1920s, the neighboring Anglican mission (the Universities' Mission to Central Africa, or UMCA) attempted to accommodate initiation and male circumcision against fierce criticism from their own ranks and other denominations, but African evangelists (Knak 1931, 281–82; Lucas 1950; Ranger 1972) pushed for these forms of acceptance. The Catholic mission followed in the 1930s (Hokororo 1961; Hölzl 2016a).

Heckel noted that after thirty years of work in the area, the missionaries had not even begun to comprehend or appreciate the depth of local culture. The first Benedictine missionaries had arrived in the region in 1887 as part of German colonization efforts. An early mission station to the west of Dar es Salaam was destroyed during the colonial war of 1888–89, after which the German Empire conquered the territory of today's mainland Tanzania, Rwanda, and Burundi. The Benedictine mission expanded throughout the southern half of Tanzania and into some areas of central Tanzania during the 1890s. Even though most of the stations were destroyed during the Maji Maji War in 1905–6, Catholicism became the majority creed in southwest Tanzania during the first half of the twentieth century. It remained in a minority position in the southeast and other regions. The Benedictine mission retained its position despite some difficulties during both world wars, and remained under the influence of European missionaries, Germans, and German-speaking Swiss throughout the colonial period. From the late 1940s onward, however, an African clergy gradually took over parishes, and from the late 1960s, African bishops directed the church organization. A Benedictine monastic culture has remained active in the area until today, with branches in Zambia and Kenya.

The focus of this chapter is the period from the 1920s to the 1960s, when mass conversion characterized many areas of East Africa, and signs of an "Africanization" of the local Catholic churches became manifest, including:

the expansion of the mission education system driven by African teachers and catechists; the emergence of lay organizations; and the ordination of African priests, monks, and nuns (Napachihi 1998; Baur 2005, 389–94). The process of missionary decolonization is often portrayed as an almost natural evolution from colonial to independent, or from a missionary to a local branch of the worldwide Catholic Church. Yet, by focusing the lens on the life stories of local actors, experiences of contention, even pain and suffering, become apparent.

In the 1920s, as Heckel noted, European missionaries isolated themselves from the African population, and were in no way "at home" in their mission fields. The results were problematic from the mission's point of view. Mass conversions in some regions contrasted with other localities, where parishes laid waste and new Christians seemed to "lapse" in large numbers. Heckel and his fellow missionaries were hardly isolated in a physical sense; they were not prototypical missionaries in a rowboat, who could only speculate about the surprises that might await them after the next river bend. At least in a material sense, they had settled and established a mission field.

I argue here that missionary anxiety deepened after settling in, when Christian communities took root and a network of local Christian activists (catechists, evangelists, teachers, priests, or nuns) carved out roles and took initiatives (Pirouet 1978; Summers 2002; Mukuka 2008; Stornig 2013; Volz 2014; Hölzl 2016b). In fact, these actors were seen as embodiments of African culture, a notion that at the time made them immensely valuable as local experts, but also a primary source of missionary anxiety. The deeper African activists penetrated the mission's organization (e.g., as priests), the stronger the anxiety about the unfathomable depth of the culture took hold of European missionaries.

Madness Is Better Than Defeat (Ned Beauman) is the catchy title of a recent novel that suggests a headline for the life story of the protagonist at the center of this chapter. Father John was one of the first Africans consecrated as a Catholic priest in 1943 in southern Tanganyika. His early years in the mission organization are tangible in the personal diary of his teacher (Hofbauer 1926–55), Father Severin Hofbauer (1868–1955), who arrived as a missionary in Tanzania in 1895 and stayed until his death, with the exception of the years 1917–26 (Egger 2016, 231–42).[5] Around 1926, Hofbauer began to teach Latin to students at the mission's school in Peramiho (southwest Tanzania); or rather, he was persuaded by a number of boys who wished to become priests. Among them was the fifteen-year-old John.

Shortly afterward, Hofbauer started a makeshift preparatory seminary, where he taught prospective candidates for priesthood. John is mentioned as an assistant teacher in 1928. The students also received training in Swahili, English, history, geography, and mathematics. In addition to ordinary secondary school examinations, which the candidates took at the mission's central school, the seminary required them to prepare written translations from Caesar and Ovid, as well as an improvised free address in Latin. By Father Hofbauer's account, John was an outstanding student: he excelled in Latin and passed all the standard exams required of the colonial secondary school system of Tanganyika Territory. The education continued at the ordinary seminary with courses in philosophy and theology, both taught in Latin. Advanced students would take periodic leave in order to assist missionaries in the parishes in the countryside, and successively took the necessary steps toward full priesthood (becoming lectors, acolytes, subdeacons, deacons, etc.). Father John was ordained in 1943 at the age of thirty-two, after having completed seventeen years of seminary education.[6] By that time, he was conversant in at least four languages (Kingoni, Swahili, English, and Latin), philosophy, theology, and church law, as well as the rituals and liturgy of the Catholic Church.

Father John overcame another obstacle that was much more obscure than proficiency in ancient and modern languages or school curricula. African priests were liminal figures, crisscrossing the worlds and expectations of European missionaries and local societies, including their own families. Terence Ranger has argued that this made them "vulnerable to mental breakdown" (Ranger 1981, 268–69). At the very least, this difficult position made them a source of suspicion in either of the communities. Father John had to navigate several lines of expectations, namely those of his immediate family, his siblings, and his widowed mother, but also those of the leading members of local society. He belonged to one of the important Sukuma families of the Songea area and stood close to ruling the Ngoni clan of Nkosi Usangira Gama (on his clan, see Ebner [1987] 2009, 214–15; on the Sukuma, see Redmond 1985, 6). European missionaries expected him to keep his distance from family, society, and in particular the vernacular cultural practices that reproduced local societies, while at the same time drawing clear boundaries to the European monastic sphere of the mission. On several occasions, John's family and local leaders attempted to orient John's path toward a secular career, possibly in the colonial administrative sector (Hofbauer 1926–55, 1:72). This road was taken by the majority of seminarians during the first decades of the Benedictine seminary: often, the seminary teachers directed candidates to other careers when they seemed unfit for a celibate, clerical life.[7] Even more often, candidates chose to leave for economic and social reasons, taking up new and prestigious jobs (e.g., as post office clerks, railway managers, or central school teachers), which allowed them to build a family life. Of eighty students who entered the seminary between 1926 and 1931, only four were ultimately consecrated. Many turned to teaching or an administrative career. One of John's fellow students, Sebastian Chale, became an activist in a teachers' union and subsequently entered parliament and the leading circles of the Tanganyika African National Union (TANU), Tanzania's ruling party. Another former Benedictine seminarian, Benjamin Mkapa (1938–2020), was president of Tanzania from 1995 to 2005. John, however, "remained steadfast," as Father Hofbauer noted in his diary (Hofbauer 1926–55, 1:72). Most likely, John had his own hopes of a social and cultural climb, expectations that formed into strong convictions the more he invested in his education and the more he was invested with the insignia of priesthood during the 1930s and 1940s. After all, Catholicism was emerging as a new and increasingly strong cultural force in southwest Tanganyika's colonial situation, though not so much in other regions of East Africa.

Father Hofbauer and Abbot-Bishop Gallus Steiger were both impressed by the crowd that the ordination of Father John and three other African priests drew to Peramiho Abbey on a Sunday in the summer of 1943 (Hofbauer 1926–55, 3:48).[8] Four thousand Christians had found space to watch the ceremony in the abbey church, while about four thousand more assembled in the churchyards. Two bishops, one former arch abbot, and thirty-eight European priests took part in the ordination of the four. Even though descriptions framed the ordination as a paternal-filial event (with the elder priests laying their hands on the candidates' heads), it was obviously a critical caesura in local church history. People claimed their church, and so did the new priests. Father John had been particularly aware of his new status and position within the religious community. The diary of Father Hofbauer also contains a description of Father John's ordination as a deacon, only a few weeks earlier, when he expressed his "gratitude" to the Lord by performing a full proskynesis, to the surprise of the other priests and missionaries. There is a symbolic and spatial quality to this ritualistic gesture, which has the person in prayer lie face down with outstretched arms and legs in front of the altar, since it claims a large share of the inner area of a church's ritual space. Its inward-focused, meditating stance proclaims an exclusive though devoted relation to God. Father Hofbauer noted ironically that the bishop quickly jumped out of the way (Hofbauer 1926–55, 3:38).

The intensity and insistence by which the thirty-two-year-old Father John entered the space of the church and claimed his priesthood requires some explanation. A priest of the Catholic Church is ordained in direct succession of the apostles. This extraordinary position is reflected in the material interior space of churches, rituals, and liturgy. The process of claiming the center space in front of the altar in the church building, the central position during service and within the religious life of parishes, is key to becoming a priest and constructing clerical, celibate masculinity. In the Benedictine mission of East Africa, it began even before a seminary was established. Candidates for baptisms carried consecrated medals of St. Benedict and small crosses. Mission teachers wore white tunics, while many also sported a rosary around their wrists (these beads could be counted in public prayer) and were often seen with a prayer book under the arm. Mission teachers also led parish prayers and performed baptisms in cases of emergency.[9]

Yet, the clerical space of the mission remained racially segregated. Young candidates in the early years of the Peramiho seminary, such as John, had to overcome obstacles regarding proper training in the ritual and liturgy, as they were denied access to the altar room of the abbey church. After several years of insistent inquiries and "downheartedness" among the African seminarians, the abbot granted them a small chapel that included a proper altar (including a saint's remains). Later they would acquire a tabernacle, and still later the right to hold a Sunday Eucharist (Hofbauer 1926–55, 2:128, 130, 165, 182). While the clerical space of the mission remained segregated by racial and colonial divide, the seminarians received access to some rituals and functions of priesthood and would undoubtedly have experienced some progress in their path toward full acknowledgment. This situation seems to have made the not-infrequent expressions of disrespect, racism, and inequality characterizing relations between African seminarians and some European missionaries even more blatant. The rector of the seminary, Father Hofbauer, feared the seminarians would lose their calling, since they would realize that they might never be fully respected. "Racial divide of Black and White also within monastery walls," he wondered skeptically (Hofbauer 1926–55, 2:184). Any white missionary could order seminarians to perform tasks, use harsh and disrespectful language before them, and sometimes apply physical violence as punishment, while a blunt reply or insistent verbal protest by African students and seminarians would lead to expulsion. The latter had to endure a strict control of their social life. Contact with local communities was frowned upon, while traditional dances were strictly prohibited (Hofbauer 1926–55, 2:190). The mission leader Abbot Gallus Steiger put forward a strict policy of segregation and in two directions. On the one hand, seminarians had to make a wide berth around the cultural practices of their local societies, which Steiger regarded as "heathen" or "primitive dirt (Shenzi-Dreck)."[10] On the other hand, he demanded clear boundaries between African and European priests. Father Hofbauer noted that Steiger announced that he would "never allow black and white clerics in the choir together, every form of European style clothing, shoes, hats, etc. is anathema to him, priests and clerics were to remain natives like their countrymen. . . . Blacks on one side—whites on the other" (Hofbauer 1926–55, 2:185).

The observations in Father Hofbauer's diary may be regarded as part of racist practices in everyday colonialism. But I suggest that there is more to it. The conflicts and injuries Father John and other seminarians suffered during their years at the seminary were rooted in the twofold effect of missionary anxiety. In the eyes of the majority of European missionaries, and certainly the mission's leadership, seminarians needed to be "isolated" from the "dangers" of the vernacular, of African culture and tradition, in order to prevent lapsing. Valentin-Yves Mudimbe (1997, 53–56) describes the seminary in Africa along the lines of Foucault's concept of discipline: as a panoptic institution directed toward eradicating the "pagan" and isolating candidates from their cultural and social environment. Mudimbe also describes the rigid physical regime that the "docile bodies" of seminarians had to undergo in the Catholic seminary in Africa, which was modeled after monastic regimes and their long hours of alternate periods of study, meditation, and prayer. No doubt this was also the case in the Benedictine seminary at Peramiho, combined with poor sanitary conditions and times of malnutrition during the 1920s.[11] Material conditions here were compounded by an attitude that physical suffering would strengthen the resolve of seminarians. On the other hand, European missionaries felt that the inner sanctum of the mission in the material and in the spiritual sense, the buildings, the ritual, and the hierarchy, had to be guarded from African seminarians. This left seminarians, and to a lesser extent teachers and church activists, in a liminal position or a double-bind situation.

The contradictions of missionary ideology were tangible from the start, and they were criticized time and again by missionaries who saw practical difficulties, like preaching the gospel while following a policy of strict monastic seclusion.[12] The material boundary work may be deduced from the built environment of the mission stations, which to some extent followed classical European monasterial traditions that envisioned a monastery as walled, with an inward-looking, self-sufficient architectural structure. The ideological work of boundary-making becomes visible in the mission's policies toward the question of African priesthood. During the early years of mission work, requests by religious activists could be easily discouraged, since there was a lack of precedence, and Roman guidelines were vague or nonexistent. In the 1920s, however, the policies of the Holy See changed, as both Benedict XV ("Maximum illud," 1919) and Pius XI ("Rerum ecclesiae," 1926) urged missions around the world to set up seminaries and establish an indigenous clergy. Pius XI even admonished mission leaders not to interfere with the calls to priesthood of indigenous Christians. The apostolic delegate in East Africa, Archbishop Arthur Hinsley of Mombasa, followed up this call with individual missions, and encouraged them strongly to speed up their efforts in seminary education.[13] Yet, the Benedictine mission remained reluctant and anxious.

Father John did not commit to a parish but remained a teacher in the seminary after his ordination in 1943. In 1949, a major conflict occurred in the mission's seminary, with Father John at its center. The sources do not reveal the nature or cause of this conflict. However, the mission called in medical expertise, an assistant to the district doctor. Father John was diagnosed with hereditary syphilis, "allegedly," as Father Severin Hofbauer added in brackets in his diary. It is not clear how the hereditary syphilis condition was diagnosed, or whether blood tests were done, or which ones. At the time in colonial Tanganyika, they were not very conclusive and false positives were common (Sadock 2013). The Indian physician who was sent to the abbey was hardly familiar with the social environments of a Catholic seminary, neither the constraints on and aspirations of African priests, nor the particular prejudices and anxieties of European Catholic missionaries. Moreover, he was not a trained (or experienced) venereal disease specialist, nor was he a psychiatrist. These were only found in less remote areas of the colony. The colonial administration first initiated a coordinated approach to venereal diseases in Tanganyika only in 1945 (Sadock 2013). Still, as Sloan Mahone argues, one effect of the colonial "East African School of

Psychiatry" was the dissemination of medical vocabulary and a trend toward conceptualizing the colonial population in psychological ("African mind") or psychiatric terms (Mahone 2007). Hofbauer—an experienced medical amateur who had taken a nurse exam, briefly headed a training facility for missionary doctors, and "practiced" missionary medicine in the field for years—had his doubts. He faulted Father John for being "proud, and academically overblown, lacking devoutness," but took him as merely a "hysteric." "Helping by prayer, would be better than cold-hearted criticism," he wrote. Father John was put under surveillance and received medical treatment (Hofbauer 1926–55, 4:11). The standard method at the time in colonial Tanganyika was six injections of bismuth, with penicillium only gradually substituting for the less effective treatment (Sadock 2013).

Whether or not the diagnosis of the physician was correct is not of great importance to my argument. More relevant are its social consequences, which put the spotlight on the origins and processes underlying missionary anxiety. In the mission's seminary in 1948, Father John's superiors reacted with the kind of moral panic that was typical of missionary anxiety. Not only did they isolate the priest under suspicion, they also put into question the whole recruiting system and launched inquiries into the psychohygienic conditions of vernacular (supposedly ethnic) communities in the mission field suspected of being subject to endemic syphilis. The seminary itself purged many students who were suspected of being afflicted with hereditary STDs and/or some kind of traditional cultural predestination for immorality.

At the time, syphilis was regarded as a social disease, to which specific social groups (e.g., sex workers, the working and lower classes), but also certain ethnic groups (in Tanganyika, matrilineal societies like the Makonde, Makua, or Mwera), allegedly were particularly susceptible. It was social because doctors, commentators, and administrators saw an intimate connection of the disease to allegedly immoral and group-specific lifestyles. While syphilis and other STDs were supposed to be endemic in certain groups, infections would not infrequently spread to others, and the proponents of social hygiene would warn of large-scale degeneration within the population as a whole. During the 1920s and 1930s, syphilis often became connected to social Darwinism, with only a short step to eugenics and even euthanasia (Sauerteig 1999, 41–52). Historians see a trend toward rationalization and pragmatism among medical experts and large proportions of the German public in the late Kaiserreich and the Weimar period. However, religious groups continued to highlight allegedly deviant and sinful lifestyles as the cause of STDs (Sauerteig 2003). This chain of cultural associations is exemplified by the development of events at Peramiho seminary, which Father Hofbauer described as "night of Bartholomew" and the "Nürnberg trials." Abbot Gallus issued the order that new seminarians had to endure background checks concerning the cultural traditions of their clans and societies, as well as the health and morals of their immediate families. The rector of the seminary, Father Eberhard Spiess, made an inquiry into the family and ethnic backgrounds of all graduate students. Rather than suspect acute psychiatric conditions among students, the missionaries inquired into the "sanitary and psychological conditions" of entire societies. The inquiry led to the expulsion of more than a dozen advanced seminarians. Particularly troubling for mission leaders were initiation processes during which—they suspected—children were "prematurely and indiscreetly educated about sexual matters," a fact that they feared would have the "gravest moral consequences," just like in Europe; "prospective priests and nuns need no introduction to things which they will later abstain from voluntarily by the grace of God."[14] The Benedictine fathers opposed both liberal education strategies and violent eugenic policies. Following a conservative Catholic line of argument, they strictly proposed monogamous marriage or abstention as the only means to prevent the feared moral and physical degeneration.

The 1949 case of Father John reactivated cultural fears that had fueled missionary anxieties since before World War I, namely that deeply ingrained traditions and deviant intimacies may taint the fundamentals of the Christian faith and organization. During the 1920s, Abbot Gallus had routinely blocked applications from candidates who belonged to the matrilineal societies of southeast Tanzania. He regarded them as contaminated by sex education during initiation procedures, with male circumcision as the physical sign. The priesthood, expectations of absolute devotion to God, authority and aloofness within the parish, and an aura of celibate masculinity: all of these were contributing to the intense missionary anxiety. It was regarded as a difficult calling in European Christian societies. The dangers suspected but hidden in African cultures seemed to put even more onus on individual candidates. The Cameroonian philosopher and Catholic priest Fabian Eboussi-Boulaga (1934–2018) has explained the conundrum of theological, moral, and cultural visions of the missionary perspective on African societies in the following way: "The obliteration or absence of the correct understanding of god as he is either entails the degradation of the human being or is its nefarious consequence." Losing the perspective on God will result in the loss of values, and vice versa. Consequently, "paganism is not a neutral state, a lack to be made up. It is a state of guilt, of rebellion against God, and of a fall beneath the threshold of humanity. . . . Because it is against nature it is inhuman. Inevitably it is accompanied by slavery, infanticide, cannibalism, polygamy, and all manner of other aberration and imperfection" (as cited in Mudimbe 1997, 58–59). From the viewpoint of theology, as criticized here by Eboussi Boulaga, the anxious and disproportionate reaction toward Father John's alleged disease becomes explicable to some extent. Syphilis, an STD associated with "unnatural, deviant" behavior and "pagan society" if diagnosed in a priest, was the embodiment of a fall or lapse and of sinfulness through the generations and across whole ethnic groups. It would potentially endanger whole parishes and the local church. The fact that Father John's alleged condition was hereditary did nothing to exonerate him but connected his case to the depth of culture and tradition.[15] Still, colonial missionary theology is not all there is to Father John's case.

Apart from a few characteristic actions noted in Hofbauer's diary, Father John's perspectives and intentions have remained obscure in this narrative so far. There are no records available to provide self-representations of this priest prior to 1960, when he wrote a series of letters to the apostolic delegate for East Africa, Archbishop Guido del Mestri, in Nairobi, and in 1963 to the bishop of Bukoba, Cardinal Laurean Rugambwe. These letters enable a new and political interpretation of his case. There are some grounds for believing that the views Father John expressed in the early 1960s had already been guiding his actions in the late 1940s, and had formed in the 1930s when mission activists began to call for equality within the parishes. Father Hofbauer noted in his diary, that African teachers and students were "watching the actions of Europeans closely and with suspicion. Both groups want equal treatment and rights in everything. It will be difficult to explain the 'certi denique finem'" (Hofbauer 1926–55, 2:211–12).[16] In the neighboring Benedictine mission province of Ndanda, backlash against conditions in schools (with discrimination and violence against pupils by European priests) and at workplaces led to student protests and labor strikes in 1956 and 1957 (Hertlein 2017, 204).

Father John had not yielded to the pressure of European missionaries and their reaction to his diagnosis. After several months, he escaped his apparently involuntary confinement and medication at the monastery and traveled several hundred miles to Dar es Salaam. It is unlikely that an educated person such as Father John would simply have denied an infectious disease if there were proper diagnostics and conditions of treatment. As Michael Tuck shows for local colonial elites in Uganda, syphilis was regarded as a serious problem and treatment for the disease was highly sought after (Tuck 2003). More likely, it was the political momentum within the mission— Father John's several-months-long isolation from the parish and seminary, as well as the targeting of whole ethnic groups—that provided the motive for resistance. After a brief period in the colony's capital, he returned to Peramiho and started applying for positions at other African dioceses that were already under African leadership and jurisdiction. He succeeded in 1957, when he received an invitation from a Black South African bishop, Bonaventure Dlamini (Mukuka 2009), and his home diocese granted him leave, as the abbot-bishop believed a change of "climate" would improve Father John's condition.[17] When he returned to Tanganyika in 1960, he was referred to a large parish in Mbinga (to the east of Lake Nyassa/Lake Malawi), where he worked as an assistant parish priest.[18] From that time on, he remained a priest in his original diocese until the end of his life.

During the early 1960s, Father John, very much in line with the rest of the colony—which became independent from Britain in 1961 and unified with the island state of Zanzibar in 1964—pursued his convictions with a new sense of vigor. For instance, he petitioned the Catholic Building Society of London for funds to independently step up missionary efforts in his home region.[19] His letters to del Mestri and Rugambwe attest to both the strong urge he felt to achieve material and social equality among European and African priests within African dioceses, and his conviction that only Pan-African or Black solidarity could bring this about. In 1960, he wrote to Archbishop del Mestri: "I thank very much the Holy See for giving us African bishops, without them, perhaps I could not be a priest again, as I was left alone. May the Good Lord increase their number and bless our African bishops."[20] This conviction may also have been reinforced by his experiences in Bishop Dlamini's South African dioceses. Conflicts with the European missionary organization had accompanied the erection of the local church in 1954, and European Christian settlers protested against being subjected to the jurisdiction of a Black bishop throughout the 1950s. In combination with severe administrative difficulties, lack of funds after the mission's withdrawal, and poor health, all this led to the resignation of Bishop Dlamini in 1968 (Mukuka 2009).

A letter from Father John to Cardinal Rugambwe began with the invocation of a *"Great African* era . . . both *religiously* and *politically"*: "Your eminence, allow me to meet you in our modern times, positions, and difficulties. Your eminence, we all in Africa and in the whole *Negro* world have been greatly edified by your very great actions and consultations in the II Vatican Council as regarding the *African Church*."[21] By the early 1960s, Rugambwe had become a well-known public figure in Tanganyika and beyond. He was emblematic of two emerging trends: a future self-confident role of Africans within the Catholic Church, and a coalition between an African Catholic Church and the new government in independent Tanganyika/Tanzania's new government, the latter of which was led by a Catholic and former mission teacher, Julius K. Nyerere. Rugambwe had not only performed a leading role in the discussions during the Second Vatican Council concerning a new missionary encyclical. He also had publicly endorsed independence and the new TANU government in 1961 by leading prayers when a new flag was raised in the National Stadium on the day of independence and by conducting High Mass on the day Tanganyika became independent in the presence of Catholic members of government and parliament, including President Nyerere (Mbogoni 2004, 122–25).[22]

In the same letter to the cardinal, Father John addressed several grievances in his own diocese, which was still led by a missionary, Abbot Eberhard Spiess, the former rector of the seminary. Father John argued that German missionaries refused "change in a changing country," and had been following an unusual policy for many years without reform. The whole organization lacked "brotherly mutual understanding" and a will for "Christian cooperation among European and African priests." Father John saw "general misunderstanding" and "dissatisfaction in our Christian life." Many decades ago, the Germans had come to a "primitive" country and had held all the power in their hands ever since. But the situation had changed. There were thirty-two Black priests as well as a Black auxiliary bishop in the diocese. Twenty years had gone by since the ordination of the first African priest. Still, African priests did not receive proper salaries, and mass stipends (sent by European parishes for commemorative prayers) were withheld from them against the stipulation of church law. Material support for mission and parish work was scarce, yet European missionaries received cars and had the support of nuns. Europeans filled all senior positions in the church administration and hierarchy. African priests led only five parishes because of a strict policy for white superiority: "No European can be a cooperator under an African superior, no African can be superior, where European missionaries are stationed." Finally, many a calling was lost because of "colour discrimination and misunderstanding between European superiors and students." As a consequence, Father John demanded that the church hierarchy (i.e., bishop, general vicar, seminary rector and prefect, and headmasters) become African, and that European missionaries address "old attitudes and prejudices."[23]

This extensive and vociferous indictment was met with a fierce counter-attack by the leadership of the Benedictine mission at Peramiho. The psychiatric diagnosis—by then almost fifteen years old—served to discredit Father John's claims. In direct response, Abbot-Bishop Spiess marked him out as "our problem priest" and "in fact a psychological case."[24] In further letters, Spiess described Father John as a "psychopath,"[25] as "suffering from hereditary syphilis with all its consequences (lack of self-control, unbalanced [!] state of mind)," and of "megalomania, as the doctor says," "a case of psychoneurosis." Yet, to be named a priest full of "self-importance and independence" who "cannot be controlled" was an ambivalent verdict in 1963 Tanzania.[26] Father John put forward a number of factual claims that Spiess could hardly disprove. African priests did not receive decent salaries, nor were they equipped with cars like their European counterparts, nor were European missionaries subordinated to senior African priests. Spiess mentioned several seminarians who had been sent to Europe to study and could possibly hold senior positions at a later date.[27] He also denied claims about a late-runner status in Tanzania regarding the Africanization of the church. Still, pressure to change and speed up efforts to transfer power to African seminarians was already mounting within the East African Bishops Conference and from the Tanzanian government (Hertlein 2017, chap. 16).

Bishop Spiess's freewheeling use of psychiatric labels warrants a closer look at his biography. He was born in 1902 and grew up in Germany during World War I and the immediate postwar period. He entered the Benedictine Congregation of St. Ottilien in 1925 and received his ordination in 1930. Two years later he arrived in Tanganyika, where he spent the rest of his life as a teacher and later abbot at Peramiho. As Paul Frederick Lerner demonstrates, the concept of trauma (and related psychiatric concepts of male hysteria and neurosis) became an important agent within medical and public discourse in Weimar Germany regarding the legacies and experiences of war. In fervent medical and political debates, trauma was "constructed, contested, and ultimately overturned in the encounters between veterans and psychiatrists and psychiatrists and general practitioners" (Lerner 2003, 226; see also chap. 8). The question of whether the many sick war veterans were traumatized or hysteric was ultimately a political one. It made a difference whether war was traumatizing to ordinary soldiers or turned weak men into hysterics needing not material compensation but hardened minds through psychiatric treatment. Tobias Weidner (2012, 329–63) has demonstrated that these were not expert discourses, or discourses of doctors and patients, but highly public affairs. Spiess himself was no medical or psychiatric expert, but a theologian who likely gathered his superficial psychiatric insights and vocabulary from newspapers and public journals. Moreover, such psychiatric labels intermingled with theological concepts of heathen sinfulness and further ethnocentered some of the concepts outlined above.

The Black priest—invested with ancient, evangelical authority, with rhetorical clarity, and a thorough knowledge of church law—could not and would not be muted. Yet he might be rendered a madman. His fifteen-year-old diagnosis had now been transformed—from a theological to a political matter. Initially, Father John's alleged illness had triggered moral panic among European missionaries, and it became rooted in missionary anxiety about the purity of faith and church before deep "African culture." Fifteen years later, amid Tanganyika's decolonization, his named illness served to discredit a political struggle for independence, self-government, and full equality among priests of one and the same church. One other thing had changed: an obscure feeling of anxiety about cultural isolation had developed into a quite open isolation of European missionaries within an independent, self-confident state and society. The ideas of uhuru (Swahili for freedom, independence), a key political term in Julius Nyerere's government, resonated strongly in Father John's letters and thinking. Moreover, Father John's ideas about African self-government within the church were resonant with the encyclicals and letters of the Holy See going back to 1919, as well as demands for material equality argued along the lines of church law, which Father John had studied and knew well. The framing of his demands within the story of his actual or alleged personal and sexual health issues may have rendered his immediate efforts unsuccessful. Records on his further life story have not been available for this analysis. However, his positions and ideas were part of a larger movement within the church toward Africanization and decolonization. In 1956, the Cameroonian Jesuit priest and cultural anthropologist Meinrad Hegba (1928–2008), for example, denounced the "arrogant nationalism in the religious sector, which Africans realize with astonishment." According to Hegba, missions sought a clean "break" with the African past and its traditions. As a consequence, Christianity lacked an "African underpinning." Christianity increasingly appeared to be an "export article and an assisting force of imperialism." He went on to ask: "Can we be sure that even we as African priests can fend off feeling that within God's Church, we are merely the poor relatives?" (Hegba 1960, 136–37; my translation). His essay is part of a collection of similar statements by African and Caribbean priests that was published in Paris in close proximity to the Negritude movement.

With the onset of missionary decolonization, an increasing number of African priests and seminarians became the focus of moral fears concerning celibacy, sexuality, and intimacy—fears related to a deep-rooted and primitivist anxiety about the "uncanny" qualities of African cultures. More than any other group, members of the Black clergy stood for the potential success or failure of the mission's endeavor, for the proliferation of faith, and for compromising the fundamentals of the gospel. Within these boundaries to a missionary culture of anxiety, Father John negotiated his path between madness and self-assertion.

There is another question this chapter needs to answer: How can—and how should—such a life story be situated and narrated as part of larger political and psychopathological processes? Father John's story is surely much more than a singular psychiatric case, with all suffering and insecurity only present or expected within that place and time. Rather, it allows us to examine the anxieties and psychopathologies of late colonialism and decolonization through the lens of a Catholic missionary church, an underrated force in the twentieth-century history of colonial empires. Missionary anxieties were an important source of conflict and rule within local societies, especially so in the countryside where colonial rule was often aloof and very mediated. Father John's life story, and his alleged madness, helped to highlight three key aspects of the transformation from the colonial to the postcolonial order of the missionary church. One was the cultural and racist boundary-making of a colonial mission church. Another was the faltering transformation of such boundaries during decolonization. A third was the violence and brutality against agents of decolonization during such processes of transformation within these church milieus. Father John, as the protagonist, experienced racial segregation and discrimination, then confinement and involuntary medication, and finally the discrediting of his ideas and convictions by his superiors. The sources of these violent acts lay in unspecific anxieties about the depth and persistence of vernacular African cultures, but they also related to specific fears concerning the corruption of faith, the fundamentals of scripture and theology, and a contamination of church hierarchy by morally unreliable priests and bishops. "Hereditary syphilis" as a diagnosis played a key role here. From a sociocultural vantage point, the disease linked a temporal line from "pagans" to converted Christians, with an ethnocentrism that characterized all society as morally deviant, with the deviant "character" passed on through initiation and other rituals, and an unyielding belief in the sinfulness of the "pagan" fueling missionary anxieties.

Linking up an individual life story with political and sociocultural sea changes surely provides a reflection of society in an individual person. Studied in this manner, a biography enables us to demonstrate how social boundaries can be embattled and reworked by a concert of individual actors over time. Father John had not a "docile body" (Foucault 1977; Mudimbe 1997, 50–56), even though he had learned a lot over a long period of time. He had undergone deprivations of food and health, strict schedules with long hours of alternating prayer, work, and study, and he acquired much linguistic and theological knowledge. He had grown intimate with the rituals and habits of the Catholic liturgy and gained experience as a teacher. Yet, after completing the seminary and receiving his ordination, he dared to speak up against racist segregation and discrimination. He demanded material equality for Africans and African self-government within the church hierarchy. His few self-representations strongly show how the Tanzanian independence movement resonated among some African clergy, how currents of decolonization reshaped individual experiences of discrimination with political demands for equality, self-government, and transition within the Catholic Church.

For the Benedictine mission of southern Tanganyika, Father John was one of the first African priests, and he was also one of the first to demand decolonization of a local church. This process proved painful and contentious. It would be wrong to portray it as a more or less natural transition. By 1969, the diocese had come under the authority and guidance of an African bishop, James Komba. In 1971, Hanga Abbey became the first independent Benedictine monastery in Africa, led by Prior Father Gregory Mwageni. In 1985, African monks were admitted to Peramiho Abbey, and in June 2020 Laurenti Mkinga became the first African abbot of the abbey.

This mission's uncanny urge to make its home in Tanzania was increasingly being fulfilled, but not in the way that European colonial missionary activists had intended. At times, they bitterly and violently opposed the process. The discord exposed tendencies toward white supremacist ideologies and tremulous shades of disquiet to a point suggesting missionary psychopathologies. Within the ongoing global process of a decolonizing Catholic Church, the particular history shared here—of anxiety, violence, and psychopathology within a missionary realm and phase—remains important for future histories of decolonization and madness.

Notes

1 Connecting "the madness of colonialism to the madness of the mad," as Megan Vaughan writes, is a classic line of argument in the history of colonial psychiatry; it dates back to a *locus classicus* of postcolonial theory, Frantz Fanon (Vaughan 2007, 1).

2 Hunt (2016) employs the term "nervous state" to analyze the intersection of the medical and the colonial state's violent politics of domination and suppression.

3 The insecurity about what conversion might mean is also problematic for research: "However, if one wishes to avoid the confusion of word and concept and concept and practice, it would be better to say that in studying conversion, one was dealing with the narratives by which people apprehended and described a radical change in the significance of their lives. Sometimes these narratives employ the notion of divine intervention; at other times the notion of a secular teleology" (Asad 1996, 266).

4 Benno Heckel to Gallus Steiger, June 6, 1922, Archives Erzabtei St. Ottilien (hereafter ArchOtt) Z.1.16; my translation.

5 Hofbauer's diary is complemented by the Notes to the Chronicle of Abbot Gallus Steiger, Archives Peramiho Abbey (hereafter ArchPera) A11, A12, A13. Abbot Gallus's note provides an official account of the stages of education and gradual development of the seminary, without mentioning conflicts or differences of opinion among European missionaries. See Steiger's biography (Doerr 2014).

6 Father John's steps toward priesthood are recorded in the abbot's Notes to the Chronicle, ArchPera A13, 166, 221, 258, 261, 315, 319, 348, 397, 465, 472.

7 Julius K. Nyerere, for instance, had toyed with the idea of entering a seminary and becoming a priest, but was probably discouraged by his erstwhile mentor Father Richard Walsh (Molony 2014, 178).

8 Steiger, Notes to the Chronicle, ArchPera A11, 421–22.

9 See, for instance, the life story of Pauli Holola (1935) and the reports of Cassian Homahoma Gama, Chronicle Lituhi, ArchPera A46, 1–3.

10 Minutes to the Regional Pastoral Conference Ungoni-Matengo, May 31, 1937, ArchOtt Z.1.24. A teacher at the seminary put out the following line: "Segregation and perfect supervision is an absolute necessity. . . . The lack of a Catholic family life, the lack of the sample [!] and of the prayer is hardly [dearly!] felt . . . , it is necessary to insulate them during the years of preparation." Küsters to Hinsley, December 22, 1932, ArchOtt Z.1.20.

11 Some seminarians protested "being exploited" and the poor quality of food (Hofbauer 1926–55, 1:53, 2:166). Hofbauer described the early years of the seminary as "camp life," and reported both a lack of food and illnesses of students due to food poisoning and bad sanitation.

12 See the critical memorandum of Beda Danzer, *Mission und Benediktinertum*, Typoskript, ArchOtt Z.1.30. A dozen missionaries protested tightening the monastic regulations in 1927; see the letter by Beatus Iten, Pirmin Fleck, Trudbert Mühling, January 11, 1927, ArchOtt Z.1.14.

13 Hinsley visited Peramiho in 1928 and 1932.

14 Steiger to Ammann, September 27, 1933, ArchOtt Z.1.27.

15 This is different from other schools of ethnocentric or race-centered psychiatry, which located the source of illness in the contact of the "primitive" with modern society, such as the "British East Africa school," or speculated on the predisposition to mental illness or crime caused by long-term biological/racial and environmental conditions, such as the "Algiers school" (Keller 2007; Mahone 2007).

16 This reference (to Horace's *Satires*) about certain limits to equality bears a strong resemblance to Homi Bhabba's dictum "almost but not quite, almost but not white" (Bhabha 1997, 156).

17 Spiess to del Mestri, February 16, 1960, ArchOtt Z.1.20.

18 See Spiess to del Propaganda Fide Congregation, August 30, 1963, ArchOtt Z.1.20.

19 See del Mestri to Spiess, March 3, 1963, ArchOtt Z.1.20.

20 Father John to del Mestri, August 22, 1960, ArchOtt Z.1.20.

21 Father John to Bishop Rugambwe, January 10, 1963, ArchOtt Z.1.20.

22 The influence of the Catholic Church on or via Julius Nyerere, and whether this worked to the detriment of the large share of Muslims among Tanzania's population, has long been a point of discussion among historians of Tanzania.

23 Father John to Bishop Rugambwe, January 10, 1963, ArchOtt Z.1.20.

24 Spiess to del Mestri, February 16, 1963, ArchOtt Z.1.20.

25 Spiess to Catholic Building Society, London, May 3, 1963, ArchOtt Z.1.20.

26 Spiess to del Mestri, Nairobi; and Spiess to State Secretariat, Holy See, August 30, 1963, ArchOtt Z.1.20. The letters were written in response to a letter by the secretary of state of the Holy See to Father John (which Spiess would not deliver, in order not to "strengthen the feeling of self-importance and independence").

27 Spiess to del Mestri, February 16, 1963, ArchOtt Z.1.20.

Sources

Archival Material

Archives Erzabtei St. Ottilien, St. Ottilien, Bavaria, Germany (ArchOtt).
Archives Peramiho Abbey, Tanzania (ArchPera).

Literature

Asad, Talal. 1996. "Comments on Conversion." In *Conversion to Modernities: The Globalization of Christianity*, edited by Peter van der Veer, 263–73. New York: Routledge.

Baur, John. 2005. *2000 Years of Christianity in Africa: An African Church History*. Nairobi, Kenya: Paulines Publications.

Benedikt XV. 1919. "Maximum illud." In *Acta Apostolicae Sedis* XI. Rome: Typis Polyglottis Vaticanis.

Bhabha, Homi K. 1997. "Of Mimicry and Man: The Ambivalence of Colonial Discourse." In *Tensions of Empire: Colonial Culture in a Bourgeois World*, edited by Frederick Cooper and Ann Laura Stoler, 152–60. Berkeley: University of California Press.

Doerr, Lambert. 2014. *Abbot Bishop Gallus Steiger O.S.B. (1879–1966): Life and Work of an Outstanding Missionary Pioneer*. St. Ottilien, Germany: EOS Edition.

Ebner, Elzear. (1987) 2009. *The History of the Wangoni*. Ndanda, Tanzania: Benedictine Publications.

Egger, Christine. 2016. *Transnationale Biografien: Die Missionsbenediktiner von St. Ottilien in Tanganyika 1922–1965*. Cologne: Böhlau Verlag.

Fischer-Tiné, Harald, and Christine White. 2016. "Introduction: Empires and Emotions." In *Anxieties, Fear, and Panic in Colonial Settings: Empires on the Verge of a Nervous Breakdown*, edited by Harald Fischer-Tiné, 1–23. New York: Palgrave Macmillan.

Foucault, Michel. 1977. *Discipline and Punish: The Birth of the Prison*. New York: Pantheon Books.

Guha, Ranajit. 1997. "Not at Home in Empire." *Critical Inquiry* 23, no. 3: 482–93.

Hegba, Meinrad. 1960. "Christentum und Negertum." In *Schwarze Priester melden sich*, edited by Alioune Diop. Frankfurt: Main Verlag. First published in 1956 as *Des pretres noires s'interrogent*. Paris: Éditions de Cerf.

Hertlein, Siegfried. 2017. *Ndanda Abbey, Vol. III: From Mission to Local Church 1950–1972*. St. Ottilien, Germany: EOS Edition.

Hofbauer, Severin. 1926–55. *Diary*. 4 vols. Library of Peramiho Abbey, typescript.

Hokororo, Alias M. 1961. "The Influence of the Church on Tribal Customs at Lukuledi." *Tanganyika Notes and Records* 54:1–13.

Holola, Pauli. 1935. "Mein Leben." *Missionsblätter* 39:11–15, 34–40.

Hölzl, Richard. 2016a. "Arrested Circulation: Catholic Missionaries, Anthropological Knowledge, and the Politics of Cultural Difference in Imperial Germany, 1880–1914." In *Anxieties, Fear, and Panic in Colonial Settings: Empires on the Verge of a Nervous Breakdown*, edited by Harald Fischer-Tiné, 307–44. New York: Palgrave Macmillan.

Hölzl, Richard. 2016b. "Educating Missions: Teachers and Catechists in Southern Tanganyika, 1890s to 1940s." *Itinerario* 40, no. 3: 405–28.

Hunt, Nancy R. 2016. *A Nervous State: Violence, Remedies, and Reverie in Colonial Congo*. Durham, NC: Duke University Press.

Keller, Richard C. 2007. "Taking Science to the Colonies: Psychiatric Innovation in France and North Africa." In *Psychiatry and Empire*, edited by Sloan Mahone and Megan Vaughan, 17–40. Basingstoke, UK: Palgrave Macmillan.

Kennedy, Dane. 2016. "Minds in Crisis: Medico-Moral Theories of Disorder in the Late Colonial World." In *Anxieties, Fear, and Panic in Colonial Settings: Empires on the Verge of a Nervous Breakdown*, edited by Harald Fischer-Tiné, 27–47. New York: Palgrave Macmillan.

Knak, Siegfried. 1931. *Zwischen Nil und Tafelbai: Eine Studie über Evangelium, Volkstum und Zivilisation, am Beispiel der Missionsprobleme unter den Bantu*. Berlin: Heimatdienst-Verlag.

Lerner, Paul Frederick. 2003. *Hysterical Men: War, Psychiatry, and the Politics of Trauma in Germany, 1890–1930*. Ithaca, NY: Cornell University Press.

Lucas, William V. 1950. *Christianity and Native Rites*. London: Central Africa House Press.

Mahone, Sloan. 2007. "East African Psychiatry and the Practical Problems of Empire." In *Psychiatry and Empire*, edited by Sloan Mahone and Megan Vaughan, 41–66. Basingstoke, UK: Palgrave Macmillan.

Mbogoni, Lawrence Ezekiel Yona. 2004. *The Cross versus the Crescent: Religion and Politics in Tanzania from the 1880s to the 1990s*. Dar es Salaam: Mkuki na Nyota.

Molony, Tom. 2014. *Julius Nyerere: The Early Years*. Woodbridge, UK: James Curry.

Mudimbe, Valentin-Yves. 1997. *Tales of Faith: Religion as Political Performance in Central Africa*. London: Athlone Press.

Mukuka, George S. 2008. *The Other Side of the Story: The Silent Experience of the Black Clergy in the Catholic Church in South Africa (1898–1976)*. Pietermaritzburg, South Africa: Cluster.

Mukuka, George S. 2009. "Bonaventure Dlamini." *Dictionary of African Christian Biography*. Accessed October 5, 2020. https://dacb.org/stories/southafrica /dlamini-bonaventure/.

Napachihi, Sebastian Wolfgang. 1998. *The Relationship between the German Missionaries of the Congregation of St. Benedict from St Ottilien and the German Colonial Authorities in Tanzania, 1887–1907*. Ndanda, Tanzania: Mission Press.

Pirouet, Louise. 1978. *Black Evangelists: The Spread of Christianity in Uganda, 1891–1914*. London: Rex Codings.

Pius XI. 1926. "Rerum ecclesiae." In *Acta Apostolicae Sedis* XVIII. Rome: Typis Polyglottis Vaticanis.

Ranger, Terence O. 1972. "Missionary Adaptation of African Religious Institutions: The Masasi Case." In *The Historical Study of African Religion*, edited by Terence O. Ranger and Isaria N. Kimambo, 221–51. Berkeley: University of California Press.

Ranger, Terence O. 1981. "Godly Medicine: The Ambiguities of Medical Mission in Southeast Tanzania, 1900–1945." *Social Science and Medicine* 15B, no. 3: 261–77.

Redmond, Patrick M. 1985. *The Politics of Power in Songea Ngoni Society 1860–1962*. Chicago: Adams Press.

Sadock, Musa. 2013. "Government and the Control of Venereal Disease in Colonial Tanzania, 1920–1960." In *The Sexual History of the Global South: Sexual Politics in Africa, Asia, and Latin America*, edited by Saskia Wieringa and Horacio Sívori, 83–98. London: Zed Books.

Sauerteig, Lutz D. H. 1999. *Krankheit, Sexualität, Gesellschaft: Geschlechtskrankheiten und Gesundheitspolitik in Deutschland im 19. und frühen 20. Jahrhundert*. Stuttgart: Steiner Verlag.

Sauerteig, Lutz D. H. 2003. "'The Fatherland Is in Danger! Save the Fatherland!' Venereal Disease, Sexuality, and Gender in Imperial and Weimar Germany." In *Sex, Sin, and Suffering: Venereal Disease and European Society since 1870*, edited by Roger Davidson and Lesley A. Hall, 76–92. London: Routledge.

Sharkey, Heather J., ed. 2013. "Introduction: The Unexpected Consequences of Christian Missionary Encounters." In *Cultural Conversions: Unexpected Consequences of Christian Missionary Encounters in the Middle East, Africa, and South Asia*, 1–26. Syracuse, NY: Syracuse University Press.

Stornig, Katharina. 2013. *Sisters Crossing Boundaries: German Missionary Nuns in Colonial Togo and New Guinea, 1897–1960*. Göttingen, Germany: Vandenhoek and Rupprecht.

Summers, Carol. 2002. *Colonial Lessons: Africans' Education in Southern Rhodesia, 1918–1940*. Portsmouth, NH: Heinemann.

Tuck, Michael W. 2003. "Venereal Disease, Sexuality, and Society in Uganda." In *Sex, Sin, and Suffering: Venereal Disease and European Society since 1870*, edited by Roger Davidson and Lesley A. Hall, 191–204. London: Routledge.

Vaughan, Megan. 1993. "Madness and Colonialism, Colonialism as Madness: Re-Reading Fanon; Colonial Discourse and the Psychopathology of Colonialism." *Paideuma* 39:45–55.

Vaughan, Megan. 2007. "Introduction." In *Psychiatry and Empire*, edited by Sloan Mahone and Megan Vaughan, 1–16. Basingstoke, UK: Palgrave Macmillan.

Volz, Stephen C. 2014. "African Evangelism and the Colonial Frontier: The Life and Times of Paulo Rrafiing Molefane." *International Journal of African Historical Studies* 47, no. 1: 101–20.

Weidner, Tobias. 2012. *Die unpolitische Profession: Deutsche Mediziner im langen 19. Jahrhundert*. Frankfurt: Campus Verlag.

Mr. Tanka and Voices

A Cameroonian Patient
Writing about Schizophrenia

On March 19, 1968, at eight o'clock in the evening, Benedict Nta Tanka heard voices for the first time, haunted as he was by "shadowy figures" and the "whispering" of the Cameroonian prime minister and his personal secretary. At the same time, Tanka suffered from gnawing, piercing pain in his head and skull (Tanka 1980, 18–19). The "voices" became "spirits" and "flies" entering his body and causing "unusual feelings," so Tanka later wrote his German psychiatrist, Dr. Alexander Boroffka (Boroffka 1980a, 11). The "voices" did not disappear the next day. Rather, they grew louder and seemed more "severe." They gave Tanka orders about how he should behave. They shouted at him, criticizing his personal and professional skills, and they warned that his family, friends, and colleagues were "devils" who oversaw him to "take good care" of his life (Tanka 1980, 18–19).

I came to know of Tanka, his life, and psychological experiences from his writings published in 1980 in a West German medical series called

"Medicine in Developing Countries" (Tanka 1980). Boroffka was a German psychiatrist and World Health Organization (WHO) visiting professor at the University Hospital, Ibadan University, Nigeria, from 1961 to 1973 (Binitie 1988, 145–54; Asuni and Williams 2006, 3–4; Boroffka 2006, 8), and it was he who edited Tanka's autobiographical writings (Parin 1983). Boroffka met Tanka as his patient in late September 1970 at the University Hospital and worked with him until Tanka's discharge on December 22, 1970, and again in several consultations in Ibadan until Boroffka returned to Germany in 1973 (Boroffka 1980c, 13–14). The WHO supported this publication series, which aimed to illustrate medical phenomena in the Global South through individual cases. Boroffka persuaded Tanka to write and then publish his writings and encouraged him to continue writing about his "illness." With Tanka's knowledge and approval, Boroffka added some case reports to another book written by psychiatrists Dan N. Lantum and Josef Schwarz, district medical officers at Tiko Hospital in English-speaking southwestern Cameroon following their individual auditions and examinations of Tanka (Boroffka 1980c, 13).

The first European-trained psychiatrist of Nigeria—probably the first African in sub-Saharan Africa, and the most famous—was Thomas Adeoye Lambo, then-deputy-director-general of the WHO, who wrote an introduction for Tanka and Boroffka's book (Lambo 1980). Lambo had previously established a widely praised, exemplary psychiatric clinic in Ibadan that was equally opposed to colonial practices of locking psychiatric patients away in prisons and to the labeling of mental illness as "witchcraft." In a decidedly reformist and humanitarian approach, Lambo sought to classify psychiatric illness according to European standards while also taking seriously vernacular experiences and ways of thinking (Heaton 2011, 2013). In his foreword, Lambo praised Tanka's writing as a "document of considerable significance," exposing the "inner dialectics of a personality" confronted by mental illness (Lambo 1980). Lambo claimed that Tanka's writings represented a "cosmology, not a story," structured by the "illness itself," that "internalizes systems of beliefs, attitudes and norms" of an African man from southwestern Cameroon (Lambo 1980). In concluding this chapter, I will reflect on some ethical questions in relation to this unusual book, jointly authored by a German psychiatrist and his Cameroonian patient.

When Tanka first had his experiences of hearing voices, he was twenty-five years old and a modest clerk in Cameroon's Department of Education.

He lived in Kumba, the capital of Cameroon's Southwestern District. Tanka's family belonged to the Menka, subsistence farmers, but the Tankas also produced palm oil and sold it on the market (Boroffka 1980a, 7; Tanka 1980, 110–20). His parents converted from so-called animism to Roman Catholic Christianity as adults, and all their children were baptized. It was quite exceptional that Tanka found a way out of farming into a position in a government office, particularly considering that he had twice failed the West African school certificate for higher education. In July 1966, Tanka received a promotion to second-class clerk (Boroffka 1980a, 6–8).

At first, as Tanka's account relates, he tried to fight against his "mysterious voices" with Christian rituals. He was praying, reading the Bible, and confessing his sins to gain absolution and redemption (Tanka 1980, 18–19). However, during some church services, the whispering and shouting in his head became stronger and more intense (Tanka 1980, 19–20). In the following weeks, he reacted to the worrying sounds somehow "in between" cultural and social spaces. He described the spaces as "traditional African" and as "modern Western" worlds. He also reflected on rational reasons for his illness yet confessed believing in "witchcraft"—that jealous and evil people from his office, family, and among his friends had caused his suffering by attacking him through "satanic" rituals. He tried to fight these "evil curses" not just with Christian prayers, but through consulting healers (Tanka 1980, 17–45; Boroffka 1980b, 139–40).

His district medical officer, a European-trained Cameroonian physician, diagnosed him with "paranoid schizophrenia," and referred Tanka to the psychiatric ward in a nearby mission hospital (Boroffka 1980a, 9). Following the diagnosis, Tanka's life changed completely: his family withdrew from him, disappointed that he could not work and did not send money home anymore. His girlfriend broke up with him (Boroffka 1980a, 6–8).

Tanka spent months in several lunatic asylums in Cameroon. One day he traveled across the border to Nigeria, a country well known for its advanced psychiatric infrastructure as a result of Lambo's work in the Aro Mental Hospital in Abeokuta and the University College Hospital in Ibadan (Tanka 1980, 18–19; for Lambo, see Sadowsky 1999; Heaton 2011, 2013). For the last four months of 1970, Tanka received treatment at the psychiatric unit of the University College Hospital in Ibadan (Boroffka 1980a, 12–13). Tanka later praised his stay there as "successful." After these four months, he returned to Cameroon and began working again, and also married a young woman from his home village (Boroffka 1980a, 14).

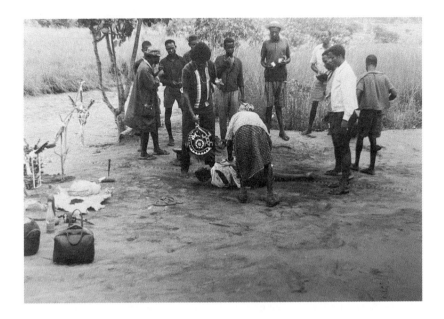

3.1 Healing ritual against "witchcraft" and "mental disturbance," Menka area of Cameroon. (Photograph by Alexander Boroffka, 1970, Alexander Boroffka Papers, Iwalewa House, Bayreuth.)

In a sense, this brief account of Tanka, about his life and illness, suggests nothing special. Millions of people all over the world have shared similar experiences of hearing voices, of being diagnosed under this now-controversial term (Henckes 2019), *schizophrenic*, and of seeking care or reacting as they and their kin thought best. Yet Tanka's case is exceptional because he wrote about it so extensively.

Breaking the Silence: Mr. Tanka's Writings

In February 1969, before leaving for Nigeria, Tanka sketched out the first part of his illness autobiography. In his view, such writing would be a way to put the sounds and incidents in his head in order, control his suffering, and prepare useful reports for his doctors (Tanka 1980, 18). Within a couple of days, he produced around fifty handwritten pages with detailed descriptions of his experiences, their circumstances, and his reactions. Between February and April 1970, Tanka also wrote a play, bringing his former girlfriend and some priests, colleagues, and physicians onto his imagined stage as angels, evils, and devils (Boroffka 1980c, 3; Tanka 1980, 46–93). In September 1970, he sketched eighty short statements summarizing his previous writing and preparing for his trip to Ibadan (Boroffka 1980c, 3). He was seemingly afraid that his future psychiatrist might not have sufficient time to read all forty thousand words he had written down (Tanka 1980, 94–104). At the request of the Cameroonian district medical officer, Tanka produced thirty-eight "dream protocols," conceptualized in a Freudian way and extensively described. In 1979, he added twenty more (Tanka 1980, 105–9).

All of his texts and communications with his physicians were very important to Tanka, so much so that he regularly hired professional typists, who made his handwritten texts seem official and readable (unlike another African typist, clerk, and writer in colonial times described by Vaughan [2005]).

In September 1970, after Tanka's arrival in Ibadan he handed over all his writings to his psychiatrist Boroffka who was convinced of the therapeutic importance of this patient's autobiographical notes. At the same time, he recognized the spectacular singularity of self-testimony from the hands and mind of an African patient diagnosed as schizophrenic, which could also teach much about global differences in schizophrenia and its experiences. Thus, he claimed, "The writings of the first literate member of an illiterate society, of which he gives a vivid description, might help the reader to form his own answer to the question if there are more similarities or dissimilarities in the symptomatology of paranoid schizophrenia between this case and cases from Western culture" (Boroffka 1980b, 141).

Boroffka recalled in 1980 that he kept asking Tanka to continue his writing. At some point Boroffka also decided, with Tanka's permission, to publish his text as a case study speaking to the symptoms, treatment, cure, and recovery of this one case of a literate African schizophrenic (Boroffka 1980c, 3). For the editing of the "first autobiography of an African schizophrenic, or of any patient from outside the Western world" (Boroffka 1980b, 144), Boroffka thought to offer Tanka some inspiration.

After his studies and psychiatric specialization in Germany and Czechoslovakia, Boroffka had worked for one year in Kansas City, Missouri's psychiatric research hospital, a leading center for psychological treatment and Freudian therapy (Krahl and Schröder 2015). One central piece of Sigmund Freud's approach was his famous analysis of the memoirs of Daniel Paul Schreber (Schreber 1903, 1955; Freud 1911, 2003; for critical psychoanalytic or historical reflections on Freud's Schreber case, see Allison et al. 1988; Santner 1996; Dalzell 2011).

Schreber was a German judge diagnosed with dementia praecox in 1884, the diagnostic category later known as schizophrenia (Bleuler 1908, 1911). In his book, Schreber (1955, 18, 24) described extensively his suffering from "divine miracles" and "orders." Boroffka had an English translation of Schreber's memoirs (1955) in his Ibadan library and loaned it to his patient Tanka. Tanka became fascinated to follow Schreber's example and to write his own book about schizophrenic experiences, responding to the presentation with the claim that he would have "enough material now" for "making a full publication" (cited after Boroffka 1980b, 144). Therefore, the Schreber text became a model and source of inspiration for Tanka as he wrote about his experiences, self-diagnoses, and observations of medical phenomena around him (Boroffka 1980b, 5, 139).

Tanka's writings may be the only detailed autobiographical notes published by an African patient with schizophrenia. They remain an exceptionally rich source for studying the history of psychiatry and schizophrenia in Africa, exposing as they do the perceptions and experiences of an individual patient. This chapter explores stories that are locally and globally connected to—and behind—Tanka's text. The idea is to investigate how Tanka described his mental experiences and, through his engaging narratives, built up communications and relationships with his doctors, nurses, and his imagined audience and readers. Finally, I discuss how Tanka's texts corresponded with global discourses on schizophrenia in and beyond Africa.

Ego-Documents and Vernacular Histories of Psychiatry

Tanka's autobiography offers authentic, rare, and deep insights into the perceptions, experiences, and feelings of a psychiatric patient in Africa, and as these relate to vernacular idioms. These insights are instructive regarding the effects of Western psychiatry and the everyday struggles of African patients searching for help from traditional healers and Western-trained psychiatrists, some of whom were Europeans. Tanka's texts, therefore, are precious for writing an African history of psychiatry "from below"—an approach promoted by historians since the 1980s that has tended to make visible and audible patients long ignored or silenced by historians (for structural silencing, see Caminero-Santangelo 1998).

Indeed, the history of psychiatry was for a long time "history from psychiatrists about psychiatrists for psychiatrists" (Micale and Porter 1994, 3). Publications by (former) patients of lunatic asylums, such as the memoirs of Schreber (1955), became well known because psychiatrists discussed them—in Schreber's case, by Freud himself—as they documented their own diagnostic efforts (Freud 2003). Similarly, the German psychiatrist Karl Birnbaum (1920) published patients' writings under the title *Psychopathologische Dokumente*. German psychiatrist Wilhelm Lange-Eichbaum (1928) also published a collection of texts written by those diagnosed with dementia praecox, and the US psychologist Bert Kaplan published a collection of patient narratives: *The Inner World of Mental Illness* (1964).

Frantz Fanon was perhaps the first to publish the "voices" of African psychiatric patients in his postcolonial classic *The Wretched of the Earth* (1961). This book investigated and revealed the psychopathological effects of colonial subjugation and a colonial war for liberation. Awareness of patient self-perceptions, their suppression by a psychiatric establishment, as well as their agency and resistance, all these were important issues in Fanon's work, even though in a sense he was a part of the Algerian psychiatric establishment, though from a dissenting stance (see Keller, chapter 8 in this volume).

Quite the same form of institutional belonging with distancing seems to apply to Boroffka of Ibadan. He published Tanka's notes to offer up a case study on the experience of schizophrenia in a patient from Africa. The book would be accessible to a large audience and was not solely intended to give a patient an opportunity to "speak" (Boroffka 1980c).

This clinical way of making patient "voices" available did not change, even with the emergence of critical research about psychiatry as a system of oppressive knowledge and institutionalization, like that carried out by Michel Foucault (2006a, 2006b) and Erving Goffman (1961) in the early 1960s. Foucault demonstrated how psychiatry served as a myth and social construction that worked to marginalize people whose behavior and whose conception of the world seemed "abnormal," thus not in line with the majority of society (Foucault 2006a, 2006b). Yet Foucault also construed these persons as silent and paralyzed, as victims, and he in a sense also marginalized their perceptions for a second time.

The manner in which scholars have dealt with psychiatric patients as objects for scientific observation and evidence slowly changed in the 1980s. At the same time, many historians developed a strong interest in the "everyday-life of ordinary people," revitalizing an older Marxist approach to "people's history" (Thompson 1966; see also the approach of German Alltagsgeschichte [history of the everyday] in the 1980s, Lüdtke 1995). Ego-documents—autobiographies, letters, diaries, and objects—became central kinds of evidence for interpreting the experiences, perceptions, discourses, and practices of historical subjects and actors. The history of medicine also discovered a more self-confident and active perspective on patients and their experiences in these same years (on Alltagsgeschichte, see Presser 1969, 277–82; Peterson 1982; Porter 1985; Dekker 2002a, 2002b; for theoretical and methodological questions regarding ego-documents, see Schulze 1996; von Greyerz, Medick, and Veit 2001).

"History from below," therefore, became a buzzword in Roy Porter's famous studies of medicine (1985) and psychiatry (1987). There is now considerable research on the experiences, perceptions, and agency of psychiatric patients, in all kinds of settings, and based on their words and remarks (Micale and Porter 1994; Brückner 2006; Berkenkotter 2008; Ledebur 2013).

The extraordinarily rich and extensive writings of some patients diagnosed with schizophrenia have been analyzed as forms of "life writing," as well as being reflections on and adaptations to worlds outside and inside lunatic asylums (Wood 2013). The structural silencing of patient voices within the bureaucratic framings of psychiatry, and the limitations of patient records, clinical reports, and diagnoses, remain evident. Ego-documents of patients were not and usually are not kept in institutional archives if they had not been used as evidence yielding a diagnosis (Caminero-Santangelo 1998).

This structuring is true for studies of insanity and psychiatry in the so-called Global South and also in (former) colonies in Africa. The largely Western epistemic culture that medicalizes the mind as it creates its psychiatric objects appears to have compounded the silencing of colonial and postcolonial African patients as if, to follow Spivak (1988, 313), they were subalterns who cannot speak.

Thus, it is important to highlight findings and assumptions about (post) colonial societies as located in psychiatric archives. The "Black," mad individual was—is—usually not allowed to speak, even if patients were able to express their perceptions and needs in writing, crafting via forms of acting, from affirmative obedience to resistance, thus embracing refusal, rejection of therapies, escape attempts, and suicide.

Jonathan Sadowsky's *Imperial Bedlam*, a history partially about colonial lunatic asylums in southern Nigeria, includes writing by African inmates. His analysis is an exception: it builds on rich archival material not then typical of research about psychiatry in Africa (Sadowsky 1999). Yet, in general, "psychiatry from below" for regions of the Global South had largely remained a blind spot or at best a desideratum because of these preconditions and limitations.

But this wish goes with some aspects not shared in this chapter, namely the idea that it might be possible to trace outpatient self-perceptions from their writings. I rather refer here to ego-document studies that analyze such sources as a complex product of genre, customs, and active adaptations experienced by individuals. In Tanka's case, this line of thinking means attending to the perception and negotiation of transcultural knowledge of his diagnosis, together with the role of schizophrenia therapeutics and forms of self-positioning within the whole complex and fraught process in an early postcolonial situation, promixate to major global schizophrenia research at the time (WHO 1973; for analyzing transcultural experiences in general, see Ulbrich, Medick, and Schaser 2012; Antić 2021, 2022). A turn to ego-documents involves a methodological perspective that places the writings of an individual within the context of their time and place, but also shows micro–macro links—or as Roland Robertson (1995) would say "glocalizations"—which transform the patient's text into a psychiatric case study corresponding to global discourses and practices (Andrande 2010; Epple 2010; Gerritsen 2012; Medick 2016).

Tanka's text was constantly changing within a "micro zone of global entanglement" (Büschel and Speich 2009, 22) as a product of, and triggering factor for, constructing, negotiating, and manifesting epistemic knowledge about schizophrenia. That entailed the self-positioning of a subjective patient who was suffering as key to these micro–macro links.

Analyzing Tanka's writings as significant microscopic traces, useful in relation to the global politics of bringing evidence into a knowledge system about schizophrenia, has been inspired here by "historical epistemology." Lorraine Daston defined this approach as a "history of emergence," suggesting the constant rise of historiographical questions about how hypotheses, assumptions, controversies, as well as epistemic concepts and certainties, become possible in a specific place and time (Daston 1994;

Daston 2007, 807). Locating Tanka's autobiography in such a context, I ask how his writing can be seen in correlation with "possible" thinking about schizophrenia by psychiatrists in Africa. As important is to investigate how Tanka translated what he learned about his specific diagnosis in his specific time and place into the texts he wrote. Taking processes of the making and editing of his writing into account, Tanka's text may be analyzed as an "epistemic thing," as coined by Hans-Jörg Rheinberger (2010). Self-labeled as a testimonial by a young, literate, partially westernized Cameroonian schizophrenic, Boroffka selected, annotated, and edited Tanka's autobiographical text. The claim of being an original patient's writing and "true evidence" of one individual's experiences of schizophrenia remained and transformed Tanka's piece into a psychiatric epistemological object (Rheinberger 2010, 2).

Reading the exceptional narratives of this schizophrenic from Cameroon "along the archival grain" (Stoler 2010) of psychiatric epistemic culture paves the way for an analysis of Tanka's text as a product *and* an engine of a global shift: a time of negotiating the codification, diagnosis, and prognosis of schizophrenia in Africa (see Henckes 2019).

The diagnosis of schizophrenia in Africa has a special dimension with a long colonial history. As early as 1991, Megan Vaughan pleaded for studying colonial and postcolonial psychiatry in Africa through historical commitments to singular psychiatric "illnesses." Research into the historical epistemic culture of a diagnosis could be useful in tracing the shadows of humanitarian or other discourses and practices (Vaughan 1991, 108, 125). Matthew Heaton (2011, 2013), Ursula M. Read, Victor C. K. Doku, and Ama De Graft Aikins (2015) have shown how central the diagnosis of schizophrenia was as an etiquette for the "insufficiently Other" of colonial times (Vaughan 1991, 125).

Such otherness fundamentally changed with decolonization. In the 1960s and 1970s, the diagnosis of schizophrenia became an urgent and highly controversial issue in Africa and beyond. One could say, in the words of Ian Hacking (1999, 58), that schizophrenia had become, of all mental diagnoses, the psychiatric disorder par excellence within laboratories of "knowledge, belief, evidence, good reason, objectivity, probability." Schizophrenia still functions today, even if the word is under question, as a partial lens for global reasoning on the prosperity, sustainability, and development of African societies. It remains oriented toward the shift from colonial oppression to postcolonial freedom, and is often construed in terms of "traditional backwardness" and "modern uncertainties."

The Most Frightening Mental Illness:
Schizophrenia in the 1960s

In the 1960s, schizophrenia was central to debates about diagnosis, treatment, and care, as well as extremely controversial within causes and therapies (Henckes 2019, 456). What was not controversial was the idea that schizophrenia could serve as a label for a sample of those psychiatric "illnesses" seen as serious and dangerous, including for epidemic reasons. Scholars claimed that schizophrenia might be less caused by physical, neurological, and genetic factors but more by social psychological factors like loneliness, social isolation, and stress. Therefore, schizophrenia could spread out like an epidemic contagious illness triggered by the effects of modernization and its destruction of family structures and accustomed way of life (for the most comprehensive summary of state-of-the-art debates during the 1960s, see Arieti 1974).

It was widely accepted that schizophrenia, though partially treatable from the 1950s, was nearly incurable, depriving patients of regular jobs as well as social and family lives for the rest of their days (Mayer-Gross, Slater, and Roth 1969, 33–35; Arieti 1974). Since the early attempts to conceptualize schizophrenia, it has been seen as a "peculiar destruction of the inner connection of the psychic personality with predominant damage to the life of the mind and of the will," as the German psychiatrist Emil Kraepelin wrote in 1899 when describing a set of mental "disturbances" with the term *dementia praecox* (Kraepelin 1899, 667; for the historical conceptualization of schizophrenia see Gottesman 1991; Shorter 1997, 241–45; Shorter 2005, 267–75; Gilman 2008; Bernett 2013; McNally 2016).

It was this "split" within an individual's personality that led Eugen Bleuler to decide in 1908 to rename Kraepelin's dementia praecox as schizophrenia, with references to the ancient Greek phrase "splitting the mind" (Bleuler 1908, 1911).

Since the 1920s, Bleuler's four A-syndromes have been used to standardize the diagnosis of schizophrenia, as (flattened) affect, autism, the (impaired) association of ideas, and ambivalence (Stotz-Ingenlath 2000;

McNally 2009). There was a division between "primary" symptoms (like the deterioration of the logical capacity of a patient, usually connected to a psychotic break with "reality") and "secondary" symptoms (dissociation in social relations or the loss of an ability to organize everyday life) (Shorter 2005, 267). In sum, it has long been common knowledge in Western psychiatry that schizophrenia can be diagnosed when patients hear voices, or suffer from sleeplessness, fear, emotional instability, and extreme personality splits, and disorders of thinking, memory, and perceptions (McNally 2016, 11–21).

As with other psychiatric diagnoses, scientists long thought that schizophrenia was not widespread in regions outside the Global North—and certainly not in the so-called underdeveloped areas of tropical Africa. Like depression (Sadowsky 2020 and chapter 5 in this volume), scientists thought schizophrenia was linked to "higher civilization" and "cultural development." It was, in a sense, seen as a "Western culture-bound syndrome." Some colonial psychiatrists held the view, surely racist at that, that paranoid schizophrenia would be rare or even absent in illiterate, so-called primitive societies, simply because African minds were too "simple" (Carothers 1940, 99; Carothers 1954, 140–42; see also Gaines 1992; Heaton 2013, 106–8).[1] Still, some psychiatrists working in colonies in Africa repeatedly pointed out that they encountered African patients with all the symptoms attributed to schizophrenia in Europe, including the repeatedly observed "split" as found in the "affected smile of da Vinci's Mona Lisa" (Vyncke 1960).

In the 1960s, statistical Western psychiatric evidence indicated that schizophrenic disorders were epidemic in many settings and that the number of patients so diagnosed seemed to be constantly growing. These statistics suggested that schizophrenia usually broke out in early adolescence, with a small male majority, with a clear link to high intelligence and academic education (McNally 2016, 11–21). This "mental disorder" was seen from Europe, therefore, to affect precisely that part of a population considered central to economic, social stability, and the growth of economies. The fear that schizophrenia could threaten a key portion of a society's population, through which it was hoped development would be achieved, suggested profound social, political, and economic damage in the process. In addition, also alarming was the fact that the majority of patients diagnosed with schizophrenia lived permanently, or at least for several years, in lunatic asylums and closed psychiatric wards, where they received intensive and costly care (Arieti 1974, 385–440). So it was that of all mental disorders, schizophrenia became the focus of governmental reasoning at national and increasingly transnational levels (Foucault 1991, 87–104). The question became how this "most frightening mental illness" (Picchioni and Murray 2007, 91) could be controlled. Early diagnosis would prevent wasteful investments in the education of young people, who would never be able to give back to society what they had received. Research on the most unclear trigger factors to schizophrenia would help to stop the epidemic spread of the disease. And, last but not least, the need for new therapies would minimize the cost of hospital care and speed up recovery (Arieti 1974; Henckes 2019).

In the 1950s, schizophrenia was only partially defined as a genetically conditioned, hereditary disorder.[2] Increasingly from this decade, the assumption prevailed that the disease could also be caused by living conditions and lived experiences (Gilman 2008, 461–86). Schizophrenia was progressively debated as a mental disease caused and pushed forward by experiences of fundamental cultural and social change. Given the colonial assumption that schizophrenia did not occur in "traditional" and "primitive" societies, combined with statistical evidence of a worldwide increase in schizophrenic disorders during the late colonial or early postcolonial decades, it was increasingly thought that the number of diagnosed cases of schizophrenia in Africa would increase with decolonization and a growing degree of Westernization (Corin and Murphy 1979; Jablensky and Sartorius 1975).

The WHO referred extensively to colonial studies, as it demonstrated the general thought that "the rapid changes of cultural patterns" would cause the epidemic spread of mental disease, noting that "mental health problems" that "arose from technical change were likely to take on increasing significance not only in communities where industrialization had just begun to develop, but also in countries which were already highly developed economically," and still in the process of "modernization" (WHO 1958, 330). The World Federation for Mental Health, a nongovernmental organization close to the WHO that promoted mental health issues at national and international levels (Brody 2004, 54–55; Opaku and Biswas 2014, 3–4), took the same line. As early as 1955, the famous American anthropologist Margaret Mead, soon to become the World Federation for Mental Health's third president, declared that modernization, development, and "rapid social and cultural changes" would cause "serious mental illnesses, including even schizophrenia" (Mead 1955, 6–7).

Research about the causes, diagnosis, and treatment of schizophrenia became in the 1930s a central element of what Michel Foucault (Foucault

1994, 73; Foucault 1997, 242) later called "biopolitics," with its wide range of societal technologies with national and transnational agendas focusing on creating and stabilizing a "sane and productive population" (Foucault 1997, 242).

Scholars pushed schizophrenia into the attention of psychiatrists, but also into those of psychologists, anthropologists, economists, and politicians (Scott 1998). The disease seemed to threaten "modernization," its implementation and development, and also seemed to have been caused by these factors. Countless scientists attested to a kind of vicious cycle that should be broken to prevent a shutdown of entire national economies.

Undergoing decolonization, the African continent entered this stage due to fears of future forms of alienation in postcolonial states, with thousands of costly patients debilitated by schizophrenia and kept from the economic systems of their societies (Akyeampong, Hill, and Kleinman 2015, 3–4; Read, Doku, and Aikins 2015). To argue here with Foucault, fear and suspicion were getting rationalized with several biopolitical techniques (surveys, statistics, field studies) from anthropology, tropical medicine, and psychiatry. These techniques were intended to avoid a potential loss of labor and economic productivity or a feared "degeneration" of African societies in the presumed processes of decolonization and "modernisation" (for the conceptual approach, see Foucault 1994, 73; Foucault 1998, 25).

The first wave of biopolitical initiatives focused on containing psychiatric disease in Africa. Anthropologists funded by the British Colonial Office carried out these initiatives and discovered that empire had to be stabilized via psychology focused on "ruling the minds" of "natives" (see Linstrum 2012, 2016). Probably the most influential study in this respect was that of Meyer Fortes and Doris Y. Mayer, who looked into the mental health of the Tallensi in the Gold Coast (Ghana) in the 1930s and 1963, respectively. They found a significant increase in cases of mental illness over the thirty years between their two field trips (Fortes and Mayer 1966). These highly respected anthropologists interpreted this increase as a result of Westernization and modernization. They noted that, among psychiatric patients encountered in 1963, were those who could be classified "simply" as "paranoid schizophrenics," and, according to Western repertoires, they concluded that the disease seemed mild (Fortes and Mayer 1966, 39–40).

The anthropologists and psychiatrists included Geoffrey Tooth for the Gold Coast, Margaret Field for colonial Gold Coast (then newly independent Ghana), and the first African psychiatrist to work in Ghana, Emmanuel Forster (see Hunt, chapter 10 in this volume). They all reported to the Colonial Office, and later to the WHO, that rapid social changes caused by colonial and postcolonial "modernization" were causing stress for numerous "native" Africans with mental illnesses like psychosis and schizophrenia (Tooth 1950; Field 1958, 1960; Forster 1962; Büschel 2015). Tooth warned the Gold Coast administration of the growing number of schizophrenics, with adverse effects on productivity in the colony. Schizophrenia seemed rare among "bush people," but was growing rapidly in the "developed centers" of the country. The forms and numbers seemed close to those in European cities (Tooth 1950, 49). Field found during the first years of Ghanaian nationhood that literacy went with psychosis with an "outburst of acute schizophrenia" significantly above average. Such psychoses were compounded by the stress experienced in educational development programs (Field 1958; Field 1960, 7–11, 201–74; Field 1968; see also Hunt, chapter 10 in this volume).

Forster delivered statistics to several British development agencies on lower rates of schizophrenia among Ghana's "native population" in the remote and "less developed" areas of the country. He claimed that the destruction of "tribal community life," or at least of individuals' ability to preserve their "traditional lifestyle," was causing "psychic reactions," while schizophrenia was spreading "like an epidemic" among Ghanaians living in "intermediate worlds" between "imported Western culture" and "African tradition" (Forster 1962, 13, 22). Clearly, in his view, "primitive people" would "present less schizophrenic disorders" (Forster 1962, 9). The growing number of schizophrenics in Ghana was alarmingly threatening the job market, it seemed, especially as people from less "developed" regions became mentally ill after migrating to the cities. The work regimens that they were experiencing would "very often and rapidly" lead to "catastrophic psychosis and schizoid disease," and on a scale that damaged the national economy, and thereby jeopardized the prosperity of the newly independent country as a whole (Forster 1960, 49).

Overall, a recognition gradually emerged that it was less increasing Westernization that caused schizophrenia, than the clash of two cultures, each with different systems of values, perceptions, and feelings. So it was that the view of Tanka's German doctor in Ibadan, Boroffka, was in sync with this kind of thinking, that continuous living "in between" and in "divided worlds" could foster the splitting of a "soul" (Boroffka 1980b, 142; Staewen and Schönberg 1970). In the Gold Coast, as in Nigeria and Ibadan, findings made the problem of schizophrenia seem urgent in the 1960s and 1970s. This interpretation of this psychiatric psychosis seemed to have an impact on all psychologists, psychiatrists, and development experts who, in this time of decolonization and development, were supposed to play a role in promoting prosperous futures in these decolonizing African societies.

The WHO and Uncertain Epistemic Cultures

These considerations carried much uncertainty about diagnoses, causes, treatments, prognoses, and the dangers of the epidemic spread of mental illness in general. In the 1950s, the global diagnostic tools in the West, used by psychiatrists, other clinicians, researchers, health insurance companies, pharmaceutical regulatory agencies and their lawyers, and policymakers, were found in the tenth edition of the WHO's *International Statistical Classification of Diseases and Related Health Problems* and the first edition of the *Diagnostic and Statistical Manual of Mental Disorders*, published in 1952 by the American Psychiatric Association. Both sets of guidelines carried huge uncertainty in relation to diagnostic categories, and they were highly controversial as well due to their ethnocentric tendencies and implicit assumptions (Good 1996; Lewis-Fernández 1996; Lewis-Fernández and Aggarwal 2013).

Similarly, even stronger uncertainties prevailed regarding treatment, chances of recovery, and the epidemiological dimensions of schizophrenia. Since the mid-1950s, psychiatrists tried to cure schizophrenia, or at least ameliorate its symptoms, with the psychotropic chlorpromazine, though with limited success as studies have shown (Turner 2007). But there were indications that schizophrenia in "traditional" societies, like in Africa, would have a milder course and faster recovery in comparison to the societies we now call the Global North (Fortes and Mayer 1966).

The continuing uncertainty about schizophrenia prompted the rhetorical question already raised by the WHO in 1973: "Why is a concept of schizophrenia necessary at all?" The answer to this question seemed simple: "Because we have the term. The word schizophrenia has come into such widespread use that it is necessary to have a practical definition" (WHO 1973, 17).

In response to the fatal combination of such lack of knowledge and the fear of an epidemic spread of schizophrenia, the WHO convened a first study group as early as 1957. It addressed the lack of knowledge about this mental disorder and demanded further empirical research (WHO 1957, 9–14). In 1959, the WHO formed a committee of experts on the epidemiology of mental disorders to develop research on psychiatric epidemiology and to reflect on the possibilities and limits of this new field, epidemiology, for research on mental disorders in areas of the Global South (WHO 1960). Since that time, the advantages and results of applying epidemiological research to psychiatry have been widely promoted (Reid 1960; Lin and Standley 1962; Morris 1964; Kramer 1969; Cooper 1999, 14–18).

Likewise, in terms of "current urgent social issues that are relevant to the entire world—such as development efforts in Africa," the WHO called for more schizophrenia studies from a comparative global perspective to comprehend the social and economic effects of a possible spread of this psychiatric illness (WHO 1964). Questions about the possibilities for, frequency of, and time of recovery from schizophrenia were central when the WHO began its first cross-cultural international pilot study on schizophrenia in 1968 investigating 1,202 patients in nine countries—Colombia, Czechoslovakia, Denmark, India, Nigeria, China, Union of Soviet Socialist Republics, the United Kingdom, and the United States (WHO 1973; Leff et al. 1992). As a result of the pilot study, by 1973 the WHO was arguing that schizophrenia, as the "most serious, least-researched, socially and economically most damaging disease," called for an extended cross-cultural, comparative pilot study under the umbrella of its core social-psychiatric and epidemiological programs (WHO 1973).

The first pilot study and its results were highly controversial for principal investigators for three reasons: first, scholars criticized the lack of clear evidence for reasons behind the demonstrated differences between recovery in "developed" and "development countries." A second point of critique was that the Third World settings were located in "developing societies," where "modernization, Westernization and partly industrialization," as typical phenomena of Western "civilization," had already taken hold. There was no clear evidence for a revision of previous assumptions about schizophrenia as a civilizing illness, whose danger of spreading via development in Africa served as a counterproductive side effect of the prosperous development of postcolonial African states. Third, the evidence for Africa—the continent labeled at this time as the most problematic for future "development" and epidemic psychiatric diseases, and the most significant for "primitive" societies—seemed quite small and, in regard to being representative of Africa, weak. For these reasons, and taking the overall critique into account, there was an urgent plea for studying individual castes and self-reports—like those of Tanka (Fuller Torrey 1980, 1987a, 1987b; Lin and Kleinman 1988; Jablensky et al. 1992; Sass 1994, 99; Jablensky and Satorius 2008).

So it is that this global detour returns us to Tanka's and Boroffka's microscopic world as doctor–researcher and patient–writer, as well as the contents and import of their writings.

Tanka's Writing as Self-Empowerment

Beyond the many uncertainties (Henckes 2019), most psychiatrists all over the world routinely diagnosed and treated schizophrenia. The same was the case when the Cameroonian district medical officer, after just a short consultation, labeled Mr. Tanka as schizophrenic (Boroffka 1980a, 9). There is little evidence in Tanka's writings about his experiences in lunatic asylums in Cameroon before he came to Ibadan, though the attending doctors and nurses repeatedly appeared in these early stories as devils and demons (Tanka 1980, 23–34, 47–93).

This psychiatric staff frightened him, motivating Tanka to seek better psychiatric care through making his six-hundred-mile-long journey from Kumba to Ibadan in summer 1970. Writing became a key means by which he established a communication structure with his doctors and made his points. Tanka was, in a sense, already familiar with biographical and reflexive life writing. As a second-rank clerk in a branch office of the Cameroonian Ministry of Education, he came across discourses on societal and economic development on the one side and the epidemic dangers of schizophrenia on the other, since psychiatric problems were a frequent problem among students (see Heaton, chapter 6 in this volume). He also was introduced to autobiographical texts written by applicants for school teaching positions. His task was to file the curricula vitae of teachers submitted before they could be hired. Tanka was also responsible for training courses for teachers and students, and they had to submit autobiographical essays as well as undergo psychological testing and consultation (Boroffka 1980a, 6; for those tests for teachers and experts in late colonialism and the process of decolonization, see Linstrum 2016, 83–115, 189–216).

In the literary sense we can see inspirations from the Bible, from missionary literature, and Onitsha market publications—narratives full of lively individual case studies and storytelling (Boroffka 1980b, 144; for Onitsha

publications, see Beier 1964; Obiechina 1971, 1972). Tanka was also familiar with educational dramas about development, used by the British mandate administration (as films or live onstage) as well as local development
experts to "educate" and "teach" colonized and illiterate Cameroonians in
"modern" agriculture, hygiene, and medicine. These development experts
also used dramatic narrative representations to teach (Büschel 2014, 165,
209, 468).

Tanka wrote such a "play" in this genre as a supplement to his autobiographical notes, translating, even perverting, the prototypical development message of these plays, which derived from discourses about the
stultifying and paralyzing psychic dangers of animistic witchcraft beliefs
often found in schizophrenic experiences. In his "play," Tanka portrayed
judges, government representatives, priests, and psychiatrists as either
good or evil demons. He depicted himself as a person fighting within a
network of relationships including the actors in the play, and also as an
archetypal schizophrenic persecuted by "voices" and devils, but who ultimately succeeds in becoming "healthy" again. One can read this play
as a developmental parable and drama, intended by Tanka to stage the
experience of schizophrenia and how to cope with it. It seems, therefore,
that Tanka came to see himself as a typical schizophrenic by reproducing
the global psychiatric devices (*dispositifs*) of the WHO, while providing evidence of his exemplary nature. Moreover, it should not be forgotten that
in these times when numerous scholars were sharing their opinions that
schizophrenia was a disease of the "educated" and "civilized" (Forster
1962, 9), a schizophrenia diagnosis provided Tanka with a clear instru-
ment to demonstrate that he belonged to the "civilized" and was no longer
"primitive" like his family.

The WHO Pilot Study, Tanka, and Schizophrenia
as a Stress Disorder

It was in September 1970, after being admitted to the University College
Hospital in Ibadan, that Tanka met Boroffka for the first time. Boroffka was
already involved in collecting data for the WHO's pilot study on schizophrenia
(Boroffka 1980a, 12–13), which began in the Ibadan hospital research unit in
April 1968. Most probably, Ibadan in Nigeria was chosen for the study because
of the influence of Lambo in his position as WHO deputy-director-general.

Lambo hired Boroffka to collect the data because of his "extensive experiences in Africa" and his "pre-eminent" attitude in "his diagnosis and total therapeutic management of the African patients" (Lambo 1980).

It appears that Tanka knew enough to try to become an active patient who could influence the epistemic cultures of the Ibadan hospital, a human laboratory for schizophrenia research. Regardless, Boroffka recalled Tanka presenting his autobiographical writings during several of their consultations. Although individuals were not given explicit roles in epidemiological research or forms of data collection, Boroffka became interested in this unconventional, engaged patient as an "exemplary character" (Boroffka 1980b, 143) for WHO's findings and strategies. The psychological strain experienced by office clerks, nurses, and teachers in tropical Africa in the course of "development" became a central theme for governmental experts, as well as in public debates on the epidemiological danger, spread, and context of schizophrenia emerging following stress. The initial spark was a series of WHO articles that appeared in the *Cameroon Times* in December 1968. These discussed the thesis that schizophrenia—similarly to the so-called brain fag syndrome (Prince 1960, 1985; see also Heaton 2013, 120–29 and chapter 6 in this volume)—resulted from stress disorders that coincided with "civilizing missions," development efforts, and education, thus with a profound immersion in "modernization" or Westernization of some kind (WHO 1968).

Tanka thought it obvious that his suffering came from the social pressures of office work amid profound societal change. Several times in his notes the secretary to the prime minister of Cameroon "Mr. Andela" appears, often with Dan Lantum, the area medical officer of Kumba who had been responsible for Tanka. Tanka recalled how Andela addressed him in an authoritarian way, with a whispering voice that penetrated Tanka's whole body: "Do not speak to me. I will speak to you" (Tanka 1980, 18, 36). These "voices" peaked in their intensity during Tanka's commute to his office and also when he was "inside the office." Sometimes he had to stop working and go home because of this constant "whispering of the voices." One time, on the way home, he saw a "girl on a Mobyllete and one of the voices told [him] that the girl was a devil and she once had been a girlfriend to Mr. Andela" (Tanka 1980, 21).

Andela met Tanka on several occasions and protected him in his official capacity. According to Tanka, Andela and Lantum were schoolmates. This network of two important bureaucrats took on a critical dimension when

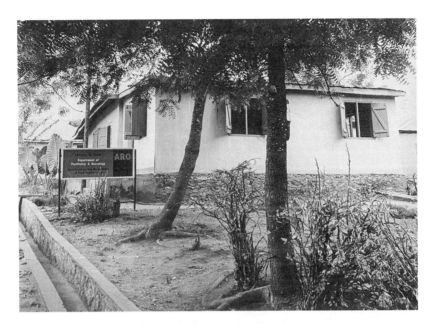

3.2 University of Ibadan Hospital, Aro Field Research Unit for the WHO study on schizophrenia. (Photograph by Alexander Boroffka, 1970, Alexander Boroffka Papers, Iwalewa House, Bayreuth.)

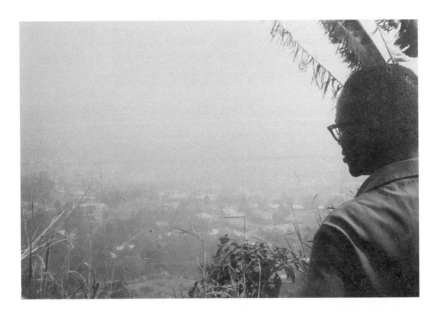

3.3 Benedict Nta Tanka in Menka country, Cameroon. (Photograph by Alexander Boroffka, 1984, Alexander Boroffka Papers, Iwalewa House, Bayreuth.)

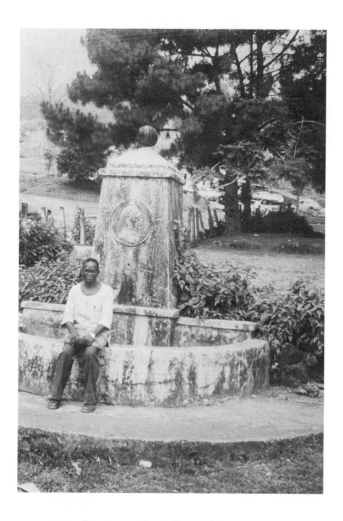

3.4 Benedict Nta Tanka in front of the Bismarck memorial in Buea, Cameroon. (Photograph by Alexander Boroffka, 1984, Alexander Boroffka Papers, Iwalewa House, Bayreuth.)

Lantum ordered Tanka released from his office duties with the accusing diagnosis of paranoid schizophrenia. The move might have disappointed Andela, who had always supported Tanka in his career as an office clerk (Boroffka 1980d, 121).

In his writing, Tanka situated these social pressures and the emergence of his schizophrenia in a wider context of triggering political upheavals.

Cameroon became independent in 1960. One year later, the southwestern part of Cameroon where Tanka had been born and raised—previously administered by the British mandate government—became a part of the nation, a process that entailed continuous administrative, social, and political changes (Tanka 1980, 115–16). When Tanka heard "voices" for the first time in 1968, he recalled, debates about restructuring and reunifying the country persisted. Menka representatives—like Tanka—were central actors, as they were supposed to mediate among traditional structures, Menka's village-based self-government, and administrative reforms. The negotiation of local political structures played a role, as did questions of modernization and "civilization" in relation to "witchcraft," "traditional customs," or religiousness (Chilver and Kaberry 1970).

There was a prominent role model for Tanka within this mix. In describing his schizophrenia as caused by work stress and social pressures, he revealed that he had encountered the writings of Schreber, given to him by his doctor Boroffka. Though completely different, there are striking biographical similarities between the Tanka and Schreber texts. It seems that Tanka read an English translation of Schreber, offered to him by Boroffka. Both Schreber and Tanka were at important stages in their careers when diagnosed with dementia praecox or schizophrenia: Schreber had just been appointed senate president of the Higher Regional Court in Dresden in 1893 when he was overcome with "mental delusions" and "crazy dreams" (Santner 1996), while Tanka had been appointed second-class clerk in the Department of Education less than two years prior to when his suffering became so dominant he could not ignore it any longer (Boroffka 1980a, 6). Both men assumed that schizophrenia could be triggered by stress and biographical upheavals. Like Tanka, Schreber was institutionalized at least twice. Both suffered from religious experiences, like hearing church music and whispering angels, and described their experiences and suffering extensively (Tanka 1980, 22–23, 95; Schreber 1955, 56, 66).

While Schreber wrote to convince doctors and lawyers that he was not insane but in fact a victim of "divine-supernatural miracles" that put him at the "center of the universe" (Santner 1996, 7–9), Tanka did not write down his notes to resist or oppose his doctors, medical officers, or psychiatrists. Rather, he constructed himself as a prime example of an African schizophrenic suffering from civilizing stress disorders, in order to become part of the WHO research laboratory located in Ibadan. For example, he wrote about suffering during his office work:

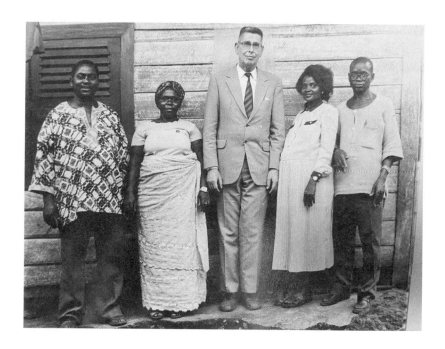

3.5   Psychiatrist Alexander Boroffka towers over Benedict Nta Tanka and his wife (*left*) and two Tanka family members (*right*) during a visit some years after their initial work together. (Photographer unknown, 1984, Alexander Boroffka Papers, Iwalewa House, Bayreuth.)

I signed the attendance register and went straight to my table. I took three letters to register and the voice . . . was severe on me. [The voice] was so hot and did not want me to work. My head was heavy and was full of vibrating air which swept in with great force through my ears and pores on my head. After thirty minutes, I was not able to register one of the letters. I was weak, tired and my head was sweating. I went up to my boss who said he would not let me go. . . . But I had to go home. There was no need sitting down in such an agony from mysterious voices. I left the office without a word and went home. (Tanka 1980a, 21)

Yet it was not only work stress and social pressure that Tanka proposed as the triggers for his disease, as we will now see.

"Living In-Between" and Splitting the Mind

Another core cause of schizophrenia discussed by the WHO and subsequently taken up by Tanka entailed living between traditional and modern worlds. Called a "split life situation and split living condition," the report noted that this in-betweenness could catalyze a pathological split of the human mind and in the form of schizophrenia (WHO 1973, 17–21).

Coming from a family of farmers, yet at the same time a civil servant for the Ministry of Education, Tanka consistently presented himself as an expert on living between different cultural and social worlds, and also as an exemplary patient who suffered from the division of his life between the vernacular or the traditional and modernity (Boroffka 1980a, 6). He often described how he sought out traditional healers as well as Western doctors (Tanka 1980, 17), and worked his way through experiences of illness with witchcraft. He also wrote that he was well aware of the extent to which Cameroon, and Menka society in particular, were "underdeveloped in medical terms." "Witchcraft" played a central role in the lives of the Menka, and Tanka situated himself as an insider and an outsider in relation to this sphere: "I have never believed there is something existing like [witchcraft], but I was forced by a supernatural occurrence to believe that there exists witchcraft" (Tanka 1980, 17).

Some scenes are striking within Tanka's self-description of his psychological tensions due to living between the worlds. At the very beginning of his autobiography, he wrote about how two days after hearing "voices" for the first time, this was his "Christian birthday," the anniversary of his Roman Catholic baptism. He described preparing himself for the church service by reading his book of hours and the holy vita of his patron saint, St. Benedict. He fervently hoped that these exercises and prayers would make the "mysterious voices" disappear. But instead the opposite happened: during mass and the following celebrations the "voices became louder and louder and more pressing" (Tanka 1980, 19). A few days later, when he went to bed countless butterflies appeared, whispering in his ears. Finally, the British queen Elizabeth II appeared: "a transparent, majestic appearance, quite silent," but also "terribly frightening" because her appearance was accompanied by a white board on which her name was written in blood (Tanka 1980, 23). The queen, one could argue, represented a double-faced sphinx: colonial suppression on the one side, and development and civilization on the other.

Following these experiences, Tanka wrote, he became stuck in a "traditional" African world of faith yet fighting against this condition. He believed that he had been "bewitched" by envious evil colleagues from his office, by his family, and by supposed friends, all of whom had caused him to be attacked by the devil in rituals. After all, he had tried to alleviate "evil forces" through Christian prayers and also through the healers whom he consulted several times. After such healing failed, and rather seemed to provoke even more frequent and louder voices, Tanka turned to the district medical officer, a Western-trained Cameroonian doctor, who made his diagnosis of "paranoid schizophrenia" and transferred Tanka to the psychiatric ward of a nearby missionary hospital (Tanka 1980, 23, 42–43).

Self-Construction as a Typical "Patient"

In all his storytelling, Tanka vividly depicted scenes and experiences full of color, sound, and feelings. One message of his text was quite clear: he was speaking from first hand experience. His text makes claims of authenticity and also demonstrates the enrichment of global discourses on schizophrenia in Africa. A specific form of patient agency develops that was communicating with Western psychiatric knowledge on schizophrenia. Considering Tanka's text itself as a "global actor," in Bruno Latour's sense, suggests an important "difference," away from uncertainties toward truthfulness in knowledge production within the contested global epistemic culture of schizophrenia (Latour 2005, 52; for some examples, see Daston 2004). Tanka propelled himself into being an exemplary prototype of a silenced, missing African patient who exposed his authentic voice. He also seems to have tried to deliver evidence from the perspective of a real patient and eyewitness regarding the deep uncertainties in knowledge about the global dimensions of schizophrenia.

Although we cannot know for certain, it is reasonable to assume that Tanka entered into dialogues and debates with his doctors about the nature of his schizophrenia and its manifestations. His autobiographical narrative suggests as much, especially since large passages of Tanka's text are structured as an exemplary case study (Boroffka 1980a, 11). It seems that Tanka at least learned about the pilot study and its assumptions through his many conversations with Boroffka (Boroffka 1980b). For Boroffka, Tanka wrote not only to process, negotiate, and accept his illness; his work was full of "literary

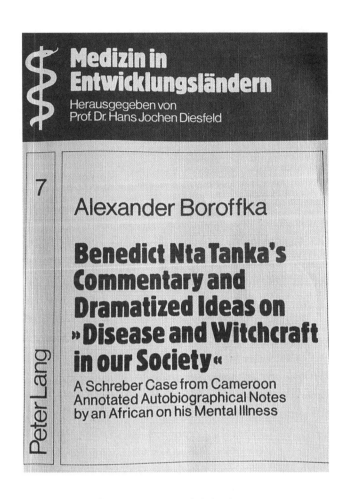

3.6   Cover of Benedict Nta Tanka's book.

quality" he wished to communicate (Boroffka 1980b, 144). It is remarkable that
Boroffka never left behind his medical hierarchical and asymmetrical perspective. On the one hand, he provided Tanka with writings like Schreber's and had
countless conversations with his patient, including about the WHO work in
Ibadan in general (Boroffka 1980b, 142–44). His "fascination as observer"
(Boroffka 1980b, 145–47)—as he wrote—always remained, however, in the
medical gaze: in the perspective of a psychiatrist on his suffering patient.
On the other hand, Boroffka could not or did not want to recognize how
much Tanka established his case for the WHO within the epistemic culture
of studying—consciously or unconsciously—psychiatry at a global scale.

Probably it was Boroffka's medical persistence regarding his patient and his view of Tanka's document as a pure, authentic patient testimonial that enabled Tanka's case to become evidence in the WHO pilot study, including its findings that patients in "developing countries" were recovering more quickly from schizophrenia. The study concluded that Nigerian patients "had a considerably better course and outcome than patients in developed countries. This remained true whether clinical outcomes, social outcomes, or a combination of the two was considered" (WHO 1973, 386–99). The study presented the remarkable fact that more than 50 percent of all schizophrenic patients in Nigeria were without any "pathological symptoms at the end of five years." In 58 percent of the Nigerian patients, a single schizophrenic episode was followed by a full recovery. In contrast, the same was the case in only 6 percent of Danish patients. Only 7 percent of the Nigerian patients were seen as "chronically ill" with a "frequent revolving episode" versus 50 percent in Denmark (WHO 1973, 386–99; Warner 1985, 156; Jablensky 1987).

When comparing "developing countries," scholars concluded that gradual differences between "developed" India and less "developed" tropical Africa were clear evidence for a correlation between the level of modernization and a pathological course of schizophrenia with less chance of recovery (Warner 1985, 148–55). Nigeria became one of the most interesting countries examined for schizophrenia and psychiatric disease during these years. Tanka's autobiography was full of clues about an exemplary correlation between schizophrenia in Africa and the relatively quick recovery of patients. Although he was not one of the patients who had just a single schizophrenic experience in their lives, Tanka was released from hospital treatment in December 1970 after just three months and he began to work again. He also married and raised a family (Boroffka 1980b, 145–46).

Conclusion

It would be reductive to see the deeper meanings of this patient's writing as simply providing individualized evidence for the WHO pilot study. Rather, Tanka inserted himself into an epistemic culture that joined WHO-funded research with the experiences of African schizophrenics. Like many once diagnosed within such a spectrum of psychotic disorders throughout the world, Tanka sought creative self-expression as he worked through his illness (Wood 2013). There was hope in his writing: to escape common vernacular diagnoses and practices surrounding mental illness, sometimes with violent and cruel dimensions. Tanka's fear of both vernacular and modern mental healing was not without reason. He feared witchcraft, and he was not wrong. Boroffka left many pictures in his papers from psychiatric asylums in Nigeria from the 1960s and 1970s, showing patients interned, chained, and physically abused.[3] Through his attempts to provide patient-based evidence regarding his malady as defined within Western psychiatry, Tanka clearly hoped that psychiatrists would not abandon him but rather care for him in the future. Core motifs of his messages aimed at attracting the attention of modern, even progressive psychiatrists like Lambo and Boroffka and thereby escaping the violent conditions of conventional psychiatric care.

With Boroffka, Tanka's hopes seemed rewarded. The German doctor constantly wrote to Tanka, and he continued to provide his special patient with schizophrenia medications. After Boroffka's death in 2014, Dr. Wolfgang Krahl (Krahl and Schröder 2015; Tesfaye, Krahl, and Alemayehu 2020), another German physician of tropical medicine and psychiatry, took over this clinical task in keeping with Boroffka's instructions.

Through his writing and his relationship with Boroffka, Tanka became a part of a global research laboratory, with effects on his upper-middle-class status in postcolonial Cameroon. Tanka effectively empowered himself, away from being a passive patient to being an active agent of global knowledge production with all its evidence, doubts, and questions. And he did so through the autobiographical, through writing, and through his special relationship—of which we know not enough—with one doctor, Alexander Boroffka.

Let me conclude with an important detour: into some retrospective ethics emerging from this case. Tanka's schizophrenia diagnosis raises ethical questions (Micale and Porter 1994), ones that relate to the accuracy or harm of such routine labeling at the time (Micale and Porter 1994; Henckes 2019). This chapter has interpreted Tanka's texts and his materialized agency, as he inscribed himself within global debates about schizophrenia in Africa and beyond, and precisely when the WHO launched its international pilot study of schizophrenia globally and in Ibadan (WHO 1973; Leff et al. 1992; Henckes 2019).

I first came to know of Tanka, his life, and psychological experiences from his autobiographical writing published in 1980 (Tanka 1980). The German psychiatrist Alexander Boroffka edited and published Tanka's writings, supplementing them with excerpts from Tanka's patient case records from his previous examinations, auditions, and the history of his diagnosis as a schizophrenic (Boroffka 1980a). Ethical questions arise when working with and analyzing such intimate sources, as surely they did in that different time of the 1970s before the creation of institutional ethics boards (in the United States from 1979 and from 1991 in Europe).

Thus, we may pose questions: Was Tanka dependent on his doctor? And how did Boroffka use his medical authority and power? Was it even possible for Tanka, in such a psychiatric patient–doctor relationship, to freely allow—to give consent for—Boroffka to publish his writings? Is it possible that Tanka's rights as a human subject were in any way violated by this process or their medical relationship? Was he always treated justly, with respect and beneficence? These are daunting questions before a thin set of documentary clues. Yet all the evidence from slender but compelling strands in the Boroffka and Tanka texts—including suggestions of kind, parallel dialogues between patient and doctor—suggests that this relationship joined what was rapidly fading from fashion in Nigeria and Germany: psychoanalytic therapeutic approaches. The psychoanalytic may be witnessed in Boroffka's choice of Schreber as an appropriate example and as reading material for his patient. At the same time, the full record suggests scientific rigor mixed with considerable humanity, leaning toward affection and affability, as witnessed in the quite private letters and Christmas cards exchanged after Boroffka returned to Germany. Affection is, of course, an ambiguous term. It might embrace avuncular compassion or cross-racial desire. A retrospective interpretation of the sentiments and ethics at play would be impossible, given the scanty evidence on hand. Still, there were surely colonial hues to this patient–doctor relationship, mixing fondness with suspicion.

What is most striking in this case is the overpowering impression that Tanka voluntarily—indeed eagerly—worked with and beside Boroffka. This patient, who wanted to be seen as civilized, released to his German doctor his autobiographical texts, authored in part for explicit clinical use and publication. There may have been condescension, identification, or residues of ambivalence from colonial hierarchies and dreams, but Boroffka was pleased by this African patient willing to write and share in textual form such publishable products (Newell 2018). Tanka, the prized patient, surely achieved plenty out of his suffering and authorial labors, namely a special form of fame: his writing anchored a published book with his name indicated as the author on the cover. For Cameroonian, Nigerian, and WHO audiences, it told of a new form of global entangled with vernacular authorship and a clinical register.

Acknowledgments

I am grateful to Nancy Rose Hunt, as well as Rebekka Habermas, Karolin Wetjen, and the participants at the "Global Histories of Psychiatry" conference, November 7–8, 2018, at the University of Groningen, for their important comments. I also thank Finn Patrick Bourke, Elena Olmedo Viana, Tancrede Pages, Sebastian Skutta, and Neele Rother for additional editorial assistance. I thank Dr. Wolfgang Krahl for his advice and assistance, as well as Dr. Nikolaus Boroffka for his and his family's generosity, kindness, and guidance in loaning me important archival papers of his father, Dr. Alexander Boroffka, regarding Benedict Nta Tanka, the history of psychiatry in Nigeria, and the WHO study on schizophrenia of the 1960s and 1970s. With his permission, I arranged the donation of this material to the Iwalewa House in Bayreuth, Germany, as the Alexander Boroffka Papers.

Notes

1   The concept of "primitivism" goes with racist devaluations and subordinations in the sense of "less civilized." Its meaning was "closer to the roots of human existence." This idea was connected with an admiration for "noble savages," and even envy of supposedly traditional, intact social life—as well as because many anthropologists, missionaries, and psychiatrists shared skeptical thoughts on European forms of modernization. Reflections on the "negative" outcomes of industrialization and urbanization were common, and civilizing mental illnesses became a booming field of research. Last but not least, "primitivism" carried heuristic potential for research on the human mind. It seemed that conscious elements of the mind would be more visible and traceable because they were not covered by modernity's "civilization." The assumptions of Sigmund Freud, that studying the "mental conditions of the savages" might help track down "neurotics" in Africa, thus functioning in the words of Helen Tilley as a "living laboratory" for many anthropologists and psychiatrists (Fabian 1983, 17–18; Freud 1919, 2000; Tilley 2011, 217–59).

2   Notably, twin studies provided strong evidence since the 1940s that if one twin develops schizophrenia, the other will develop a schizophrenic disorder as well (Gottesman 1991, 104–32).

3   Alexander Boroffka Papers, Iwalewa House, Bayreuth, Germany.

Sources

Archival Material

Alexander Boroffka Papers, Iwalewa House, Bayreuth.

Literature

Akyeampong, Emmanuel, Allan G. Hill, and Arthur Kleinman. 2015. "Introduction: Culture, Mental Illness, and Psychiatric Practice in Africa." In *The Culture of Mental Illness and Psychiatric Practice in Africa*, edited by Emmanuel Akyeampong, Allan G. Hill, and Arthur Kleinman, 1–23. Bloomington: Indiana University Press.

Allison, David B., Prado de Oliveira, Mark S. Roberts, and Allen S. Weiss, eds. 1988. *Psychosis and Sexual Identity: Toward a Post-Analytic View of the Schreber Case*. Albany: State University of New York Press.

Andrande, Tonio. 2010. "A Chinese Farmer, Two African Boys, and a Warlord: Toward a Global Microhistory." *Journal of World History* 21, no. 4: 573–91.

Antić, Ana. 2021. "ERC Starting Grant: Decolonising Madness? Transcultural Psychiatry, International Order and the Birth of a 'Global Psyche' in the Aftermath of the Second World War." University of Copenhagen. https://cultmind.ku.dk /research/decolonising-madness/about-the-project/.

Antić, Ana. 2022. "Decolonizing Madness? Transcultural Psychiatry, International Order and Birth of a 'Global Psyche' in the Aftermath of the Second World War." *Journal of Global History* 17, no. 1: 20–41.

Arieti, Silvano. 1974. *Interpretation of Schizophrenia*. New York: Basic Books.

Asuni, Tolani, and Folahan Williams. 2006. Foreword to *Psychiatry in Nigeria: A Partly Annotated Bibliography*, edited by Alexander Boroffka, 1–4. Kiel, Germany: Brunswiker Verlagsbuchhandlung.

Beier, Ulli. 1964. *Public Opinion on Lovers: Popular Nigerian Literature Sold in Onitsha Market*. Ibadan, Nigeria: Mbari.

Berkenkotter, Carol. 2008. *Patient Tales: Case Histories and the Uses of Narrative in Psychiatry*. Columbia: University of South Carolina Press.

Bernett, Brigitta. 2013. *Schizophrenie: Entstehung und Entwicklung eines psychiatrischen Krankheitsbildes*. Zurich: Chronos.

Binitie, Ayo. 1988. "Outstanding Contributions to Nigerian Psychiatry." *Nigerian Journal of Psychiatry* 1, no. 3: 145–54.

Birnbaum, Karl. 1920. *Psychopathologische Dokumente*. Berlin: Springer.

Bleuler, Eugen. 1908. "Die Prognose der dementia praecox (Schizophreniegruppe)." *Allgemeine Zeitschrift für Psychiatrie* 65, no. 6: 436–63.

Bleuler, Eugen. 1911. *Dementia Praecox oder Gruppe der Schizophrenien*. Leipzig: Franz Deuticke.

Boroffka, Alexander. 1980a. "Clinical Notes." In *Benedict Nta Tanka's Commentary and Dramatized Ideas on "Disease and Witchcraft in Our Society": A Schreber Case from Cameroon; Annotated Autobiographical Notes by an African on His Mental Illness* by Alexander Boroffka, 6–16. Frankfurt: Peter Lang.

Boroffka, Alexander. 1980b. "Psychiatric Comments." In *Benedict Nta Tanka's Commentary and Dramatized Ideas on "Disease and Witchcraft in Our Society": A Schreber Case from Cameroon; Annotated Autobiographical Notes by an African on His Mental Illness* by Alexander Boroffka, 127–46. Frankfurt: Peter Lang.

Boroffka, Alexander. 1980c. Introduction to *Benedict Nta Tanka's Commentary and Dramatized Ideas on "Disease and Witchcraft in Our Society": A Schreber Case from Cameroon; Annotated Autobiographical Notes by an African on His Mental Illness* by Alexander Boroffka, 3–5. Frankfurt: Peter Lang.

Boroffka, Alexander. 1980d. "Annotations to 4." In *Benedict Nta Tanka's Commentary and Dramatized Ideas on "Disease and Witchcraft in Our Society": A Schreber Case from Cameroon; Annotated Autobiographical Notes by an African on His Mental Illness* by Alexander Boroffka, 12–16. Frankfurt: Peter Lang.

Boroffka, Alexander. 2006. *Psychiatry in Nigeria: A Partly Annotated Bibliography*. Kiel, Germany: Brunswiker Verlagsbuchhandlung.

Brody, Eugene B. 2004. "The World Federation for Mental Health: Its Origins and Contemporary Relevance to WHO and WPO Policies." *World Psychiatry* 3, no. 1: 54–55.

Brückner, Burkhart. 2006. "Psychiatriegeschichte und Patientengeschichte: Eine Literaturübersicht zum Stand der deutschsprachigen Forschung." *Sozialpsychiatrische Informationen* 36, no. 4: 26–30.

Büschel, Hubertus. 2014. *Hilfe zur Selbsthilfe: Deutsche Entwicklungsarbeit in Afrika 1960–1975*. Frankfurt: Campus.

Büschel, Hubertus. 2015. "'Die Moderne macht sie geisteskrank!' Primitivismus-Zuschreibung, Modernisierungserfahrung, Entwicklungsarbeit und globale Psychiatrie im 20. Jahrhundert." *Geschichte und Gesellschaft* 41, no. 4: 685–717.

Büschel, Hubertus, and Daniel Speich. 2009. "Einleitung: Konjunkturen, Probleme und Perspektiven der Globalgeschichte von Entwicklungszusammenarbeit." In *Entwicklungswelten: Globalgeschichte der Entwicklungszusammenarbeit*, edited by Hubertus Büschel and Daniel Speich, 7–32. Frankfurt: Campus.

Caminero-Santangelo, Marta. 1998. *The Madwoman Can't Speak: Or Why Insanity Is Not Subversive*. Ithaca, NY: Cornell University Press.

Carothers, John C. 1940. "Some Speculations on Insanity in Africans in General." *East African Medical Journal* 17, no. 3: 90–105.

Carothers, John C. 1954. *The African Mind in Health and Disease*. Geneva: WHO.

Chilver, Elisabeth M., and Phyllis M. Kaberry. 1970. "Chronology of the Bamenda Grassfields." *Journal of African History* 11, no. 2: 249–57.

Cooper, John E. 1999. "Towards a Common Language for Mental Health Workers." In *Promoting Mental Health Internationally*, edited by Giovanni De Girolami, Leon Eisenberg, David P. Goldberg, and John E. Cooper, 4–46. London: Gaskell.

Corin, Ellen, and Henry B. M. Murphy. 1979. "Psychiatric Perspectives in Africa Part I: The Western Viewpoint." *Transcultural Psychiatric Research Review* 16, no. 2: 147–78.

Dalzell, Thomas. 2011. *Freud's Schreber between Psychiatry and Psychoanalysis*. London: Routledge.

Daston, Lorraine. 1994. "Historical Epistemology." In *Questions of Evidence: Proof, Practice, and Persuasion across the Disciplines*, edited by James Chandler, Arnold I. Davidson, and Harry D. Harootunian, 282–89. Chicago: University of Chicago Press.

Daston, Lorraine, ed. 2004. *Things That Talk: Object Lessons from Art and Science*. New York: Zone Books.

Daston, Lorraine. 2007. "The History of Emergences." *Isis* 98, no. 4: 801–8.

Dekker, Rudolf. 2002a. Introduction to *Egodocuments and History: Autobiographical Writing in Its Social Context since the Middle Ages*, 7–20. Hilversum, Netherlands: Verloren.

Dekker, Rudolf. 2002b. "Jacques Presser's Heritage: Egodocuments in the Study of History." *Memoria y Civilización* 5:13–37.

Epple, Angelika. 2010. "New Global History and the Challenge of Subaltern Studies: Plea for a Global History from Below." *Journal of Localitology* 3:161–79.

Fabian, Johannes. 1983. *Time and the Other: How Anthropology Makes Its Object*. New York: Columbia University Press.

Fanon, Frantz. 1961. *The Wretched of the Earth*. New York: Grove Press.

Field, Margaret J. 1958. "Mental Disorder in Rural Ghana." *Journal of Mental Science* 104, no. 437: 1043–51.

Field, Margaret J. 1960. *In Search for Security: An Ethno Psychiatric Study of Rural Ghana*. London: Faber and Faber.

Field, Margaret J. 1968. "Chronic Psychosis in Rural Ghana." *British Journal of Psychiatry* 114, no. 506: 31–33.

Forster, Edward B. 1960. "A Short Psychiatric Review from Ghana." In *Mental Disorders and Mental Health in Africa South of the Sahara: CCTA/CSA-WFMH-WHO Meeting of Specialists on Mental Health, Bakavu 1958* (CCTA Publications 35), edited by Scientific Council for Africa South of the Sahara, 7–27. Bakavu, DRC: Nelson.

Forster, Edward B. 1962. "The Theory and Practice of Psychiatry in Ghana." *American Journal of Psychotherapy* 16, no. 1: 7–51.

Fortes, Meyer, and Doris Y. Mayer. 1966. "Psychosis and Social Change among the Tallensi of Northern Ghana." *Cagier d'Études africaines* 21, no. 6: 5–40.

Foucault, Michel. 1991. "Governmentality." In *The Foucault Effect: Studies in Governmentality*, edited by Graham Burchell, Colin Gordon, and Peter Miller, 87–104. Chicago: University of Chicago Press.

Foucault, Michel. 1994. "The Birth of Biopolitics." In *Ethics: Subjectivity and Truth*, vol. 1 (*The Essential Works of Foucault 1954–1984*), edited by Paul Rabinow, 73–80. New York: New Press.

Foucault, Michel. 1997. *Society Must Be Defended: Lectures at the Collège de France, 1975–1976*. New York: Picador.

Foucault, Michel. 1998. *The History of Sexuality*. Vol. 1, *The Will to Knowledge*. London: Penguin.

Foucault, Michel. 2006a. *Madness and Civilization: A History of Insanity in the Age of Reason*. New York: Taylor and Francis.

Foucault, Michel. 2006b. *Psychiatric Power: Lectures at the Collège du France 1973–74*. New York: Palgrave Macmillan.

Freud, Sigmund. 1911. "Psychoanalytische Bemerkungen über einen autobiographisch beschriebenen Fall von Paranoia (Dementis paranoides)." In *Jahrbuch für psychoanalytische und psychopathologische Forschungen III. Band, 1. Hälfte*, edited by Eugen Bleuler and Sigmund Freud, 9–68. Leipzig: Franz Deuticke.

Freud, Sigmund. 1919. "Das Unheimliche." *Imago: Zeitschrift für Anwendung der Psychoanalyse auf die Geisteswissenschaften* 5, no. 5/6: 297–324.

Freud, Sigmund. 2000. "Totem und Tabu: Einige Übereinstimmungen im Seelenleben der Wilden und Neurotiker (1913)." In *Fragen der Gesellschaft, Ursprünge der Religion* (Sigmund Freud, Studienausgabe 9), edited by Alexander Mitscherlich, 287–444. Frankfurt: S. Fischer Verlag.

Freud, Sigmund. 2003. *The Schreber Case*. New York: Penguin.

Fuller Torrey, Edwin. 1980. *Schizophrenia and Civilization*. New York: Jason Aronson.

Fuller Torrey, Edwin. 1987a. "Prevalence Studies in Schizophrenia." *British Journal of Psychiatry* 150, no. 5: 598–608.

Fuller Torrey, Edwin. 1987b. "Incidence Worldwide of Schizophrenia." *British Journal of Psychiatry* 150, no. 1: 132–33.

Gaines, Atwood D. 1992. "Ethnopsychiatry: The Cultural Construction of Psychiatries." In *Ethnopsychiatry: The Cultural Construction of Professional and Folk Psychiatries*, edited by Atwood D. Gaines, 3–50. Albany: State University of New York Press.

Gerritsen, Anne. 2012. "Scales of a Local: The Place of Locality in a Globalizing World." In *A Companion to World History*, edited by Douglas Northrop, 213–26. London: Wiley-Blackwell.

Gilman, Sander L. 2008. "Constructing Schizophrenia as a Category of Mental Illness." In *History of Psychiatry and Medical Psychology: With an Epilogue on*

Psychiatry and Medical Psychology, edited by Edwin R. Wallace and John Gach, 461–83. New York: Springer.

Goffman, Erving. 1961. *Asylums: Essays on the Social Situation of Mental Patients and Other Inmates*. New York: Anchor.

Good, Byron J. 1996. "Culture and DSM-IV: Diagnosis, Knowledge and Power." *Culture, Medicine and Psychiatry* 20, no. 2: 127–32.

Gottesman, Irving. 1991. *Schizophrenia Genesis: The Origins of Madness*. New York: W. H. Freeman.

Hacking, Ian. 1999. "Historical Meta-Epistemology." In *Wahrheit und Geschichte: Ein Kolloquium zu Ehren des 60. Geburtstages von Lorenz Krüger*, edited by Wolfgang Carl and Lorraine Daston, 53–77. Göttingen: Vandenhoeck and Ruprecht.

Heaton, Matthew M. 2011. "Thomas Adeoye Lambo and the Decolonization of Psychiatry in Nigeria." In *Science and Empire: Knowledge and Networks of Science across the British Empire, 1800-1970*, edited by Brett M. Bennett and Joseph M. Hodge, 275–96. London: Palgrave Macmillan.

Heaton, Matthew M. 2013. *Black Skin, White Coats: Nigerian Psyc Knowhiatrists, Decolonization and the Globalization of Psychiatry*. Athens: Ohio University Press.

Henckes, Nicolas. 2019. "Schizophrenia Infrastructures: Local and Global Dynamics of Transformation in Psychiatric Diagnosis-Making in the Twentieth and Twenty-First Centuries." *Culture, Medicine and Psychiatry* 43, no. 4: 548–73.

Jablensky, Assen. 1987. "Multicultural Studies and the Nature of Schizophrenia: A Review." *Journal of the Royal Society of Medicine* 80, no. 3: 162–67.

Jablensky, Assen, and Norman Sartorius. 1975. "Culture and Schizophrenia." *Psychological Medicine* 5, no. 2: 113–24.

Jablensky, Assen, and Norman Satorius. 2008. "What Did the WHO Studies Really Find?" *Schizophrenia Bulletin* 34, no. 2: 253–55.

Jablensky, Assen, Norman Sartorius, Gunilla Ernberg, Martha Anker, Ailsa Korten, John E. Cooper, Robert Day, and Aksel Bertelsen. 1992. "Schizophrenia: Manifestations, Incidence and Course in Different Cultures: A World Health Organization Ten-Country Study." *Psychological Medicine Monograph Supplement* 20:1–97.

Kaplan, Bert. 1964. *The Inner World of Mental Illness: A Series of First-Person Accounts of What It Was Like*. New York: Harper and Row.

Kraepelin, Emil. 1899. *Psychiatrie: Ein Lehrbuch für Studierende und Ärzte*. Vol. 2. Leipzig: J. A. Barth.

Krahl, Wolfgang, and Ekkehard Schröder. 2015. "In Memorian: Dr. Alexander Boroffka (1920–2014)." *Transcultural Psychiatry* 52, no. 6: 2–6.

Kramer, Morton. 1969. *Applications of Mental Health Statistics*. Geneva: WHO.

Lambo, Thomas Edoye. 1980. Preface to *Benedict Nta Tanka's Commentary and Dramatized Ideas on "Disease and Witchcraft in Our Society": A Schreber Case from Cameroon; Annotated Autobiographical Notes by an African on His Mental Illness* by Alexander Boroffka. Frankfurt: Peter Lang.

Lange-Eichbaum, Wilhelm. 1928. *Genie, Irrsinn und Ruhm*. Munich: Reinhardt.

Latour, Bruno. 2005. *Reassembling the Social: An Introduction to Actor-Network-Theory*. Oxford: Oxford University Press.

Ledebur, Sophie. 2013. "Sehend schreibend, schreibend sehen: Vom Aufzeichnen psychischer Phänomene in der Psychiatrie." In *Krankheit schreiben: Aufzeichnungsverfahren in Medizin und Literatur*, edited by Yvonne Wübben and Carsten Zelle, 82–108. Göttingen: Wallstein.

Leff, Julian, N. Sartorius, A. Jabalensky, and G. Ernberg. 1992. "The International Pilot Study of Schizophrenia: Five-Year Follow-Up Findings." *Psychological Medicine* 22:131–45.

Lewis-Fernández, Roberto. 1996. "Cultural Formulation of Psychiatric Diagnosis." *Culture, Medicine and Psychiatry* 20, no. 2: 133–44.

Lewis-Fernández, Roberto, and Neil K. Aggarwal. 2013. "Culture and Psychiatric Diagnosis." *Advances in Psychosomatic Medicine* 33:15–30.

Lin, Keh Ming, and Arthur Kleinman. 1988. "Psychopathology and Clinical Course of Schizophrenia: A Cross-Cultural Perspective." *Schizophrenia Bulletin* 14, no. 4: 555–67.

Lin, Tsung-Yi, and C. C. Standley. 1962. *The Scope of Epidemiology in Psychiatry* (Public Health Papers No. 16). Geneva: WHO.

Linstrum, Erik. 2012. "The Politics of Psychology in the British Empire, 1898–1960." *Past and Present* 215, no. 5: 195–233.

Linstrum, Erik. 2016. *Ruling the Minds: Psychology in the British Empire*. Cambridge, MA: Harvard University Press.

Lüdtke, Alf, ed. 1995. *The History of Everyday Life: Reconstructing Historical Experiences and Ways of Life*. Princeton, NJ: Princeton University Press.

Mayer-Gross, Willy, Eliot Slater, and Martin Roth. 1969. *Clinical Psychiatry*. London: Tindall and Cassell.

McNally, Kieran. 2009. "Eugen Bleuler's Four A's." *History of Psychology* 12, no. 2: 43–59.

McNally, Kieran. 2016. *A Critical History of Schizophrenia*. Basingstoke, UK: Palgrave Macmillan.

Mead, Margaret. 1955. Preface to *Cultural Patterns and Technical Change*, edited by Margaret Mead. New York: New American Library.

Medick, Hans. 2016. "Turning Global? Microhistory in Extension." *Historische Anthropologie* 24, no. 2: 241–52.

Micale, Mark Stephen, and Roy Porter. 1994. "Introduction: Reflections on Psychiatry and Its Histories." In *Discovering the History of Psychiatry*, edited by Mark Stephen Micale and Roy Porter, 3–36. New York: Oxford University Press.

Morris, Jeremy Noah. 1964. *Uses of Epidemiology*. Edinburgh: Livingstone.

Newell, Stephanie. 2018. "Narrative." In *Critical Terms for the Study of Africa*, edited by Guarav Desai and Adeline Masquelier, 245–59. Chicago: University of Chicago Press.

Obiechina, Emmanuel. 1971. *Literature for the Masses*. Enugu, Nigeria: Nwankwo-Ifeljika.

Obiechina, Emmanuel. 1972. *Onitsha Market Literature*. London: Heinemann.

Opaku, Samuel O., and Sanchita Biswas. 2014. "History of Global Mental Health." In *Essentials of Global Mental Health*, edited by Samuel O. Opaku, 1–10. Cambridge: Cambridge University Press.

Parin, Paul. 1983. Review, "Boroffka, Alexander: Benedict Nta Tanka's Commentary and Dramatized Ideas on 'Disease and Witchcraft in Our Society'. A Schreber Case from Cameroon; Annotated Autobiographical Notes by an African on His Mental Illness." *Psyche: Zeitschrift für Psychoanalyse und Ihre Anwendungen* 37, no. 3: 285–87.

Peterson, Dale. 1982. *A Mad People's History of Madness*. Pittsburgh, PA: University of Pittsburgh Press.

Picchioni, Marco M., and Robin M. Murray. 2007. "Schizophrenia." *British Medical Journal* 335, no. 7610: 91–95.

Porter, Roy. 1985. "The Patient's View: Doing Medical History from Below." *Theory and Society* 14, no. 2: 175–98.

Porter, Roy. 1987. *A Social History of Madness: Stories of the Insane*. London: Weidenfeld and Nicolson.

Presser, Jacques. 1969. "Memoires als geschiedbron (1958)." In *Uit het werk van dr. J. Presser*, edited by Maarten Brands and Jan Haak, 277–82. Amsterdam: Polak and van Gennep.

Prince, Raymond H. 1960. "The 'Brain Fag' Syndrome in Nigerian Students." *Journal of Mental Science* 106, no. 443: 559–70.

Prince, Raymond H. 1985. "The Concept of Culture-Bound Syndromes: Anorexia Nervosa and Brain Fag." *Social Science and Medicine* 21, no. 2: 197–203.

Read, Ursula M., Victor C. K. Doku, and Ama de-Graft Aikins. 2015. "Schizophrenia and Psychosis in West Africa." In *The Culture of Mental Illness and Psychiatric Practice in Africa*, edited by Emmanuel Akyeampong, Allan G. Hill, and Arthur Kleinman, 73–111. Bloomington: Indiana University Press.

Reid, Donald D. 1960. *Epidemiological Methods in the Study of Mental Disorders* (Public Health Papers No. 2). Geneva: WHO.

Rheinberger, Hans-Jörg. 2010. *On Historicizing Epistemology: An Essay*. Stanford, CA: Stanford University Press.

Robertson, Roland. 1995. "Glocalization: Time–Space and Homogeneity–Heterogeneity." In *Global Modernities*, edited by Mike Featherstone, Scott Lash, and Roland Robertson, 25–44. London: Sage.

Sadowsky, Jonathan. 1999. *Imperial Bedlam: Institutions of Madness in Colonial Southwest Nigeria*. Berkeley: University of California Press.

Sadowsky, Jonathan. 2020. *The Empire of Depression: A New History*. Cambridge, UK: Polity.

Santner, Eric L. 1996. *My Own Private Germany: Daniel Paul Schreber's Secret History of Modernity*. Princeton, NJ: Princeton University Press.

Sass, Louis A. 1994. "Civilized Madness: Schizophrenia, Self-Consciousness and the Modern Mind." *History of the Human Sciences* 7, no. 2: 83–120.

Schreber, Daniel Paul. 1903. *Denkwürdigkeiten eines Nervenkranken, nebst Nachträgen und einem Anhang über die Frage: "Unter welchen Voraussetzungen darf eine für geisteskrank erachtete Person gegen ihren erklärten Willen in einer Heilanstalt festgehalten werden?"* Leipzig: Mutze.

Schreber, Daniel Paul. 1955. *Memoirs of My Nervous Illness*. New York: Macalpine and Hunter.

Schulze, Winfried, ed. 1996. *Ego-Dokumente: Annäherungen an den Menschen in der Geschichte* (Selbstzeugnisse der Neuzeit, vol. 2). Berlin: Akademie.

Scott, James. 1998. *Seeing Like a State: How Certain Schemes to Improve the Human Condition Have Failed*. New Haven, CT: Yale University Press.

Shorter, Edward. 1997. *A History of Psychiatry: From the Era of the Asylum to the Age of Prozac*. New York: Wiley.

Shorter, Edward. 2005. *A Historical Dictionary of Psychiatry*. Oxford: Oxford University Press.

Spivak, Gayatri Chakravorty. 1988. "Can the Subaltern Speak?" In *Marxism and the Interpretation of Culture*, edited by Cary Nelson and Lawrence Grossberg, 271–333. Basingstoke, UK: Macmillan Education.

Staewen, Christoph, and Friderun Schönberg. 1970. *Kulturwandel und Angstentwicklung bei den Yoruba Westafrika*. Munich: Weltforum.

Stoler, Ann Laura. 2010. *Along the Archival Grain: Epistemic Anxieties and Colonial Common Sense*. Princeton, NJ: Princeton University Press.

Stotz-Ingenlath, Gabriele. 2000. "Epistemological Aspects of Eugen Bleuler's Conception of Schizophrenia in 1911." *Medicine, Health, Care* 3, no. 2: 153–59.

Tanka, Benedict Nta. 1980. "Writings." In *Benedict Nta Tanka's Commentary and Dramatized Ideas on "Disease and Witchcraft in Our Society": A Schreber Case from Cameroon; Annotated Autobiographical Notes by an African on His Mental Illness* by Alexander Boroffka, 17–120. Frankfurt: Peter Lang.

Tesfaye, Elias, Wolfgang Krahl, and Selamawit Alemayehu. 2020. "Khat Induced Psychotic Disorder: Case Report." *Substance Abuse Treatment, Prevention, and Policy* 15. 10.1186/s13011-020-00268-4.

Thompson, Edward P. 1966. "History from Below." *Times Literary Supplement*, April 7, 1966, 279–80.

Tilley, Hellen. 2011. *Africa as a Living Laboratory: Empire, Development and the Problem of Scientific Knowledge, 1870–1950*. Chicago: University of Chicago Press.

Tooth, Geoffrey. 1950. *Studies in Mental Illness in the Gold Coast*. London: HMSO.

Turner, Trevor. 2007. "Chlorpromazine: Unlocking Psychosis." *British Medical Journal* 334, no. 1: 7.

Ulbrich, Claudia, Hans Medick, and Angelika Schaser. 2012. "Selbstzeugnis und Person." In *Selbstzeugnis und Person: Transkulturelle Perspektiven*, edited by Claudia Ulbrich, Hans Medick, and Angelika Schaser, 1–26. Cologne: Böhlau.

Vaughan, Megan. 1991. *Curing Their Ills: Colonial Power and African Illness*. Stanford, CA: Stanford University Press.

Vaughan, Megan. 2005. "Mr Mdala Writes to the Governor: Negotiating Colonial Rule in Nyasaland." *History Workshop Journal* 60, no. 1: 171–88.

Von Greyerz, Kaspar, Hans Medick, and Patrice Veit, eds. 2001. *Von der dargestellten Person zum erinnernden Ich: Europäische Selbstzeugnisse als historische Quellen (1500–1800)*. Cologne: Böhlau.

Vyncke, Julien. 1960. "L'Assistance psychiatrique en Ruanda-Burundi." In *Mental Disorders and Mental Health in Africa South of the Sahara: CCTA/CSA-WFMH-WHO Meeting of Specialists on Mental Health, Bakavu 1958* (CCTA Publications 35), edited by Scientific Council for Africa South of the Sahara, 52–55. Bakavu, DRC: Nelson.

Warner, Richard. 1985. *Recovery from Schizophrenia: Psychiatry and Political Economy*. London: Routledge and Kegan Paul.

WHO. 1957. *Report of a Study Group on Schizophrenia*. Geneva: WHO.

WHO. 1958. *The First Ten Years of the World Health Organization*. Geneva: WHO.

WHO. 1960. *Epidemiology of Mental Disorders* (Technical Reports Series No. 185). Geneva: WHO.

WHO. 1964. *Report of the Scientific Group on Mental Health Research*. Geneva: WHO.

WHO. 1968. "Report on Brain Fag Syndrome." *Cameroon Times*, December 12, 1968, 17.

WHO. 1973. *Report of the International Pilot Study of Schizophrenia*. Vol. 1, *Results of the Initial Evaluation Phase*. Geneva: WHO.

Wood, Mary Elene. 2013. *Life Writing and Schizophrenia: Encounters at the Edge of Meaning*. Amsterdam: Rodopi.

PART II

PATIENT WORDS MEET
DIAGNOSTIC CATEGORIES

Raphaël Gallien   4

Delirious Words and Social Ambition
in French Colonial Madagascar

I came into the world imbued with the will to find a meaning in things, my spirit filled with the desire to attain the source of the world, and then I found that I was an object in the midst of other objects. . . . While I was forgetting, forgiving, and wanting only to love, my message was flung back in my face like a slap. The white world, the only honorable one, barred me from all participation.

Frantz Fanon, *Black Skin, White Masks*

The psychiatrist Frantz Fanon here pointed to a central question of subjectivity within a colonial situation: how to deal with a self as the Other, given that the colonizer imposes constant limitations on you. What answer does madness provide in the face of the structural impossibility of realizing oneself, due to such ceaseless external objectification? Madness was, in Fanon's view, the last place before death, a place where an individual could radically extract themselves from colonial domination: "they know," he said of his patients, "that only this madness can remove them from the colonial oppression" (Fanon 2002, 72). Confronted with the internees of Blida, Algeria, he set himself the task of interpreting madness and resituating it within broader political and social contexts. So aiming while also interpreting madness, this chapter focuses on those barred from participation, not in Algeria but in another French colonial territory: the island of Madagascar.

From a psychiatric point of view, Madagascar was an exception within the French colonial empire. It was the very first territory to have a psychiatric hospital: that of Anjanamasina, inaugurated in 1912 in response to the law of June 30, 1838, which placed the insane under the authority of the colonial administration.[1] To compare, Indochina did not have such an institution until 1918, Algeria until 1933, and French West Africa until as late as 1956. Seventeen years after its conquest in 1895–96, the island was able to take care of mental illness in an official establishment dedicated to the issue. It is true that a few "maisons de fous" (madhouses) had already existed in Madagascar and other territories like Martinique and Guadeloupe. However, the use of an alienist template was unprecedented in France's colonies, and it entailed its own architecture and large-scale health and social policies, devised at the scale of the colony.[2] The health authorities, as well as alienists of the time, welcomed these developments, making Anjanamasina a model to be duplicated in other colonies of the French empire (Reboul and Régis 1912, 111). The number of patients grew significantly, from 91 inmates in its first year to 234 in 1936. Gradually, the establishment extended over a little more than two hectares and consisted of a dozen pavilions that separated European patients from so-called native (or indigenous) patients,[3] as well as the "agitated" from "quiet" patients,[4] and men from women.

In recent years, as historians have turned afresh to the important question of madness in the French colonial empire, Madagascar has remained conspicuous in its absence from this history. Yet, paradoxically, this asylum was quite ahead of its time (Gallien 2019). French imperial historiography has demonstrated the important role that medicine—and psychiatry—played in elaborating racial categories necessary for the colonial project. Medical knowledge made it possible to objectify individuals—and pathologize their reactions—and mobilize this information as part of a privileged tool of biomedical control (Vaughan 1983; McCulloch 1995; Sadowsky 1999; Keller 2001, 2007; Mahone and Vaughan 2007). Historians have also stressed the importance of madness as a prism through which to observe and dictate the organic constitution of a subject. The use of race to justify the alleged inferiority of the colonized (Jackson 2005; Oyebode 2006; Parle 2007; Scarfone 2014; Studer 2015) made it difficult to accept such a legacy after decolonization in the 1960s (Kilroy-Marac 2019; Pringle 2019).

Here, rather than revisit the use of medical knowledge resulting from the colonial introduction and use of psychiatry, I turn to the worlds of alienated internees. To date, the most important work on psychiatry in British colonial territories is that of historian Jonathan Sadowsky, who examined internees, their delusions and words, drawing on writings left behind by patients or the language recorded by doctors in patient files (Sadowsky 1999). In continuing this approach, the aim here is to get as close as possible to deliria and the delirious within patient stories in order to interrogate the images they mobilized, their vocabulary, and materialities to their narratives, however irrational they may be.

Of course, approaching the "words" of a patient from medical archives is not without methodological challenges. The archive is in fact never a pure reproduction of the past (Ricoeur 2000), but "debris" (Hunt 1999, 281–319), a selection partially made by the hand of the person who produced the archive, until the time it is destroyed with a degrading of its "documentality" (Ferraris 2012). Moreover, the psychiatric archive in a "colonial situation" (Balandier 1951) is situated at the intersection of at least two points of view, one with a medical filter (Artières 1998; Thifault et al. 2016; Basso and Delbraccio 2017) and another with a colonial filter (Stoler 2008). Elaborating from these two angles leads to a selection that irreparably distorts the historian's vision of medical and colonial issues. Medical records, therefore, do not tell the whole story. Very often, elements in a case file focus on an event that caused the patient to be sent to the asylum, thus being limited to the evolution of the patient's situation during internment. The historian must be modest and cautious in order not to get caught up in the doctor's language and redouble an essentializing of the patient in the process. Above all, it would be a mistake to confuse the patient's identity or fail to differentiate them from a wider, more complex social identity by summarizing the life course solely in terms of the symptoms and psychological suffering identified by a doctor.

Even if an internee's files suggest a medical rewriting, they nevertheless may "reveal" the social world from which the person emerged: "the words of the madman lodges in the discourse of the psychiatrist who transcribes it and gives it to us to read in the tight mesh of a rhetoric that we must be careful not to decode hastily, [but which] is more porous than it appears at first glance" (Murat 2013, 35).[5] With these methodological issues in mind, and without claiming to summarize from such files the totality of human experience, it is interesting to question the contents of case-based archives from the internee's point of view. By adopting their perspective from below (Thompson 1963; Porter 1985), the patient's world may be revealed. If each life trajectory is appreciated as unique and singular, in the files—and in the disorders recorded—we may glimpse vocabulary, names, desires, and fears. We should not refuse to hear these details, which provide rich insights into the internee's world and daily life.

Such trajectories can best be approached through examining case files situated in relation to other studies in order to identify commonalities or, conversely, exceptional features. I have had access to the case files of those interned at Anjanamasina between 1906 and the end of the twentieth century, some 1,100 files in all. In this chapter, I focus on the files of four patients, all interned during the 1920s. I have chosen this decade because it was pivotal in the life of the institution. By the 1930s, the asylum no longer aroused the same interest on the part of European doctors, and the material prosperity of earlier years had disappeared. In the 1920s, budgets were shrinking, and there was a shortage of nursing staff. Doctors had to refocus on the most important issue, namely, the treatment of socially problematic patients, usually those who had caused an important disturbance to the public order. More than in the 1910s, attention turned to the key reason for even having an asylum in the 1920s.

It is not a question of interpreting these files to arrive at all kinds of situations encountered at Anjanamasina. To suggest them as exemplary is rather to mobilize a fine, qualitative approach and get as near as possible to colonized subjectivities. I adopt a "case" methodology (Passeron and Revel 2005), one lying at the intersection of *microhistoria* (Ginzburg 1980) and *subaltern studies* (Guha 1983). These cases do not summarize madness. Rather, they tell of an aspect of madness through providing information about "being mad" in a colonial situation. It is a matter of taking these files for what they expose: life itineraries revealing possible horizons within everyday colonial lives. These four files trace a common political line, one regularly encountered in asylum archives: the impossibility of becoming oneself.

The four persons had in common the fact that they had fallen into madness—or at least their physicians considered it so. They did so when faced with the impossibility of reaching the social status to which they aspired, and despite their efforts to meet colonial expectations. All were

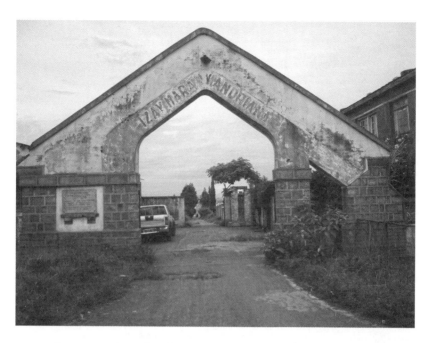

4.1   Entrance to the asylum for the insane at Anjanamasina, Madagascar, 2019. (Photograph by the author.)

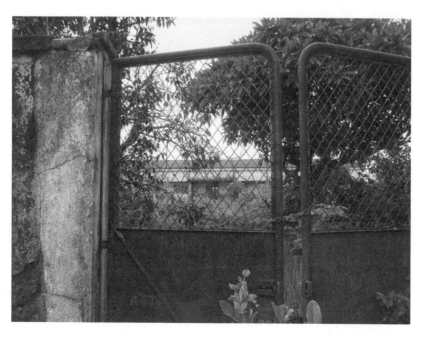

4.2   Abandoned ward of the Malagasy asylum at Anjanamasina, 2019. (Photograph by the author.)

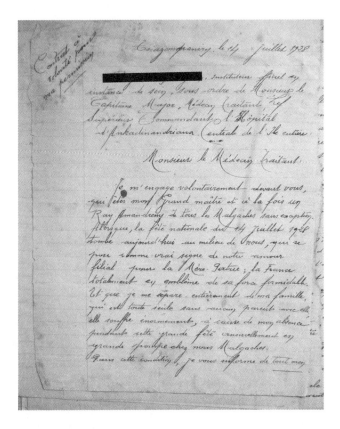

4.3 Letter by a Malagasy teacher requesting his asylum release to participate in July 14 festivities, 1928. The doctors saw in his request an additional sign of disease. The request for release was not granted. (Archives of Anjanamasina, Madagascar.)

situated on the border between the world of the colonized and that of the colonizers. At least three of them were literate and had mastered many colonial codes. All collapsed into madness at a moment when the possibility of a long-awaited social promotion seemed to disappear. Their "reason," or more precisely "the abandonment of their reason," seems to have been a response to social and racial immobilities imposed by a colonial situation that prevented any "future," and precluded projecting a present of emancipation.

This situation was a regular issue in the internment process, yet it has not been sufficiently studied in the historiography of colonial psychiatry. I have chosen these four files because of their surprising density, enabling appreciating their situations with depth and comprehensiveness. From their respective situations, madness became a performance of dignity, a last attempt to negotiate with oneself—and one's situation—before the complete destruction of subjectivity. Madness became an antechamber of death. A study of such madness allows reckoning with the indignity that a colonized individual confronted daily.

I divide my analysis into two sections. First, I detail the situations of the four internees. I then turn to what does and does not constitute the specificity of these cases, placing them in a broader medical, social, and political context. Using the work of Achille Mbembe (1996), I reflect on the "usage de la raison" (use of reason) specific to and permeating these life trajectories. Madness is revealed in its textuality. The madman is no longer synonymous with a radical destruction of subjectivity but carries a language confronting the entire colonial world. As a last attempt to preserve a dignity that colonizers refused them, such subaltern madness was ultimately a refusal to be subjected to the oppression of everyday colonial conditions.

Four Anjanamasina Patients in the 1920s

One objective is to highlight common lines running through the four life trajectories and to situate them in relation to 194 other files from the 1920s. First, a few general indications suggest common features to the four cases. All were interned after a decision taken by an administration following medical advice. This situation was typical since, out of the 194 files examined for this decade, only two did not result from involuntary internment. Of the four cases, only one was a woman. Women were a minority in Anjanamasina: they represented 21 percent of internments in the 1920s, or less than one woman for every four men. The proportion surprised the doctors, all European, since mental illness tended to be a female affliction in European representations and medical constructions since the middle of the nineteenth century (Edelman 2003). In the four cases, all were between thirty-two and forty-three years old at internment, with an average age of thirty-seven years, which was representative of the average age in the 1920s: thirty-five years old. All came from two geographical regions: Antananarivo and its province, as well as the city of Fianarantsoa, located a little farther south. This geography was also representative of the four files, with these two regions overrepresented. Anjanamasina was close to the capital, Antananarivo, and Fianarantsoa, the second largest city in the Highlands, was well connected to the capital through the existing communication infrastructure. The transport of patients to the asylum from these regions was much easier than for other territories. Two indicators distinguish these cases from others of the same period: the duration of internment and the level of education received prior to internment. The average length of internment was 2,468 days, or roughly six years and eight months. This duration, which in each ended in the internee's death, was half the average duration for those entering the asylum during the 1920s (an average of 4,317 days, or a little more than eleven years). A key question concerns educational standing. Each had a high level of education and thus a rather high social standing relative to the general colonized population. All were literate in French. Their social position at the border between two worlds—that of the colonized and that of the colonizer—enables this study of the traces these inmates left behind.

The first file is that of Joseph Rakotao,[6] married and father of one child. He was interned on April 24, 1922, and until then he had been deputy governor of Fianarantsoa Province. His delirium, according to his doctors, began a year before his internment, when this deputy governor was accused of committing multiple forgeries by signing documents in the place of French authorities. It is hard to understand what motivated such an accusation. Was it true or false, as Rakotao told his doctor? It is impossible, even from the archives, to know beyond any doubt. The doctor wrote that his patient was a "dégénéré supérieur paranoïaque" (superior and paranoid degenerate).[7] First, this colonial medical label of *dégénéré supérieur* (superior degenerate) is interesting. If the term *degenerate* is regularly used in the files, the word *superior* suggests a graduation for the deluded, based on the patient's high social position. An inmate's personal identity was socially mediated, and a delirium diagnosis was linked to social position. This high-ranking degenerate, according to the doctor, was plunged into megalomania by believing himself to be a "representative of France, in beginning to gesticulate and shout angrily. . . . He believes himself to be France" ("représentant de la France, en se mettant à gesticuler et à vociférer. . . . Il se croit la France").[8] That the doctors noted such "gesticulations" is significant. The anthropologist Malanjaona Rakotomalala has since studied the importance of such bodily manifestations. In colonial Madagascar, imitating the French colonizer, or caricaturing him, went with an attitude with gestures and loud, sometimes pretentious, speech. A Frenchman would impose his voice and body language on his audience, whereas Malagasy society prescribes discretion and restraint in vocal and physical self-expression (Rakotomalala 2009). Rakotao adopted the position of a Frenchman and denied the accusations that he issued false signatures. In short, his delusion went with a construction, a social and bodily position superimposed on a Frenchman. It is this attitude of departing from the expected that was pathologized: signing documents in the place of a French authority transgressed his expected official subaltern duties. In their physicality, it also broke with a stereotyped humility expected of Malagasy.

Originally from Ambohimandroso, Antoine Rasoarivony lived alone until his internment. On August 16, 1927, at age thirty-seven, the police brought him to the asylum. According to his file, he publicly declared to be descended from King Andriamanalina I, who ruled the whole of Madagascar before the arrival of the French. Andriamanalina I, relatively well known to historians, was a Betsileo ruler and an opponent of King Andrianamponimerina. The latter founded the Merina monarchy which, at the end of the seventeenth century, unified the island well before the arrival of the French and put up a strong resistance to colonialism. By claiming this affiliation, Rasoarivony was refusing, according to his doctors, to bow to any authority. A former student of the Frères des Écoles chrétiennes, the elite of the young Malagasy generation, he used that history, which he claimed to have learned from the Frères, to avoid the local authorities. Claiming to be a descendant of Andriamanalina was significant: it was a way to oppose the end of the Malagasy monarchy due to the French colonial presence, but above all it was an attempt to be at odds with the Merina monarchy, the first interlocutor within colonial society. At this point in his madness, those historical elements not erased by colonialism became entangled. Rasoarivony was using Malagasy history to oppose the legitimacy of the colonizer. But he also drew on a more internal history to Malagasy society—alluding to the Betsileo sovereign Andriamanalina I—to challenge the Merina monarchy that issued from Andrianamponimerina.

Through madness, history became mobilized as a last space of dignity, freed from Merina control and placed within "competitive temporalities" (Bantigny and Deluermoz 2013). Conversely, the unworthy was the colonizer denied any legitimacy and also the Merina king for collaborating with colonial powers. Rasoarivony penned in a letter that he needed a passport to reach Paris because "I will not stay here in the insane asylum."[9] He also asked for five hundred francs to pay for a dinner in Antananarivo and travel to Fianarantsoa by car.

The automobile was one of the most important symbols of modernity in Madagascar. As early as 1902, General Gallieni introduced a car during official parades. He made it a symbol of progress on the island. While claiming a royal genealogy competing with that of the Merina, Rasoarivony wished to obtain the same opportunities as any colonist: the power to move around after the education he had received and free himself from the restricted framework constraining him after his schooling by the Frères des Écoles chrétiennes. It is interesting that he explained that it was "the police who sent him here to Anjanamasina, to the parish of the insane."[10] This splendid expression, "parish of the insane," distilled Antoine Rasoarivony's perceptions of Anjanamasina. The expression deepened in importance when, in the same document, the doctor noted that his patient had a good memory and retained well notions of time, space, and places. The idiom of "this parish for the insane" also contains a religious imprint surrounding madness and the patient who ends up in an asylum after being treated by "traditional" or monotheist medicine. Antoine Rasoarivony, another document suggests, was delirious when asking for money, as if someone who was: "Not mad, but very wise. I am sorry, Mr. Director."[11] This request for forgiveness and mercy, common in Christianity, combined with that rhetoric of social order and wisdom constitutive of internment. The patient's capacity for self-discipline, morality, and following hygiene rules conditioned any possibility for exit. Rasoarivony seems to have integrated such behavior into his attitude toward the director when seeking a departure from the asylum.

Now I turn to Ramboamavo, interned on August 14, 1928, and the only woman in the four cases under discussion. She arrived at age thirty-two, the mother of three children and a French citizen, having been naturalized following her marriage to a French doctor. He had been stationed in Madagascar at the time of her internment but returned to work as a private practitioner in the French town of Avallon. The asylum doctor who first examined Ramboamavo wrote that she "had been abandoned by her husband for seventeen years and this seemed to have had a great influence on the morale of our patient."[12] He specified that her initial disorders appeared at age fourteen during her first menstruation and when she married. Married young, there are no further details on the union or the situation that followed. The doctor wrote that her troubles became manifest during menstruation, and that the rest of the time she was perfectly calm. During her moments of madness, she spent her time saying "maty aho," or "I am dying." For a while, the doctors labeled her "hysterical," though without giving any reason for this diagnostic word. After a few months, this diagnosis disappeared from the medical records. Her qualification as "mad" came after a Bible reading session at Analakely, one of the most important temples of Antananarivo. When the clerics declared her mad—perhaps as a result of an exorcism, though not named as such—Ramboamavo was committed to the asylum. In the doctors' eyes, the initial element was being abandoned by her French husband. The religious interpretation disappeared in the rest of the file, while explanation turned to the role of her marriage in her life itinerary and in triggering her disease. According to her doctors, it was her husband's abandonment that issued her into—triggering—disease.

The fourth case is Jean Rakotomanana. He entered the asylum on July 3, 1928, at age forty-three. Married and considered by medical authorities as mixed race (his father was Merina and his mother Betsileo), his disease began while working as a schoolteacher at the Ambohitrimanjaka school. When he became delirious on the morning of June 27, 1928, he asked his pupils and colleagues to kneel down in front of him and greet him. His superior, whose letter is in the file, stated that within a half hour, news of his madness spread in the village. The people, frightened, had come to look for their children. Just one hour after lessons began, the whole school had been emptied of its pupils. In short, Rakotomanana created a scandal. The doctors saw in him a "systematized psychosis," or a coherent delirium built on interpretations with a prevalent theme with affective reactions and behaviors linked. Rakotomanana's situation is interesting because, after being interned, he wrote several dozen letters testifying to his state of mind. That he was delirious is not in doubt, though his letters reveal his perceptions of the situation he confronted. Although at times disjointed, the letters express knots of tension running through him. At the beginning of several, Rakotomanana wrote: "to be opened in front of all the teachers,"[13] suggesting his wish to tell the world what was happening to him. "I was left without anything at the foot of my diploma . . . [and] you do not want to receive me in your midst. This morning I was beaten by one of the patients and received a wound on my forehead. And I don't know where I was, neither from here nor elsewhere, as if in a sense with nothing regarding my person."[14]

In another letter Rakotomanana wrote: "since I am in service of the teacher and spent the totality of my strength as a man, I have demonstrated that I have no book, nor bulletin, nor an object of government, nothing with a dose of comfort."[15] Books were a form of comfort to which he no longer had access. Using "the totality of his strength as a man,"[16] he found himself deprived of everything worthy of his profession and status, first of all books. He went on to explain that he wanted money to return home to his family in Fianarantsoa. From January 1930 onward he wrote essays in French, elaborating on what he was teaching: natural sciences, grammar, and so on. In one essay he wrote: "It is often said, wrongly and mistakenly, that other Andriana [nobles] turn into caimans; and even that among others stand aligned with the sky. I dare to summarize with precision and from the bottom of my heart that I always take the science of the learned and illustrious French as the true opening for the capacity of men."[17] In another essay, he discussed the role of Sikidy, the art of prediction in Malagasy society often practiced by Ombiasy soothsayers and healers who occupy a central place in the daily order: "The Sikidy of my own inwardly personal thought, I recognize that all that one says of them is totally illusory and deceives backward fools from other regions in the care of the most remote cause of their previous laziness in space."[18]

Rakotomanana asserted in these essays that he was a former medical school student who could treat people, dissect bodies, and examine organs. Claiming to be a medical school alumnus was not insignificant since this was the place par excellence of social success under colonialism. As the most prestigious professional path on the island, being a doctor meant belonging to the most elite category, socially and economically. The School of Medicine brought together young Merina, who stood at the interface between the colonizers and colonized, and constituted a Malagasy elite. It was from the medical school's ranks that nationalist leaders emerged in the 1910s, fighting for the French colony's independence. To claim having passed through the Antananarivo School of Medicine expressed a desire to belong to the elite.

In the first days of his internment, Rakotomanana escaped. This was not an uncommon event, rather one found in a considerable number of cases. Yet Rakotomanana's motivations were singular. He escaped on July 6, 1928, in order to attend the July 14 festivities. He was caught on July 9 and wrote a letter asking for a leave of absence on July 14 because he "could not leave [his] family without relatives on that date,"[19] the French national holiday, a day of military parades and honoring the fatherland. His letter went so far as to offer four hundred francs as a guarantee, in the hope of obtaining permission to leave. If he did not return, he affirmed, then the doctors would be able to confiscate this sum. Although he complained about his lack of means and the low consideration given him by the colonial administration so far, to not participate in this colonial version of France's national holiday was evidently unbearable for him.

Reason in a Colonial Situation,
or Madness as Language

It is difficult, if not impossible, in accounts of such situations to know their truth. However, here it is not a question of trying to invalidate or retrospectively accredit a diagnosis made by doctors regarding these four persons. The delirious in their words is not in doubt, nor a certain opacity and the disjointed character to their speech. So, how can a work in history, one seeking to reconstruct the truth of a past time from archives, make use of such "false words"? How can one claim to construct a true narrative when the specificity of the words of a mad person resides in a close relationship with delusions, with little grip on reality?[20] I wish to demonstrate that it is by studying such delusions as madness that we can glimpse from an individual's subjectivity the truth of a social and political situation. To take delusions seriously, starting with patient obsessions, is to observe the torments and anxieties of a particular era. It is also to fundamentally question the position of all actors—colonizers, mad persons, the colonized—and the imaginaries shaping their positions.

One similarity across these cases is that these four inmates all initially radically subscribed to the colonial project. One was a deputy governor general. The second was loyal to his education received from French Catholics. The woman married a French doctor, possibly for reasons of social advancement, though we cannot possibly know the reality of her feelings. The last, a schoolteacher, did not hesitate in writing to denigrate the ancestral knowledge of Sikidy or Ombiasy.

At first, they all tried to follow the colonial model while hoping for a future of emancipation. However, in each case and for apparently different reasons, the emancipation never came to be. The woman did not follow her husband to France, even though she attained French citizenship. The deputy governor general expressed his wish to sign, like a French colonial authority, acts determining local politics. An education received, even for a schoolteacher, did not enable access to a freedom fantasized about or expected. Whether it is by passing through a more or less fictitious genealogy or by asking within a school, with everyone kneeling down as a sign of deference, a demand for social recognition and status was not only denied but also interpreted as madness, or as doctors categorized it, as "megalomania." Today, "megalomania" often translates into fragility in a social and political condition articulated around the stakes of race. Since they were

Malagasy—even if citizens—they were never able to claim the same rights or recognition as the French. The psychiatrist Frantz Fanon repeatedly said about his patients in Algeria: "the first thing the native learns is to stay in his place, not to go beyond limits" (Fanon 2002, 53). But in colonial Madagascar, "staying in one's place" seems to have been learned quite late in relation to this society's colonial hierarchy. Yet most came to find themselves unable to access a status of humanity, as that dignity was aligned with the social position of colonizers and remained out of reach for those marked as *les indigènes* or as natives. Once the colonial ladder had been climbed, the so-called native was confronted with the indignity of a daily colonial life that excluded them from a status as an equal citizen in their own country. This "grammar of the unworthy" (Ajari 2020, 96) remained omnipresent. Efforts made to rise within the colonial hierarchy dominated social relations as a whole. In fact, the claims emerging in delusions demonstrate a clear political line: the right to exist like the French. To paraphrase these delusions: the right to sign official documents like a Frenchman, the right to a passport, the right to go to Paris, the right to use a car, and the right to be recognized as fully educated. Even the woman who became a French citizen, she encountered abandonment as an only option. She was not who she wished to be. It was impossible for her to follow her husband to France, and she was not able to understand the reasons for this impossibility. In any case, she remained a wanderer: morally, psychologically, and symbolically mutilated. Like the other three cases, she did not emerge alive. Indeed, all died in the asylum within a few years.

Madness is a way of formulating the structural impossibility of accessing a world out of reach, for it is those who appear most integrated in the political and social order who undermined the ambitions of the colonial project. From a negative perspective, madness is a response to the impossibility of any "future": if tomorrow is inevitable, a projection into the future suddenly becomes impossible. Thinking about what is to come is impossible, as the individual is frozen in a present articulated within an interminable competition of two laws that make any rise in status unattainable. The example of Jean Rakotomanana, who ran away to attend the July 14 ceremonies, is obvious. For him, it was vital to be present on that day, even though the festive events would obviously be held without him. We see here a full subjection of the personality in a colonial context, which, for natives, was consubstantial with the social world. Madness appears as the marker of social and political borders between the colonizing and the subjectivities of each inmate: subjectivities that might have been impossible to bear without falling into madness. Madness reveals itself as an expression of wishes, repressed to a greater or lesser degree, stemming from traumatic events of the "real"—"real" in an analytical sense, as that which emerges and that one no longer manages to apprehend—a "real" that mutilates. Madness is then the work of a fictive reality and appears as a response to those impossibilities constantly imposed on the so-called *indigènes* or natives. Delusional activity and the psychosymbolic economy underlying it—far from being asocial, situated outside of humanity, or reducible solely to the sphere of the "private"—reveals itself to be linked to the tribulations of a particular time. At stake is a struggle of constituting the colonized as a political subject. Even when it is a question of a wife abandoned by her husband, what is at stake is not of the order of a private libidinal economy, of a "conjugal crisis," but of access to a self-image.

Madness, in this situation, is therefore a profound expression of colonial order and disorder. Its world belongs to a category of transferring the imaginary of problems that are insoluble in reality. Such was illustrated by the anthropologist Gérard Althabe (1969) in relation to possession. What seems fundamental to me is to study the words and images of madness, a praxis that becomes a way of frequenting and summoning the political. A madman accomplishes an act as much political as cultural, by seeking to reactivate his capacity to control the meaning of events, while continuing to generate these same events and meanings. When in his madness Rakotomanana pondered the "exactitude of the science of the French as a window into the capacity of men,"[21] he was with words seeking a way for a colonized native to become aware of his identity as a self-interpreter and political subject. He was also seeking a way to resituate himself, through a tragic delirious affirmation regarding colonial oppression, by proclaiming an accumulation of knowledge that he supposed would enable him to affirm a place in this political economy. It was indeed an attempt at the "public exercise of reason" (Mbembe 1996), as we see in his letters, where he wrote on the front: "to be opened in front of all the teachers." From these epistolary remains emerges an intellect torn to shreds, an intellect intended to be affirmative and authorizing the analysis of letters as procedures in constituting individual and social identities, but also as political practices. To talk about school programs, as Jean Rakotomanana did, was to solve colonial conflict by exorcizing it, in a madness that depended on material determinants of everyday reality. This madness distilled a "debris" of meanings out of a colonial moment, out of a world where each signifier constantly referred to a frame bringing the delirious subject back into a field of a power of subjection from which they desperately tried to escape or to respond, experiencing it until death. Hence the idea of "systematized psychosis," acknowledged by doctors as informing more a political and social order than a medical one, invoked the impossibilities of everyday life turned into obsessions.

Let us specify all the same that the refusal to die socially—to see one's freedom, desires, and will constantly broken—often took the form of a delirious drama, which was in no way a liberation of the self. On the contrary, it was a tragic displacement leading to death. Thus, it is not surprising that patient Ramboamavo spent her time in delirious moments saying, "maty aho, maty aho," "I die, I die." Madness was not an absolute passivity of the self. To take the mad person as seriously as possible, to be attentive to what they say to us, is to penetrate the colonial social world, to sense its borders, a certain topography, and affirm the colonial necessity of apprehending mad persons as social actors: performers who came to reveal the limits of a world from a political symptomatology within their struggle for dignity and a right to exist.

Madness, a Tragic Reinvention of Reason in the Colonies

I want to move away from Madagascar for a moment and return to the significance of madness from a more theoretical point of view. In the 1960s, following his *Histoire de la folie à l'âge classique*, Michel Foucault (1961) engaged in a lively debate with Jacques Derrida. Foucault rejected the idea that madness is an objective fact making sense in itself, and insisted on medical interpretation. His view corresponded to a historical formulation situated in time and space. In fact, madness becomes, in this sense, pure exteriority. For Foucault, the madman is a truncated individual, but also a mind that has completely stopped functioning. The madman is pure unreason, with completely destroyed mental faculties. Only bodily faculties remain. Derrida, some years later, expressed a clear divergence from this viewpoint (Derrida 1963). According to him, total madness does not exist, and he developed in his response to Foucault the idea of a fundamental interpenetration between Reason and Unreason. Derrida affirmed madness as part of the cogito, a rationality in itself. It is never far from true perception, even if plunged into a narrative that Derrida saw as closer to the oneiric. Thus, for Derrida, a madman could never be deluded enough to be totally mad.

In a different manner, the psychoanalyst Octave Mannoni (1950) several years earlier questioned madness or the neuroses of Malagasy daily life. Beginning from dreams, Mannoni tried to discern their distillations, and put at their center the relationship of domination and exploitation characteristic of the colonial situation. He readily acknowledged that, in such a situation, one finds a confrontation between two types of subjectivity. This interpretive framework allows for questioning the relationship between the colonizer and the colonized and perceiving the violence taking place in a political and social structure. But Mannoni, in the course of his analysis, reduced all meanings to the problem of inferiority and superiority. The question of dependence, well known and rightly attacked by Fanon (1986), reduces matters to an individual complex aggravated by colonialism. It also emphasizes the social contextualization surrounding the native, in this case Malagasy, psyche. Dependence locks the complex into a form of oedipal return.

What seems to take shape here, arising from these four cases, is a third way of structuring the problem. By drawing on the approaches of Derrida and Mannoni and of course Fanon, I have been able to begin again from this "mad" word found in medical files, so as to examine the role of speech in society. At a theoretical level, I have focused on the processes that the words of the "mad" and their speech summon. It is a question of focusing on the apparatus surrounding madness, but also of considering at greater length the logic of madness, as read from its internal coherences. This is, a priori, a paradoxical approach because of the invention consubstantial with any madness, but it is also a perspective that allows questioning these coherences as a dynamic that made sense for the internee. It authorizes us to analyze madness as a political practice filled with meaning, but also as an imprint in the fabric of the social and psychological life of the colonized. Very often, the question of madness in the colonies was mobilized for reasons of security, from the anxious position of the colonizer. Yet, to be aware of the construction of madness from its speech, from its words, is to turn upside down the colonizer's point of view. It enables examining, above all, the anxieties of the colonized, surely more than those of the colonizer. These interned persons, who would probably never have entered into history had they not been deemed mad, manifested through their madness ambitions, anxieties, and frustrations. It is therefore an entirely vernacular, subaltern subjectivity that appears.

Madness is often seen as a "cultural" or "individual" factor: the result of a small private theater during an individual's journey. In contrast, by examining the speech and words of mad persons themselves, these four cases expose political projections: like whether it is normal to respond to and satisfy the injunctions of a colonial regime. Madness also appears as an individual link between death and agony within a social space, and as a movement of indiscipline in the colonies, reinscribed in measures of opposition, bifurcation, and the reinvention of reason. Madness was a tragic remaking of reason in the colonies, one that we should study with care.

Notes

Epigraph: Frantz Fanon (1986, 109–14).

1   The law of June 30, 1838, imposed an obligation in each French department to have an establishment for receiving the "insane." In Madagascar, the supervision of the insane was under French law, and Anjanamasina was an institution directly answerable to the colonial administration.

2   The medical model deployed in Madagascar was one of the earliest in the French colonial empire, with the creation of the *Assistance médicale indigène* as early as 1898 (Merlin, Mafart, and Triaud 2003).

3   The terms "European" and "indigenous" were legal—and also social—categories specific to this colonial situation, not geographical definitions. The term "indigenous" is a reference to the *"régime de l'indigénat"* (the Native Code).

4   It is not clear what such terms mean or by what criteria such a categorization is made.

5   "La parole du fou loge dans le discours du psychiatre qui la retranscrit et nous la donne à lire dans le maillage serré d'une rhétorique qu'il faut se garder de décoder à la hâte, [mais qui] est plus poreux qu'il n'y parait de prime abord."

6   All names have been anonymized.

7   Joseph Rakotao's medical file, Archives of Anjanamasina (hereafter ArchAn).

8   Joseph Rakotao's medical file.

9   Antoine Rasoarivony's medical file, ArchAn.

10 Antoine Rasoarivony's medical file.

11 Antoine Rasoarivony's medical file.

12 Ramboamavo's medical file, ArchAn.

13 The following quotes are in French in the files. When deemed necessary, to avoid distortions in translation, I have inserted the original French version as a note. Jean Rakotomanana's medical file, ArchAn.

14 "Je restais sans rien avoir au pied de mon diplôme . . . vous ne voulez pas me recevoir auprès de vous. Ce matin j'étais battu par un des malades et reçu une plaie au front. Et je ne sais plus où je devenais, ni d'ici ni d'ailleurs, comme en sens de rien vis-à-vis de ma personne." Jean Rakotomanana's medical file.

15 "Depuis que je suis en service d'instituteur et dépensais la totalité de ma force d'homme, j'ai démontré que j'ai aucun livre, ni bulletin, ni de quel objet de gouvernement, rien de la dose du réconfort." Jean Rakotomanana's medical file.

16 Jean Rakotomanana's medical file.

17 "On raconte souvent à tort et à travers en disant que les autres Andriana [les nobles] se changent en caïmans; et même que certains autres se dressent en alignement au ciel. J'ose en résumé comme exactitude au fond de mon cœur que je prends toujours la science des Français savants et illustres pour la vraie ouverture de la capacité des hommes." Jean Rakotomanana's medical file.

18 "Le sikidy de ma propre pensée intérieurement personnelle, j'en reconnais que tout ce que l'on en dise est totalement fabuleux pour en tromper les imbéciles arriérés dans d'autres régions en tout soin de les plus reculés cause de leur paresse antérieurement en espace." Jean Rakotomanana's medical file.

19 Jean Rakotomanana's medical file.

20 The historian, Luise White, using rumors as a starting point, asks a similar question about how to approach the truth of a social and political situation from the falsehood of rumors (White 2000, 56–86).

21 "L'exactitude de la science des Français comme ouverture sur la capacité des hommes." Jean Rakotomanana's medical file.

Sources

Archival Material

Archives of Anjanamasina (ArchAn), Madagascar.

Literature

Ajari, Norman. 2020. *La dignité ou la mort: Éthique et politique de la race.* Paris: Seuil.
Althabe, Gérard. 1969. *Oppression et libération dans l'imaginaire: Les communautés villageoises de la côte orientale de Madagascar.* Paris: Maspero.

Artières, Philippe. 1998. *Clinique de l'écriture: Une histoire du regard médical sur l'écriture*. Paris: Éditions Synthélabo.

Balandier, Georges. 1951. "La situation coloniale: Approche théorique." *Cahiers internationaux de sociologie* 11:44–79.

Bantigny, Ludivine, and Quentin Deluermoz. 2013. "Coexistence et concurrence des temps." *Vingtième siècle: Revue d'histoire* 1, no. 117: 3–250.

Basso, Elisabetta, and Mireille Delbraccio. 2017. "La psychiatrie en ses archives, entre histoire et épistémologie." *Revue d'histoire des sciences* 70, no. 2: 255–73.

Derrida, Jacques. 1963. "Cogito et histoirc de la folie." *Revue de métaphysique et de morale* 68, no. 4: 460–94.

Edelman, Nicole. 2003. *Les métamorphoses de l'hystérique: Du début du XIXᵉ siècle à la Grande Guerre*. Paris: La Découverte.

Fanon, Frantz. 1986. *Black Skin, White Masks*. London: Pluto.

Fanon, Frantz. 2002. *Les damnées de la terre*. Paris: La Découverte.

Ferraris, Maurizio. 2012. *Documentality: Why It Is Necessary to Leave Traces*. New York: Fordham University Press.

Foucault, Michel. 1961. *Folie et déraison: Histoire de la folie à l'âge classique*. Paris: Librairie Plon.

Gallien, Raphaël. 2019. *Le fou colonisé: Une histoire de l'institution psychiatrique en situation colonial. Madagascar, 1900–1960*. Mémoire de master II. Paris: Université Paris VII–Denis Diderot.

Ginzburg, Carlo. 1980. *Le fromage et les vers: L'univers d'un meunier frioulan du XVIᵉ siècle*. Paris: Aubier.

Guha, Ranajit. 1983. *Elementary Aspects of Peasant Insurgency in Colonial India*. Delhi: Oxford University Press India.

Hunt, Nancy Rose. 1999. *A Colonial Lexicon: Of Birth Ritual, Medicalization and Mobility in the Congo*. Durham, NC: Duke University Press.

Jackson, Lynette. 2005. *Surfacing Up: Psychiatry and Social Order in Colonial Zimbabwe, 1908–1968*. Ithaca, NY: Cornell University Press.

Keller, Richard C. 2001. "Madness and Colonization: Psychiatry in the British and French Empires, 1800–1962." *Journal of Social History* 35, no. 2: 295–326.

Keller, Richard C. 2007. *Colonial Madness: Psychiatry in French North Africa*. Chicago: University of Chicago Press.

Kilroy-Marac, Katie. 2019. *An Impossible Inheritance: Postcolonial Psychiatry and the Work of Memory in a West African Clinic*. Berkeley: University of California Press.

Mahone, Sloan, and Megan Vaughan. 2007. *Psychiatry and Empire*. Basingstoke, UK: Palgrave Macmillan.

Mannoni, Octave. 1950. *Psychologie de la colonisation*. Paris: Seuil.

Mbembe, Achille. 1996. *La naissance du maquis dans le Sud-Cameroun (1920–1960): Histoire des usages de la raison en colonie*. Paris: Karthala.

McCulloch, Jock. 1995. *Colonial Psychiatry and the African Mind*. Cambridge: Cambridge University Press.

Merlin, Jean, Bertrand Mafart, and Jean-Louis Triaud. 2003. "L'assistance médicale indigène à Madagascar (1898–1950)." *Médecine Tropicale* 63:17–23.

Murat, Laure. 2013. *L'homme qui se prenait pour Napoléon: Pour une histoire politique de la folie*. Paris: Gallimard.

Oyebode, Femi. 2006. "History of Psychiatry in West Africa." *International Review of Psychiatry* 18, no. 4: 319–25.

Parle, Julie. 2007. *State of Mind: Searching for Mental Health in Natal and Zululand, 1868–1918*. Pietermaritzburg, South Africa: KwaZulu-Natal Press.

Passeron, Jean-Claude, and Jacques Revel. 2005. *Penser par cas*. Paris: EHESS.

Porter, Roy. 1985. "The Patient View: Doing Medical History from Below." *Theory and Society* 14, no. 2: 175–98.

Pringle, Yolana. 2019. *Psychiatry and Decolonization in Uganda*. London: Palgrave Macmillan.

Rakotomalala, Malanjaona. 2009. "Paroles et gestes en Imerina: Quelques éléments d'éthologie humaine à Madagascar." In *Madagascar revisitée: En voyage avec Françoise Raison-Jourde*, edited by Didier Nativel and Faranirina Rajaonah, 139–50. Paris: Karthala.

Reboul, Henri, and Emmanuel Régis. 1912. *Rapport sur l'assistance des aliénés aux colonies*. Paris: Librairie de l'Académie de médecine.

Ricoeur, Paul. 2000. *La mémoire, l'histoire, l'oubli*. Paris: Seuil.

Sadowsky, Jonathan. 1999. *Imperial Bedlam: Institutions of Madness in Colonial Southwest Nigeria*. Berkeley: University of California Press.

Scarfone, Marianna. 2014. "La psichiatria coloniale italiana: Teorie, pratiche, protagonisti, istituzioni (1906–1952)." Thèse de doctorat en histoire, Université Ca' Foscari-Lyon II.

Stoler, Ann Laura. 2008. *Along the Archival Grain: Epistemic Anxieties and Colonial Common Sense*. Princeton, NJ: Princeton University Press.

Studer, Nina. 2015. *The Hidden Patients: North African Women in French Colonial Psychiatry*. Cologne: Böhlau Verlag.

Thifault, Marie-Claude, Isabelle Perreault, Alexandre Klein, and Jean Caron. 2016. "L'archive psychiatrique." *Santé mentale au Québec* 41, no. 2: 7–195.

Thompson, Edward P. 1963. *The Making of the English Working Class*. London: Victor Gollancz.

Vaughan, Megan. 1983. "Idioms of Madness: Zomba Lunatic Asylum, Nyasaland, in the Colonial Period." *Journal of Southern African Studies* 9, no. 2: 218–38.

White, Luise. 2000. *Speaking with Vampires: Rumor and History in Colonial Africa*. Berkeley: University of California Press.

Jonathan Sadowsky 5

Sickness and Symptoms as Cultural Capacities in Colonial Ideology

Onset about ten years ago. She seldom slept but lay on her mat, thinking. She was utterly miserable and often wept. When she slept she dreamt the same dream that later troubled her mother.

Five years ago she began to feel "changed" and miserable. She "couldn't go anywhere," could do no work, take no interest in anything, nor sleep. Sometimes she shed tears.

Languid . . . slow and dejected. She was perfectly accessible but too listless to talk. She said perfunctorily that she was better but could not interest herself in anything. She said it was more than three months since she had felt any pleasure in work. She was thin but said she had been fat till she became uninterested in eating.

Margaret Field, *Search for Security*

This chapter considers the problem of depression in African studies. Lethargy, insomnia, extreme sorrowfulness, loss of appetite and consequent weight loss, lack of interest in activities . . . to the psychiatrically inclined, these excerpts from case notes will be more than a little suggestive of clinical depression. That, however, is not how the women described here named their distress. They were self-accused witches. The excerpts are from Margaret Field's study of supplicants at a shrine in late colonial Ghana. As Field observed, though, self-accusation, that is, relentless preoccupation with guilty thoughts, is also a feature of clinical depression.

After American actor Robin Williams took his own life in 2014, Kenyan writer Ted Malanda wrote: "I can't wrap my mind around the fact that depression is an illness. We are stressed and depressed all the time! In fact, it is such a non-issue that African languages never bothered to create a word for it. Anybody who knows what they call depression in their mother tongue, please step forward" (Malanda 2014).[1] Malanda's commentary compressed two complications regarding depressive illness. The first is that depression is only intelligible as an illness state if the symptoms are disproportionate to the life context. People in objectively hard circumstances, in this view, can have depressed moods, but are not *clinically* depressed. The second is that, for depression to be an illness, it needs to be seen as one—it exists as sickness only when it is named as a sickness.

Malanda could be read as taking one of two positions, both of which have been richly developed in depression studies. One is that depression is not really an illness at all; in this view, the concept of depressive illness only exists as an artifact of the Western propensity to medicalize hardship. Or, Malanda may be saying that depression may well be an illness but, if so, it is not one for African people, but a Western culture-bound syndrome (Bell 2014; Dorwick 2013). If it had any currency as illness in African societies, it would have a corresponding name in African vernacular nosologies.

These debates are also dramatized in Chimananda Ngozi Adichie's novel, *Americanah*, wherein the protagonist, Ifemelu, has a prolonged period of depressed mood after coming from Nigeria to the United States for college. Her aunt, a physician, wants Ifemelu to seek medical care for depression, but Ifemelu responds that she is in objectively hard circumstances, not sick, and that depressive illness is just an example of Americans giving a medical name to all of life's problems (Adichie 2014, 150–58).

Malanda's column appeared after decades of epidemiology claiming to document ever higher rates of depression in African societies. Many observers in the first half of the twentieth century, during formal colonial rule in much of Africa, agreed with Malanda, claiming that depressive illness was rare in African societies: though, as we will see, their explanations often differed sharply from his. Research conducted in the early independence period, by contrast, often found rates of depression to be much higher than was previously recorded (Orley and Wing 1979; Pringle 2018, 188). Some more recent work in global health has found rates of depression in Africa to be as high or higher than those of Western societies (Abas and Broadhead 1997). If Malanda and those who agree with him are right, the recent epidemiology is counting a phantom.

We have by now a large literature on the colonial image of Africa and Africans as diseased (Comaroff 2003). This ideological production is not only a matter of prejudicial thought, or "implicit bias." It has worked to justify colonialism and foreign intervention. It depicted Africans as dependent and in need of outside resources.

Yet Europeans have long also considered Africans relatively immune from certain ailments, not because African environments did not induce those afflictions, but because they were afflictions of advanced races—"diseases of civilization" (Porter 1993).[2] White physicians at one time considered tuberculosis, cancer, and diabetes to be diseases from which Black people were relatively protected, because they were diseases of more advanced races (Wailoo 2009; Roberts 2011; Tuchman 2020). Another of these illnesses has been depression. As scholars of colonial psychiatry have shown exhaustively, a rise in "madness" in a broad sense was often attributed to the rapid acceleration of modernization in the early twentieth century (Vaughan 1991; McCulloch 1995). Depression was a special case though. Even as rates of madness were supposedly on the rise, rates of depression in Africa were supposedly remaining low. European observers regarded a propensity toward depression not just as a vulnerability, but as a cultural achievement.

By the 1960s, though, a shift in the epidemiology was apparent. In what was for most of Africa the early postindependence period, researchers suddenly found high rates of depression. Was this new data reflecting a real change in prevalence, or changing diagnostic fashion? Raymond Prince, a psychiatrist who did research in southwestern Nigeria, tried to sort this out in a 1967 article (Prince 1967). Prince reviewed fourteen reports on insanity from different parts of Africa during the colonial period, ranging from the

1890s to the 1960s. With one exception, they found depression to be rare or nonexistent. The exception was Field, an anthropologist with medical training who worked at a healing shrine in Ghana. Field found depression to be the commonest of mental illnesses among rural Akan women.

Prince argued that the fourteen reports he looked at did not reference one another much, so their similar findings could not be explained by mutual influence. That argument failed to consider whether they might all be equally influenced by more broadly held colonial ideologies and discourse. After reviewing the reports, Prince concluded that there were four possible explanations for the changing rates: (1) a possible "prestige factor" (i.e., a growing number of people enchanted by the "mystique" of depression); (2) the discovery of "masked depressions" (i.e., cases of depression that were initially presenting with nonaffective, mostly somatic symptoms, but which could be determined to be depressions on closer examination); (3) different catchment areas (i.e., moving away from looking only at asylum and hospital admissions, where the cases were likely to be troublesome to social order, which depression often is not); and (4) true prevalence, meaning that there was an actual rise in depression cases.

Prince did not decide definitively which explanation he thought was the strongest. The section on "mystique" and "prestige" is muddled, with a digression into psychoanalytic theory and the need for a well-developed superego in order to have depression, without explaining what this has to do with prestige or mystique, and ultimately claiming that it might simply be a matter of observers having the paradigm to notice depression. He also doubted there was a rise in true prevalence. He pointed out that Field's catchment area, rather than being a strange outlier, might be more accurate, a better reflection of actual prevalence, since it was not an institutional setting. Her findings agreed with that of his own fieldwork. Prince did not, however, consider that there might be a politics to psychiatric diagnosis.

The existence and prevalence of depression in African societies remains a fraught problem. My purpose is not to try to determine how much actual depression there is in African societies. Instead, I want to burrow deeper into the history of the diagnosis in African settings. Depression has received some mention in the historiography of madness and psychiatry in Africa, but mostly in passing.[3] The glancing attention probably reflects much of the field's reliance on colonial sources, because it is mostly mentioned in passing in them, too. The process of counting depressions was long meshed with colonial ideas about depression as a disease of civilization. Depression was considered not just an ailment, but a cultural capacity. That idea has been partly anchored in conceptions regarding guilt and guilty ruminations as symptoms of depressive illness. The notion of depression as a cultural capacity hinged on the idea of guilt itself as a cultural capacity. These ideas saturated colonial psychiatric discourse. Important dissents, though, were voiced during the colonial period—notably those of Field and of Frantz Fanon. I also explore a surprising affinity between these two dissimilar authors working in unlike contexts.

This chapter differs from most others in this volume in that, instead of being a focused case study, it zooms out to consider conceptual problems of diagnosis and cross-cultural comparison in a broad sense. Perhaps ironically, though, it also makes an indirect case for closely considered case studies and granular particularity. But first, I want to sketch out a bit more the contours of the debates about depression and cultural variation.

Depression as a Global Mental Health Conundrum

In the late colonial period, a patient admitted to Nigeria's new Aro Mental Hospital had symptoms the clinicians believed were psychosomatic in origin.[4] His symptoms included trouble concentrating, continuous headaches he described as "crushing," body shakes, feelings of paralysis, and body aches. Is it possible that this was a case of depression, expressed in somatic terms? Such a supposition could be a misguided attempt at retrospective diagnosis. But the patient himself introduced the word *depressed* into the discourse, saying he was "very tired and depressed at the weak heart." The case illustrates the challenge posed in trying to determine rates of depression. How do you know which cases count? Questions about rates of depression are never only about numbers. They are also about the definitions and cultural assumptions that shape how the numbers are collected. As Megan Vaughan (2010) has put it regarding the related problem of suicide in Africa, "The history of suicide is in part a history of subjectivity, and no history of that sort is ever going to be straightforward." Sushrut Jadhav (2000) has called depression the single most fraught psychiatric diagnosis for cross-cultural study.

According to the World Health Organization (WHO) (2017), depression is now—newly—the single biggest contributor to the global health burden. The WHO estimates that there are more than three hundred million people worldwide living with depression, with an 18 percent increase between 2005 and 2015. As Prince (1967) observed though, the meaning of these statistics is not obvious. Are more people really suffering from depression? If so, what is causing this apparent epidemic? Or are doctors simply diagnosing depression more? If so, are they catching more cases than were visible previously, or changing the criteria for diagnosis? Or is the rising currency of this particular diagnostic label influencing how people interpret their mental distress, whether it is profound psychic pain, or moderate unhappiness? How much does the mere presence of antidepressants influence the rates of diagnosis? Are we living through less an epidemic of depression than one of *calling things* depression?

Knowing the true prevalence of a disease can be challenging enough when you have a stable definition and unambiguous markers, such as a blood test. Counting by, say, hospital admissions risks omitting many afflicted people who cannot get to a hospital, or wish to avoid one, for example. You can go into communities and check for people with symptoms, but some may be asymptomatic, not eager to talk to you, or missed for myriad other reasons. With an illness like depression, it is harder still, partly because depression is hard to define. In everyday language, it can refer both to a mood anyone can have and also to a clinical syndrome, and the blurriness of the border between these meanings can lead critics like Malanda to wonder if such a border even exists. As a clinical syndrome, it has been subject to numerous revisions of the criteria for inclusion. The number of symptoms that have been named as symptoms of depression is vast. Even the core symptom most people associate with clinical depression—depressed affect—is not a necessary symptom in all definitions (though it is a common one). In many conceptions, the depressed affect must be excessive somehow. It can be excessive in time—that is, going on for longer than is normal. Or, it can be excessive in intensity, seeming out of proportion to any precipitating events. Both of these criteria for excessiveness depend on ideas of normality: What is the normal amount of time to be sad? What is a normal intensity of reaction to one's life circumstances? These are not questions that can be settled objectively, the way the presence or absence of a pathogen in the bloodstream can.

And so, some question whether it is a "real" illness at all, though in some discussions, the criteria for "realness" are mostly implicit. One criterion many have turned to is cultural universality—or lack of it. The frequent assumption is that if one can show a depression to be universal, occurring as an illness state in all cultures, then it must be real. But how do you show whether something is universal or not, if its very definition is subject to constant disputes? Debate over the universality of depression has revolved around two main questions: (1) Is depression uniquely Western—a Western culture-bound syndrome? (2) If not, do some cultures express depression in a more physical way, and less in terms of mood—and if so, what is the ground for calling it "depression"?

The case for calling depression a Western culture-bound syndrome has two typical facets—both expressed in short form in the quote from Malanda, though both have also received elaborate scholarly articulation. One is the claim that naming sad affect as a clinical problem depends on the expectation of happiness; something can only be considered pathology if it departs from a culture's norm. Cultures that see sadness as the normal course of life therefore would not recognize depression as an illness (Lutz 1985; Obeyesekere 1985). The second is that some medical cultures seem to have no word that translates as depressive illness. These are formidable positions, but they are not unassailable. The claim that only societies with an expectation of happiness have concepts of depressive illness has empirical counterexamples (Good, Good, and Moradi 1985; Behrouzan 2016). As for the lack of a vernacular diagnostic label, most of modern medical nomenclature did not exist for most of human history. Do we really want to say that people therefore did not get any of these illnesses?

As Prince observed, apparent lack of depressive illness may be explained by somatization (Sethi, Nathawat, and Gupta 1973; Racy 1980; Cheung 1982; Kleinman 1986; Tran 2016).[5] In this view, depressive illness is not absent, but presenting primarily in bodily complaints—unexplained tummy troubles or backaches, for example. To be clear, no one is saying that you can automatically pin otherwise mysterious body complaints on depression. You need to find further evidence of depressive illness, such as sad affect, on deeper investigation of the patient.[6] The idea of somatized depression, though, did not originate in cross-cultural study. The idea was expressed at least by the early twentieth century in Western psychiatry—what came to be called "masked depression."[7] And it is still used in Western contexts. People often come into primary care physicians in the United States with physical complaints and leave with a diagnosis of depression if other depressive symptoms are found in the exam. The term somatization may be inherently misleading. It assumes that the primary state of depression is emotional, and the physical aspects secondary. The fifth edition of the *Di-*

agnostic and Statistical Manual of Mental Disorders (DSM) requires five of nine listed symptoms for a diagnosis of major depressive disorder (American Psychiatric Association 2013). Depression cannot be the diagnosis without at least one somatic symptom. Purely affective ones will not reach the required threshold of five symptoms. It is telling that the DSM, the most influential document of Western psychiatry, a source you might most expect to emphasize the psychological, *insists* on a somatic dimension. Dividing the world into somatizing and nonsomatizing cultures risks stereotyping both (Kohrt, Mendenhall, and Brown 2015).

Using labels from one culture in another one always risks obscuring local experience (Watters 2010; Mills 2014). One path across this impasse is to use local categories, or "idioms of distress" (Nichter 1981; Kaiser and Weaver 2019). This essentially means using the vernacular. One idiom of distress, "thinking too much," may have particular relevance to the study of depression (Kaiser et al. 2015). Syndromes that translate into English as "thinking too much," have been documented in many places. The term shows both the appeal and the limits of using local categories. It does not mean the same thing everywhere. In some contexts, the associated symptoms overlap a lot with depressive disorder, though in other places not.[8] In Shona, the word *Kufungisisa* translates as "thinking too much" and refers to nonpsychotic mental illness, a condition with similar symptoms to depression and anxiety (Patel, Simunyu, and Gwanzura 1995). In Haiti, "thinking too much" is a syndrome marked by "troubled rumination at the intersection of sadness, severe mental disorder, suicide, and social and structural hardship" (Kaiser et al. 2014). "Thinking too much" in Haiti is considered thought that is not aimed at problem solving, but also features social withdrawal, weight loss, and insomnia. Not surprisingly, Haitians with the syndrome had high scores on a psychiatric depression inventory. Among a San group in South Africa, "thinking too much" also has a lot of overlap with depression, including "emotional and psychological problems, social withdrawal, behavioral changes, and somatic complaints" and "sadness, loneliness, 'hurting inside', worrying, stressing, losing self-worth, and suicidal thoughts" (den Hertog et al. 2016). In this case, the word for "thinking too much" covers both illness states as well as bad feelings that are not thought to rise to the level of illness—as the English term depression does. Among Kenyan Kiswahili speakers, descriptions of distress use a term that translates to thinking too much, but also to the English word *depression*. The two terms refer to similar, but not identical, clinical pictures (Mendenhall et al. 2019). Virtually all places with an idiom of "thinking too much," consider it to involve excessive rumination—as do current clinical concepts of depression. One attempt to account for the gender ratio of depression in the United States has proposed that the ratio is due to women's greater tendency toward rumination (Nolan-Hoeksema 1993).

Is it possible that many of the places thought to have no word for "depression" actually do, and the word translates more literally as "thinking too much"? Calling instances of "thinking too much" *depression* may risk losing shades of meaning particular to their contexts. The risk, though, is not limited to contexts that are remote from the origin sites of biomedicine. Using the biomedical label of depression can hide shades of meaning in contexts most influenced by Western biomedicine.

Understanding local idioms does not require us to forgo global labels—it is not an either/or. As Byron Good, Mary-Jo DelVecchio Good, and Robert Moradi (1985) pointed out: "When Topley (1970) wrote that Cantonese in Hong Kong interpret measles as caused by 'womb poisoning' and respond with elaborate ritual avoidances for one hundred days, or when Bowen wrote in her classic *Return to Laughter* (1953) of a smallpox epidemic experienced as a pestilence of witchcraft by the Tiv, none objected to their use of the disease categories measles and smallpox without placing them in quotes." Local nuance will always be lost if you do not use local words. But if we only use local words, we foreclose cross-cultural comparison, and treat the reality of cultural difference as incommensurable ideational universes. Chiara Thumiger, a scholar of madness in classical antiquity, offers a useful set of four principles for cross-cultural comparison. She proposes that (1) the human mind is based in biology, so there is going to be some measure of universality because of our common inheritance as a species; (2) the mind, mental life, are not confined to the brain, but involve other parts of the body; (3) the mind is also always a product of culture, so one can expect cultural variability; and (4) there is an irreducible individual quality to every person (Thumiger 2017, 27–29).

Western medical traditions may have given depressive illness extraordinary attention compared to others. The sources for the diagnosis's fraught quality, though, may not lie solely in its Western history. They may also lie in a universal problem that depressive illness poses: its continuity with the normal experience of life. Depressive illness is illness of excess—excessive sadness, or sadness of excessive duration. In the absence of an objective marker for what is excessive, cultural differences become heavily freighted.

Identifying, and thus counting, incidence of depressive illness in Africa has, for all of these reasons, been a challenge. One measure of the challenge can be seen in the work of the Nigerian psychiatrist Thomas A. Lambo. After training in medicine and psychiatry in the United Kingdom, Lambo returned to develop psychiatric services in Nigeria and oversee the transformation of dismal, and purely custodial, colonial asylums into therapeutic hospitals (Sadowsky 1999; Heaton 2013). He also did pioneering research on culture and mental illness, and produced important critiques of colonial psychiatric theory (Lambo 1956).

Looking at Yoruba culture, Lambo articulated three distinct positions with regard to depression in the span of less than a decade. In a 1956 article, he joined with common colonial opinion in considering depression rare in Africa. He speculated that depression might reflect the effects of a repressed society, and that Africa was spared the affliction by having less repression (Lambo 1956). In 1960, however, Lambo proposed that depression was not so much rare in Africa as it was misdiagnosed with the label neurasthenia (Prince 1967). Coined in the nineteenth century by American neurologist George Beard, neurasthenia was a diagnostic category that had substantial symptom overlap with more recent conceptions of depression: including depressed mood, mania, anxiety, irritability, impaired intellect, indigestion, malnourishment, insomnia, weakness, nerve pain, loss of faith, and fear of poverty (Schuster 2011). Beard, however, considered neurasthenia an illness with physical origins that could have psychological effects, as opposed to a mental illness that could have physical effects. As his criticism of colonial psychiatry unfolded, Lambo began to wonder whether Western psychiatrists diagnosed neurasthenia in colonial Africa instead of depression because the psychiatrists did not think Africans had a lot of inner conflict—a capacity they considered particularly Western. Then, in the early 1960s, Lambo worked with an international team of researchers on the landmark study, *Psychiatric Disorder among the Yoruba* (Leighton et al. 1963). They compared Yoruba conceptions of mental illness, and their prevalence, with those in Western contexts. No Yoruba word translated exactly as depression. Many symptoms of depression, though, came up in Yoruba descriptions of distress. They included lost vitality, crying continuously, worry, diminished appetite, and lack of interest in life. The team left it an open question whether depression qualified as an illness state for the Yoruba. Yet they found depressive *symptoms* were at least as common in southwest Nigeria as in the Western context they used for comparison. Some later research in the region also considered the low diagnosis rates to be the result of failures to recognize differences in presentation (Olatuwara 1973).

Finding and Counting Depression: Colonial Legacies

As Lambo was one of the first to point out, diagnosis is a problem not just because of cultural difference but also because of politics and ideology. The colonial belief that depression was absent or rare in Africa frequently bumped into evidence that it might not be, or that there were at least alternative explanations for why it was not being seen. In order to account for any dissonance that might have ensued, colonial authors often engaged in what Barbara Fields and Karen Fields have called "racecraft" (Fields and Fields 2014). By analogy with E. E. Evans-Pritchard's analysis of witchcraft among the Azande, Fields and Fields show that racism can function as a deeply ingrained form of "common sense" that will be resistant to logic or evidence that contradicts it, causing the holder of the racist beliefs to go through mental gymnastics in order to preserve them.

In the case of depression, the idea that Africans might, as a "race," be immune is old, predating the colonial period. During the Atlantic slave trade, European slaveholders' stereotypes of carefree Africans extended to the ideas that they were immune to melancholy and other mental illness (Smith 2014, 32). These images survived despite slave owners and slave traders seeing that slavery could cause severe melancholy. On ships carrying enslaved people, slaveholders saw that even among captives in this most dismal of settings, some extreme cases of melancholy stood out, and they even sometimes took modest medical measures to address it (Mustakeem 2016, 115–17). The stereotype survived in racist North American science well into the twentieth century. A 1962 study of American Blacks and depression exemplifies racecraft at work. The study did not show lower rates of depression in Black people than white people but offered a number of possible reasons for why rates *might* be low among Black people. The authors argued that these speculations confirmed the premise that the rates were low—still without any evidence of lower rates (Prange and Vitols 1962).

Reports from colonial Africa reflected this discourse. T. Duncan Green-lees's 1895 report from South Africa found little depressive illness among South African Blacks, saying that depression was a disorder of the "higher and latest developed . . . strata . . . [of the] mental organism" (Greenlees 1895, 72). Geoffrey Tooth in the late-colonial Gold Coast and R. Cun-yngham Brown in 1930s Nigeria both also reported low rates of depression. As Heaton has pointed out, they conceded that the hospital setting was not where you were likely to find depression, but that concession did not stop them from explaining its low incidence with alleged inherent attributes in African people. Reporting from Tanganyika's Mirembe mental hospital in the late colonial period, Cyril G. F. Smartt wrote that "In the male African, a depressed mood contrasts sharply with his normal carefree, gay and ir-responsible attitude." Smartt also acknowledged, though, that the type of illness influenced treatment patterns: "it is often an anti-social episode that brings the patient into the hospital" (Smartt 1956, 453).

John C. Carothers probably gave colonial psychiatry its most notorious expression, in his characterization of the Mau Mau rebellion as a form of mass pathology, and his comparison of the normal African brain to that of a lobotomized European. With specific regard to depression, Carothers said it was rare in Africa because it was essentially an illness of remorse and Afri-cans did not have the sense of responsibility that would induce guilt (Caroth-ers 1953; Vaughan 1991). Notorious though he may be, Carothers's historical importance lies less in the virulence of his views than in the continuity of those views with those of his colleagues (McCulloch 1995; Sadowsky 1999).

The views of Carothers and his colleagues matter not only because of their typicality for their own time. Some of their assumptions survive in crude or subtle ways. For example, a relatively recent book not only de-scribes, but *defines* depression as a Western malady (Bell 2014). The trou-ble here lies beyond the identification of depression as Western, but in the explanation. Western culture, in this explanation, is characteristically intro-spective, and a propensity for looking inward is a necessary precondition for depressive illness. If there were any doubt that we are meant to see this as a cultural accomplishment, the explanation continues to explain that various non-Western cultures may be "great" in their own way but lack the "inte-riority" of the West. Such a claim for Western distinctiveness is extraor-dinary. Written in the early twenty-first century, and not during the high noon of colonialism, it depicts depression not simply as an illness, but also a capacity, a reflection of a special, culturally distinct ability. The argument is not supported with demonstration of any lack of introspection elsewhere.

Field's *Search for Security*, Prince's outlier study, documented numerous cases that Field considered as depression (Field 1960). Aware of the widespread colonial view that Africans did not get depression, Field made a vigorous and detailed rebuttal.

The people Field labeled as "depressed" were mostly women, and mostly self-accused witches. They had come to the shrine seeking spiritual relief. In exhaustive detail, Field recounted these women's stories, emphasizing how much their presentation resembled that of English depressives—deep sorrowfulness, insomnia, and lethargy, combined with somatic complaints that were not easily explained by purely physical problems. They did not go to physicians, because they understood their distress in the idiom of witchcraft. Field went so far as to argue (dubiously, in my opinion) that if there were no depression, there would be no witchcraft either. Field's argument can be summed up as: Africa has as much depression as anywhere else if you know where to look for it—and how to see it.

How to account for Field's different conclusions? Prince based his explanation on her catchment area. He thought Field's work stood out because she worked at a shrine, while the others worked at asylums. He had a point. Colonial asylums were not for therapy. They were more like prisons for the mad. People would be unlikely to bring someone to the asylum for extreme sadness or lack of interest in life. They were likely to bring someone who was a threat to public order. At a shrine like the one Field worked near, people might go voluntarily for help in distress. Field herself supported this interpretation, pointing out that women suffering in the ways she observed at the shrine were unlikely to be confined in asylums.

With a background in both psychiatry and anthropology, Field also had better training than the other colonial observers, who were mostly asylum administrators. But she also had a less distant relationship with the people about whom she wrote, which is mostly to say that she was interested in them and listened to what they had to say about themselves, instead of simply affixing a Western diagnostic label to them (though she did that, too).

That the women from the shrine were *self-accused* witches was key to Field's argument. They came to the shrine lamenting enormous damage they believed they had inflicted on their communities and loved ones. Field considered these claims of destructive behavior to be highly implausible— but also reminiscent of the equally unrealistic guilty ruminations of English depressives. On this point, Field differed significantly from the other colonial observers. Africans, in colonial psychiatric thought, were not only incapable of depression, but also of one of its signature symptoms: guilt.

Guilt: A Symptom as Cultural Capacity

In 1947, a Nigerian asylum inmate named Ruth was diagnosed with a case of melancholia with delusions and hallucinations.[9] If one wishes to translate this into contemporary psychiatric discourse, one could call it psychotic depression. As was often the case in colonial asylums, cultural differences might have emerged regarding the meaning and proper treatment of mental illness, but not necessarily regarding the presence of illness. In this case, her uncle, a Lagos policeman, acknowledged her illness, but sought her release so she could be cared for outside of the asylum (which at that time was providing little care at all). Ruth too seemed to acknowledge that she was ill. What were notably considered delusions featured an obsessive concern that she had inadequately placated deities, who she said were responsible for her madness. This was their retribution.

Guilty rumination is now considered a common part of the symptom profile of clinical depression. Whether guilt has always been a major feature in Western conceptions of melancholic or depressive illness is debated but, by the early twentieth century, it undoubtedly was, figuring prominently in descriptions by Pierre Janet and Emil Krapaelin. In Sigmund Freud's major work on depressive illness, guilt is not only a major feature, but the symptom that unravels the etiology of this puzzling ailment (Freud 2005). In much of the psychoanalytic tradition, depression was understood as "anger turned inward," characterized by guilty thoughts that originated in rageful feelings toward others, especially loved ones, which, because they were unacceptable, were unconsciously redirected at the self. Freud did not only think guilt was central to the pathology of depression. He also saw it as the price of the repression necessary for a "civilized" society. Guilt, then, was a cultural capacity. The idea that Western culture was particularly prone to guilt was given perhaps its most famous expression in Ruth Benedict's ([1946] 2005) distinction between Japanese "shame culture" and American "guilt cultures." Benedict scholars are divided over whether she was speaking merely of difference or erecting, at least implicitly, a hierarchy. But in colonial psychiatric thought about Africa and Africans, it was certainly used to refer to a capacity of "developed" peoples, and not of Africans. For Carothers, for example, the absence of depression in Africa was a function of the lack of guilt, which in turn depended on a sense of responsibility (Vaughan 1991).

Guilty obsessions were not just present in Field's cases, but nearly omnipresent. In the majority of the people Field considered "depressed" on the basis of other symptoms—such as frequent weeping, insomnia, and lethargy—guilty obsessions were also present. They were at fault, they said, for the death of all their deceased kin, blight on crops, and traffic accidents, for example. Field saw a similarity to patients she had seen in London hospitals, who were also convinced, without good reason, that they were guilty of terrible crimes. Smartt seems to have been on the verge of the same observation in Tanganyika, though he could not quite get there: "while guilt feelings and self-reproach were absent, a feeling of bewitchment was almost universal. . . . The depressives believed their bewitchment had been brought on by themselves, while the schizophrenics blamed others" (Smartt 1956, 453). Like the presence of depression, the presence of guilt as a symptom may depend on how you look for it, and what you call it when you see the signs. Perhaps we should speak of "idioms of guilt" as we do of "idioms of distress."

Fanon saw this as well. In *The Wretched of the Earth*, Fanon observed that his French colleagues thought that Algerians were not capable of melancholia since they claimed that "There is no inner life where the North African is concerned. On the contrary, the North African gets rid of his worries by throwing himself on the people who surround him. He does not analyze . . . by definition melancholia is an illness of the moral conscience." Their presuppositions presented French psychiatrists with a challenge when they encountered patients with depressive symptoms. In an act of racecraft, they rescued the presuppositions by diagnosing the patients with a "pseudo-melancholia" (Fanon 1963, 296–310; Schiesari 1992, 236).

Fanon's long-neglected clinical writings show that he saw psychiatry as a bridge discipline, and madness always as a problem with neurological, psychological, and social dimensions (Fanon 2019). As a clinician, Fanon engaged closely with patients. He belonged to a loose tradition that believed that psychiatric practice should consist not merely of affixing labels or subduing symptoms by physical means (though he was not opposed to the use of physical treatments to control symptoms). The patients, their life histories, and their subjectivity warrant careful attention. Jean Khalfa

(2019) argues that biological psychiatry flourished in colonies because it seemed to provide racism with a scientific backing. This had relevance to native criminality. Colonial psychiatry thought that failure to confess when presented with clear evidence of wrongdoing reflected a deep-seated constitutional primitivism. Fanon—who had, like Field, observed patients with guilty ruminations while training in Europe—thought that admission of guilt is a ritual of being reintegrated into a social context, a meaningless ritual if you do not see that context as your own, as in a colonial court.[10]

In *Search for Security*, Field wrote dismissively about the meaning of Ghanaian independence: "I have turned a deaf ear to those of my English friends who demand a chapter on Self-Government. They should know that rural people the world over—in Ghana no less than England—know little and care less about any political upheaval . . . drought and blight concern them, but the birth of nations goes unnoticed" (Field 1960, 3).

The contrast with Fanon could not be greater. Fanon was famed above all for his hopes for the liberatory potential of decolonization, not just in political and economic life, but for the transformation of consciousness— though he could also be presciently apprehensive about the decolonization's pitfalls and limitations. Other contrasts between Field and Fanon run deep: Field was a white woman, trained in medicine and psychiatry in the United Kingdom. Field showed little interest in psychoanalytic theory in her pursuits. That work was ethnographic research in a rural setting, in a nonsettler colony undergoing a relatively peaceful transition to independence. Fanon, meanwhile, was a Black man, trained in medicine and psychiatry in France; a clinician working in institutional contexts in North African cities, influenced by psychoanalytic thought; and a political theorist and activist working during one of the most violent anticolonial struggles. What united Field and Fanon, and led them to similar observations, was not their politics or their "subject position." The connection between them, and with Lambo, is that they listened carefully to their positions.

Conclusion

In my 1999 book *Imperial Bedlam*, I wrote that "The idea that what is mad in one culture might be sane in another has been exaggerated by proponents and understated by its critics. It is a debate that will continue to run into dead ends as long as the question is posed as an either-or" (Sadowsky 1999, 8).

That either-or, which I obviously believe to be a false choice, continues to inflect inquiry. Some work, for example, continues to stress that use of psychiatric labels outside their culture of origin is cultural imperialism, only.

That insistence may simplify things, but it is a reasonable reaction to the real problem of "DSM hegemony." Psychiatric diagnostic manuals *do* efface cultural specificity. Even including culture-bound syndromes in a manual, while better than failure to see cultural difference at all, amounts simultaneously to a canonization of the syndromes and a sequestering of cultural difference in a way that keeps it statically exotic. In *Imperial Bedlam*, I also wrote that "a psychiatric label can itself become a place of confinement," concealing "a vast archive containing densely textured and symbolically charged transcripts of political situations, cultural predicaments, and daily trials" (Sadowsky 1999, 96). Diagnosis, by itself is flattening and, at best, is inadequate. Neither Field's nor Fanon's clinical observations would have had much power if they had consisted simply of diagnostic labels. What made those labels intelligible, and useful to any extent that they were, was their respective deep immersion in the granular particularities of people in distress.

Malanda and Adichie's Ifemelu seem to imply that the medicalization of sadness reflects a flaw in Western culture, a view many internal critics of Western psychiatry echo. But Jadhav's description of depression as particularly "fraught" for cross-cultural study is a two-way warning, against both uncritical application of the label, and reflexive rejection of it. Would we not be remiss to deny treatments for someone with an infectious disease because local understandings of the etiology or symptoms differed from those of cosmopolitan medicine?

Diagnoses in psychiatry are always imperfect, including in their culture of origin (Callard 2014; Szmukler 2014). It does not follow that the diagnoses have no practical utility. They deserve continued scrutiny, but their categorical rejection is more a reflex than real scrutiny. The prevalence of depression cross-culturally remains a hard problem to resolve definitively. Broad statistical surveys, such as those provided by the WHO, should neither be accepted uncritically nor dismissed summarily. As we examine them, we need to remember that diagnostic labels have a political history. The application of Western nosology has been considered a colonial or neocolonial gesture. In the case of depression, though, *withholding* the diagnostic label was a colonial gesture.

Notes

Epigraphs: Margaret Field (1960, 157, 159, 162).

This chapter draws on and also expands on arguments in *The Empire of Depression: A New History* (Sadowsky 2020). The arguments here overlap with one made in the book, but there is research and detail in this chapter that is not in the book.

1   Thanks to Njambe Kimani for this reference. An autopsy revealed that Williams was suffering from a neurological condition, Lewy body dementia, while he had been diagnosed with Parkinson's disease when he was still alive.

2   Porter carefully distinguished between actual epidemiological changes associated with social changes such as urbanization and "diseases of civilization" as an ideological construct stemming from evolutionist assumptions in comparing human societies.

3   Heaton (2013) is a notable exception—probably in part because it is about postcolonial history.

4   Aro Mental Hospital Case File Pt. Opd. 68, 1955.

5   Tran (2016) found that in Vietnamese hospitals, patients are now coming in expecting and preferring a neurasthenia diagnosis, while the doctors believe they have depression. The patients prefer a diagnosis that is more physical, because they feel that it carries less stigma. The doctors prefer the depression diagnosis, in part because antidepressants give them a treatment.

6   This point is sometimes missed: "The difficulty for Kleinman and others of this postmodern and culture-bound perspective is that it now becomes unclear in what sense depression can meaningfully be said to exist at all. How can lower back pain be equated with sadness?" (Lawlor 2012, 199). Kleinman was exploring cultural translatability, which is the opposite of culture boundedness. And Kleinman's argument was not "postmodern" in any way I can see.

7   Prince says the concept of masked depression in Western psychiatry can be traced back to at least 1912.

8   Among Nicaraguan women, it refers to a syndrome with pain at the base of the skull, distinct from normal headache, caused by stressful life situations (Yarris 2011, 2014).

9   "Lunatics, General Matters Affecting," Nigerian National Archives, Ibadan, Comcol 1 735/s. 1, vol. 1, [1947], 406.

10 On guilty ruminations, see Fanon (2019, 82).

Sources

Archival Material

Aro Mental Hospital Archives, Abeokuta, Nigeria.
Nigerian National Archives, Ibadan, Nigeria.

Literature

Abas, Melanie A., and Jeremy C. Broadhead. 1997. "Depression and Anxiety among Women in an Urban Setting in Zimbabwe." *Psychological Medicine* 27:59–71.

Adichie, Chimamanda Ngozi. 2014. *Americanah*. London: HarperCollins.

American Psychiatric Association. 2013. *Diagnostic and Statistical Manual of Mental Disorders*. 5th ed. Washington, DC: American Psychiatric Association.

Behrouzan, Orkideh. 2016. *Prozak Diaries: Psychiatry and Generational Memory in Iran*. Stanford, CA: Stanford University Press.

Bell, Matthew. 2014. *Melancholia: The Western Malady*. Cambridge: Cambridge University Press.

Benedict, Ruth. (1946) 2005. *The Chrysanthemum and the Sword: Patterns in Japanese Culture*. New York: Mariner Books.

Callard, Felicity. 2014. "Psychiatric Diagnosis: The Indispensability of Ambivalence." *Journal of Medical Ethics* 40:526–30.

Carothers, John Colin. 1953. *The African Mind in Health and Disease*. Geneva: World Health Organization.

Cheung, Fanny M. 1982. "Psychological Symptoms among Chinese in Urban Hong Kong." *Social Science and Medicine* 16:1339–44.

Comaroff, Jean. 2003. "The Diseased Heart of Africa: Medicine, Colonialism, and the Black Body." In *Knowledge, Power, and Practice: The Anthropology of Medicine and Everyday Life*, edited by Shirley Lindenbaum and Margaret M. Lock, 305–29. Berkeley: University of California Press.

Den Hertog, Thijs N., Marije de Jong, A. J. van der Ham, Devon E. Hinton, and Ria Reis. 2016. "'Thinking a Lot' among the Khwe of South Africa: A Key Idiom of Personal and Interpersonal Distress." *Culture, Medicine, and Psychiatry* 40:383–403.

Dorwick, Christopher. 2013. "Depression as a Culture-Bound Syndrome: Implications for Primary Care." *British Journal of General Practice* 63, no. 610: 229–30.

Fanon, Frantz. 1963. *The Wretched of the Earth*. New York: Grove.

Fanon, Frantz. 2019. *The Psychiatric Writings from Alienation and Freedom*. Edited by Jean Khalfa and Robert J. C. Young. Translated by Steven Corcoran. London: Bloomsbury Academic.

Field, Margaret. 1960. *Search for Security: An Ethno-Psychiatric Study of Rural Ghana*. London: Northwestern University Press.

Fields, Barbara J., and Karen E. Fields. 2014. *Racecraft: The Soul of Inequality in American Life*. London: Verso.

Freud, Sigmund. 2005. "Mourning and Melancholia." In *On Murder, Mourning, and Melancholia*, translated by Shaun Whiteside. London: Penguin.

Good, Byron J., Mary-Jo DelVecchio Good, and Robert Moradi. 1985. "The Interpretation of Iranian Depressive Illness and Dysphoric Affect." In *Culture and Depression: Studies in the Anthropology and Cross-Cultural Psychiatry of Affect and Disorder*, edited by Arthur Kleinman and Byron J. Good, 369–428. Berkeley: University of California Press.

Greenlees, Thomas Duncan. 1895. "Insanity among the Natives of South Africa." *Journal of Mental Science* 41:71–78.

Heaton, Matthew M. 2013. *Black Skin, White Coats: Nigerian Psychiatrists, Decolonization, and the Globalization of Psychiatry*. Athens: Ohio University Press.

Jadhav, Sushrut. 2000. "The Cultural Construction of Western Depression." In *Anthropological Approaches to Psychological Medicine*, edited by Vieda Skultans and John Lee Cox, 41–65. Philadelphia: Jessica Kingsley.

Kaiser, Bonnie N., Emily E. Haroz, Brandon A. Kohrt, Paul A. Bolton, Judith K. Bass, and Devon E. Hinton. 2015. "'Thinking Too Much': A Systematic Review of a Common Idiom of Distress." *Social Science and Medicine* 147:170–83.

Kaiser, Bonnie N., Kristen E. McLean, Brandon A. Kohrt, Ashley K. Hagaman, Bradley H. Wagenaar, Nayla M. Khoury, and Hunter M. Keys. 2014. "*Reflechi Twòp*—Thinking Too Much: Description of a Cultural Syndrome in Haiti's Central Plateau." *Culture, Medicine, and Psychiatry* 38:448–72.

Kaiser, Bonnie N., and Lesley Jo Weaver. 2019. "Culture-Bound Syndromes, Idioms of Distress, and Cultural Concepts of Distress: New Directions in Psychological Anthropology." *Transcultural Psychiatry* 56, no. 2: 589–98.

Khalfa, Jean. 2019. Introduction to Frantz Fanon, *The Psychiatric Writings from Alienation and Freedom*, edited by Jean Khalfa and Robert J. C. Young, translated by Steven Corcoran, 28–31. London: Bloomsbury Academic.

Kleinman, Arthur. 1986. *Social Origins of Distress and Disease: Depression, Neurasthenia, and Pain in Modern China*. New Haven, CT: Yale University Press.

Kohrt, Brandon A., Emily Mendenhall, and Peter J. Brown. 2015. "Historical Background: Medical Anthropology and Global Mental Health." In *Global Mental Health: Anthropological Perspectives*, edited by Brandon A. Kohrt and Emily Mendenhall, 19–36. New York: Routledge.

Lambo, Thomas Adeoye. 1956. "Neuropsychiatric Observations in the Western Region of Nigeria." *British Medical Journal* 2, no. 5006: 1388–94.

Lawlor, Clark. 2012. *From Melancholia to Prozac: A History of Depression*. Oxford: Oxford University Press.

Leighton, Alexander Hamilton, Thomas Adeoye Lambo, Charles C. Hughes, Dorothea Cross Leighton, Jane M. Murphy, and David B. Macklin. 1963. *Psychiatric Disorder among the Yoruba*. Ithaca, NY: Cornell University Press.

Lutz, Catherine. 1985. "Depression and the Translation of Emotional Worlds." In *Culture and Depression: Studies in the Anthropology and Cross-Cultural Psychiatry of Affect and Disorder*, edited by Arthur Kleinman and Byron J. Good, 63–100. Berkeley: University of California Press.

Malanda, Ted. 2014. "How Depression Has Never Been an African Disease." *The Standard*, August 18, 2014. https://www.standardmedia.co.ke/entertainment/counties /article/2000131772/how-depression-has-never-been-an-african-disease.

McCulloch, Jock. 1995. *Colonial Psychiatry and the "African Mind."* Cambridge: Cambridge University Press.

Mendenhall, Emily, Rebecca Rinehart, Christine Musyimi, Edna Bosire, David Ndetei, and Victoria Mutiso. 2019. "An Ethnopsychology of Idioms of Distress in Urban Kenya." *Transcultural Psychiatry* 56, no. 4: 620–42.

Mills, China. 2014. *Decolonizing Global Mental Health: The Psychiatrization of the Majority World*. London: Routledge.

Mustakeem, Sowande M. 2016. *Slavery at Sea: Terror, Sex, and Sickness in the Middle Passage*. Urbana: University of Illinois Press.

Nichter, Mark. 1981. "Idioms of Distress: Alternatives in the Expression of Psychosocial Distress: A Case Study from South India." *Culture, Medicine, and Psychiatry* 5:379–408.

Nolan-Hoeksema, Susan. 1993. *Sex Differences in Depression*. Palo Alto, CA: Stanford University Press.

Obeyesekere, Gananath. 1985. "Depression, Buddhism and the Work of Culture in Sri Lanka." In *Culture and Depression: Studies in the Anthropology and Cross-Cultural Psychiatry of Affect and Disorder*, edited by Arthur Kleinman and Byron J. Good, 134–53. Berkeley: University of California Press.

Olatuwara, Michael O. 1973. "The Problem of Diagnosing Depression in Nigeria." *Psychopathologie africaine* 9:389–403.

Orley, John, and John K. Wing. 1979. "Psychiatric Disorders in Two African Villages." *Archives of General Psychiatry* 36:513–20.

Patel, Vikram, Essie Simunyu, and Fungisai Gwanzura. 1995. "*Kufungisisa* (Thinking Too Much): A Shona Idiom for Non-Psychotic Mental Illness." *Central African Journal of Medicine* 41, no. 7: 209–15.

Porter, Roy. 1993. "Diseases of Civilization." In *Companion Encyclopedia of the History of Medicine*, vol. 1, edited by William F. Bynum and Roy Porter, 611–26. London: Routledge.

Prange, Arthur J., and Mintauts M. Vitols. 1962. "Cultural Aspects of the Relatively Low Incidence of Depression in Southern Negroes." *International Journal of Social Psychiatry* 8, no. 2: 104–12.

Prince, Raymond. 1967. "The Changing Picture of Depressive Syndromes in Africa: Is It Fact or Diagnostic Fashion?" *Canadian Journal of African Studies* 1, no. 2: 177–92.

Pringle, Yolana. 2018. *Psychiatry and Decolonisation in Uganda*. London: Palgrave Macmillan.

Racy, John. 1980. "Somatization in Saudi Women: A Therapeutic Challenge." *British Journal of Psychiatry* 137:212–16.

Roberts, Samuel K. 2011. *Infectious Fear: Politics, Disease, and the Health Effects of Segregation*. Chapel Hill: University of North Carolina Press.

Sadowsky, Jonathan. 1999. *Imperial Bedlam: Institutions of Madness and Colonialism in Southwest Nigeria*. Berkeley: University of California Press.

Sadowsky, Jonathan. 2020. *The Empire of Depression: A New History*. Cambridge, UK: Polity.

Schiesari, Juliana. 1992. *The Gendering of Melancholia: Feminism, Psychoanalysis, and the Symbolics of Loss in Renaissance Literature*. Ithaca, NY: Cornell University Press.

Schuster, David G. 2011. *Neurasthenic Nation: America's Search for Health, Happiness, and Comfort, 1869–1920*. New Brunswick, NJ: Rutgers University Press.

Sethi, S., S. Nathawat, and S. C. Gupta. 1973. "Depression in India." *Journal of Social Psychology* 91:3–13.

Smartt, Cyril G. F. 1956. "Mental Maladjustment in the East African." *Journal of Mental Science* 428:441–66.

Smith, Leonard. 2014. *Insanity, Race, and Colonialism: Managing Mental Disorder in the Post-Emancipation Caribbean, 1838–1914*. London: Palgrave Macmillan.

Szmukler, George. 2014. "When Psychiatric Diagnosis Becomes an Overworked Tool." *Journal of Medical Ethics* 40, no. 8: 517–20.

Thumiger, Chiara. 2017. *A History of the Mind and Mental Health in Classical Greek Medical Thought*. Cambridge: Cambridge University Press.

Tran, Allen L. 2016. "Neurasthenia, Generalized Anxiety Disorder, and the Medicalization of Worry in a Vietnamese Psychiatric Hospital." *Medical Anthropology Quarterly* 31, no. 2: 198–217.

Tuchman, Arleen Marcia. 2020. *Diabetes: A History of Race and Disease*. New Haven, CT: Yale University Press.

Vaughan, Megan. 1991. *Curing Their Ills: Colonial Power and African Illness*. Stanford, CA: Stanford University Press.

Vaughan, Megan. 2010. "Suicide in Late Colonial Africa: The Evidence of Inquests from Nyasaland." *American Historical Review* 115, no. 2: 385–404.

Wailoo, Keith. 2009. *How Cancer Crossed the Color Line*. Oxford: Oxford University Press.

Watters, Ethan. 2010. *Crazy Like Us: The Globalization of the American Psyche*. New York: Free Press.

World Health Organization. 2017. "'Depression: Let's Talk' Says WHO, as Depression Tops List of Causes." March 30, 2017. http://www.who.int/mediacentre/news/releases/2017/world-health-day/en/.

Yarris, Kristin Elizabeth. 2011. "The Pain of 'Thinking Too Much': *Dolor de Cerebro* and the Embodiment of Social Hardship among Nicaraguan Women." *Ethos* 39, no. 2: 226–48.

Yarris, Kristin Elizabeth. 2014. "*'Pensando Mucho'* ('Thinking Too Much'): Embodied Distress among Grandmothers in Nicaraguan Transnational Families." *Culture, Medicine, and Psychiatry* 38:473–98.

Matthew M. Heaton

6

Rethinking Brain Fag Syndrome

Students, Symptoms, and a
Late Colonial Survey in Nigeria

One student complained of "bad sight."[1] Another worried about what "seems like a caterpillar . . . walking from one edge of my brain to the other."[2] Still another relayed a macabre "feeling of death at all times and thinking that this world is not the place for me,"[3] while another grumbled about a "serious headache" from being "hit with a cricket ball on bridge of nose."[4]

This strange list of seemingly unrelated maladies were all responses to the same question. In the spring of 1959, five prestigious secondary schools in southern Nigeria received a questionnaire seeking information about "symptoms associated with study" from Dr. Raymond Prince, a Canadian transcultural psychiatrist from McGill University, then conducting research as a visiting psychiatrist at the Aro Mental Hospital in Abeokuta. Concerned about the possibility of an epidemic of psychiatric disorders among Nigerian students, Prince sent the questionnaire as a means of ascertaining how widespread the symptoms he treated in clinical settings were within the general student population. Ultimately, after analyzing their responses to 844 completed and returned questionnaires, Prince concluded that Nigerian students were at a significant risk of developing "brain fag syndrome," a culture-bound syndrome that Prince coined to describe a constellation of symptoms, including crawling and burning sensations in the head and body, visual disturbances, fatigue, and an inability to comprehend the written word. All could become so severe as to incapacitate (Prince 1962, 198). Prince's publications of his findings in the early 1960s helped to cement brain fag syndrome as a culture-bound disorder in psychiatric circles, leading to its inclusion in the appendix of culture-bound syndromes in the fourth edition of the *Diagnostic and Statistical Manual of Mental Disorders* (American Psychiatric Association 1994, 846).

Prince, like other psychiatrists, pathologized Nigerian students as highly vulnerable to psychological disorder. Many psychiatrists have critiqued the nosology of brain fag syndrome since the 1970s yet have identified the symptoms as being related to generalized—not culturally bound—anxiety and depressive disorders (Anumonye 1973; Morakinyo 1980; Jegede 1983; Ayonrinde, Obuaya, and Adeyemi 2015). However, as the responses above demonstrate, the symptoms that students articulated in the questionnaires can be interpreted well beyond the narrow confines of brain fag syndrome as Prince understood it. Being hit by a cricket ball is hard to interpret as pathological. Bad eyesight might be related to some psychiatric conditions, but very possibly is not. While Prince chose to interpret all the expressed symptoms in relation to his discovery of brain fag syndrome, this chapter explores what other impressions students might have been communicating in their responses, based not so much on Prince's understanding of the questionnaire's purpose but on how it might have been interpreted by the students themselves. Using the original data from the 844 returned surveys, located in the Raymond Prince Papers in the Division of Social and Transcultural Psychiatry at McGill University, I offer here alternative interpretations of the students' responses following from hermeneutic insights found in African medical history and anthropology. While some responses lend themselves to biomedical interpretation, others open avenues toward vernacular understandings of illness and disease. Some answers align more with what Murray Last has described as a position of "not knowing," that is, divorced from categorization within a system of thought, or tied to a "non-system," evasion, or secrecy (Last 2007). I suggest that the diverse, discordant, and often confusing responses of these students might reflect a generalized "nervousness" that has been associated with (late) colonial settings like Nigeria: not necessarily pathological in a medical sense, but characterized by precarity, uncertainty, danger, and varying degrees of violence that students were navigating, perhaps on an everyday basis (Hunt 2016).

These interpretive strains overlap, and none necessarily occlude or invalidate the others. As Sally Swartz has noted, even those of us who study the structures and networks of psychiatric knowledge production critically do not do so any more objectively than the medical practitioners we critique. "Just as we dream up our patients," she says, "we dream up our archive, as we interact with it in order to create a narrative" (Swartz 2018, 294). This chapter traverses such an archival dreamscape: it begins with embodied, medicalized narratives of "brain fag syndrome" and ends more with a generalized, diffuse late colonial "nervousness." In the process, it seeks to disrupt the diagnostic category work that Prince imposed on his student subjects by interpreting the questionnaires through psychiatric and transcultural lenses. We can sense what Prince thought about the "Nigerian personalities" present in these questionnaires and what they were communicating. But what did the students themselves think they were saying? We cannot know with certainty, of course, but we can decenter medicalized and psychiatric narratives and engage with the "popular, the subaltern, and the insurgent" (see Hunt, introduction to this volume) as found in the language of these Nigerian students within this late colonial psychiatric archive.

A Questionnaire

Raymond Prince arrived in Nigeria in 1957 at an exciting and tumultuous time, with the country well on its way toward a path of constitutional reforms that would lead to full independence in 1960. The 1950s were an era of investment in public services and infrastructure in Nigeria, which saw massive growth and improvement in the realms of Western education and medicine. A further aspect of decolonization was the Africanization of the civil service and other professions, previously the purview of Europeans alone (Falola and Heaton 2008, 146–48). The political, economic, and social contexts of decolonization shaped the way that the Canadian psychiatrist viewed his Nigerian patients, especially as he articulated brain fag syndrome. By the late 1950s, the burnt-out Nigerian student had become something of a stereotype. In 1957, the Nigerian psychiatrist Thomas Adeoye Lambo had been commissioned by the government of Nigeria's Western Region to study the psychological problems faced by Nigerian students in the United Kingdom (Lambo 1958). The symptoms of brain fag were widely recognized in Nigeria prior to Prince's arrival. As he noted, "one medical officer remarked to me, 'if a young man comes in with glasses and European dress, you may be sure that he will complain of burning in his head and inability to read'" (Prince 1960, 559). The nomenclature that Prince adopted—"brain fag"— was a term that Nigerian students had used to describe the symptoms they associated with mental fatigue. Prince believed brain fag to be a new culture-bound syndrome, potentially unique to the psychological conflicts of, so he said, the innately collectivistic "Nigerian personality" struggling to adapt to "the circumstances of prolonged isolated book learning and the intense individual responsibility-in-isolation inherent in the western type of 'examination' system" (Prince 1960, 568). Prince's brain fag syndrome was a rejection of "modern" European education by "traditional" African minds, an idea that had significant purchase in colonial ethnopsychiatry since at least the 1930s (Carothers 1953; Field 1960; McCulloch 1995; Heaton 2013).

Intrigued by the possibility that brain fag might be an occupational hazard for Nigerian students, Prince hastily crafted his questionnaire probing the potential prevalence of brain fag symptoms in a general population of students. Prince mailed the questionnaire to six all-male secondary schools in southern Nigeria, receiving cooperation from five. Two of the schools (King's College, Lagos, and Government College, Ibadan) were located in Nigeria's Western Region, and two (Government College, Umuahia, and Hope Waddell Institute, Calabar) were situated in the Eastern Region. It is not clear what the fifth school was: Prince did not identify it by name in his article, nor was it clearly identified in his notes. The age range of the respondents was between thirteen and twenty-one years. Ethnic affiliations were widespread, but the majority of respondents from schools in the Western Region were Yoruba, and most Igbo were undergoing schooling in the Eastern Region. Class markers are difficult to assay from the surveys. The most likely indicators would be parental occupation and literacy rates. However, answers to these questions would not necessarily convey class status in 1950s Nigeria. A student who identified his father as a "trader" or "farmer" might be relatively poor or quite wealthy, depending on the nature and scope of the activities. Parental literacy would indicate some level

It has been found that many students suffer to a greater or lesser extent from certain symptoms of a nervous nature which interfere with or are related to study and reading.

We are at present carrying out some research on the nature and causes of this disturbance with a view to obtaining some understanding of it and arriving at suitable treatment or preventive measures. It is of importance to determine how prevalent in the student population these symptoms are and we are therefore asking you to complete this questionnaire as completely and as accurately as possible to assist us in this study. The student is asked to complete the questionnaire whether he has suffered the symptoms or not.

1. Age *16 yrs 7 months*   2. Sex *MALE*

3. Tribe *SCOTTISH/YORUBA* 4. Father's Occupation *MEDICAL PRACTITIONER*

5. Mother's Occupation *Staff Nurse S.R.N .S.C.M*

6. Information about Brothers and Sisters (Same father)

Indicate whether same or different mother.	Age	Class at School	Progress at School (Good, above average, or below average)
Different	*24*	*Pharmacist just qualified*	*Good*

7. Have you ever suffered from burning or pain or other sensation in the head associated with reading or study ?
   YES _____ NO *NO*

8. Have you suffered any other unpleasant body sensations or mental difficulties that appeared to be related to study ? If so, please list them.

   NONE

9. Would you estimate the average ammount of time you spend in study (apart from lectures) *½* hour/ per day.

10. Are you satisfied with your general efficiency and retentiveness in study ? (Please check appropriate opinion)

    (a) Fully satisfied _____
    (b) Moderately Satisfied ____*✓*____ *MODERATELY SATISFIED*
    (c) Not satisfied _____

11. Do any of your brothers and sisters or your parents suffer from such symptoms associated with study ? *NO* If so please check the appropriate family member under item 4, 5 or 6 above.

6.1 Typical response by sixteen-year-old Scottish-Yoruba student in Raymond Prince's 1959 survey of Nigerian students. (Prince Papers, Division of Social and Transcultural Psychiatry, McGill University. Photograph by Todd Meyers.)

of intergenerational privilege, but many illiterate parents could have held positions of high status in their communities.

The questionnaire began by providing a significant amount of information about the nature of the study. Prince explained his purpose at the outset:

> It has been found that many students suffer to a greater or lesser extent from certain symptoms of a nervous nature which interfere with or are related to study and reading. We are at present carrying out some research on the nature and causes of this disturbance with a view to obtaining some understanding of it and arriving at suitable treatment or preventive measures. It is important to determine how prevalent in the student population these symptoms are and are therefore asking you to complete this questionnaire as completely and as accurately as possible to assist us in this study. The student is asked to complete the questionnaire whether he has suffered the symptoms or not.[5]

The questionnaire then asked for basic demographic information: age, sex, "tribe," parental occupations, and the number of siblings and their respective levels of education.

Next, the questionnaire prompted students about the primary symptoms that Prince had identified, asking if they "ever suffered from burning or pain or other sensation in the head associated with reading or study." The next question asked if the student had "suffered any other unpleasant body sensations or mental difficulties that appeared to be related to study"[6] and prodded the student to describe the nature of symptoms. This question stimulated qualitative descriptions of symptoms expressed in students' own words. Finally, the questionnaire asked students to estimate how much time they spent daily studying outside of class, and to rate their satisfaction with their studies on a scale of fully, moderately, or not satisfied.

Historians have long recognized the methodological complexity of using primary documents produced by psychiatrists, medical personnel, and other authority figures for understanding patient perspectives on mental illness and its treatment. The psychiatric case history has received a great deal of analysis from scholars in the medical humanities. Historians have deconstructed these texts layered with multiple perspectives and produced within the context of biomedical power structures (Berkenkotter 2008;

Jones, Rahman, and Everitt 2012; Schöhl and Hess 2019). Court records (Sadowsky 1996), media and literary representations (Gilman 1985), and the writings and artwork of mentally ill individuals (Hornstein 2017) have been analyzed in terms of constructions of mental illness by medical and legal authorities, as well as in terms of the negotiation and assimilation of and resistance to psychiatric categories with social consequences for patients. These scholarly efforts to parse the archival record recognize the limitations such sources pose for understanding mental illness and the experiences of psychiatric subjects (Swartz 2018).

In many ways, Prince's brain fag questionnaire is similar to other sources of psychological knowledge in terms of its assumptions and intended purpose. A medical authority created the questionnaire. Prince, driven by a desire to learn specific information related to the mental state of subjects (the respondents), construed his work as a way to achieve an accounting of symptoms. However, the questionnaire was unique in important ways. Significantly, medical personnel did not administer the questionnaires to patients. Rather, teachers and other school staff gave them to the students to fill out. Also, the questionnaire made no effort to contextualize symptoms for the respondents, though Prince's published articles on brain fag ultimately did so. As a result, the raw data remains intact: it may be accessed and interpreted separately from Prince's narratives and assumptions.

However, the uniqueness of these questionnaires carries methodological caveats. The structure of the questionnaire suggested to respondents the kinds of answers being sought. On the one hand, the questionnaire identified particular types of symptoms as appropriate answers to the questions. Some of Prince's colleagues criticized the project on these grounds. By telling students it was studying particular somatic complaints, the survey might have "reminded" students of symptoms they otherwise would not have thought significant or suggested that the "right" answers to questions were affirmative and that good students would provide useful information. In response to a letter from an unidentified colleague (found in the Prince Papers), this transcultural psychiatrist admitted that "your criticism of the questionnaire is justified re: the leading questions, etc. It may be that I suggested the symptoms to the students."[7] In his memoir, Prince noted that the principal of University College, Ibadan, declined to have his students participate out of concern that such a questionnaire might create the very syndrome it was attempting to study. Prince lamented this critical response as "disappointing" and attributed it to the discontent of this principal who, he added, was "an Englishman, not a Yoruba man" (Prince 2010, 251). Prince also admitted that he "should have formulated some of the questions more precisely" (Prince 2010, 249).

Despite the questionnaire providing direct commentary from the student population, the responses were shaped in ways that remain impossible to fathom. The questionnaires were not administered in a clinical setting but were carried out in an institutional environment: secondary schools. Teachers administered the survey, but the questionnaire offered no instructions on how to fill in the blanks or mark the boxes. It also placed no parameters or restrictions on what students might consider a symptom in the qualitative response section. Thus, while the questionnaire offered students a level of freedom to articulate highly individualized responses, the students were aware that their teachers and administrators might see their responses. It is clear that some administrators reviewed the contents of the questionnaires before returning them to Prince. Some questionnaires have handwriting from multiple people written on them, whether correcting spelling mistakes or adding omitted information about a student's family. The exact circumstances under which third parties modified answers are not clear, but the questionnaires clearly were not confidential. Nor were they anonymous: some respondents wrote their full names at the top, despite no textual prompting to do so. There may have been oral instructions to do so, of course. We will never know the exact circumstances by which the questionnaire was administered or its influence on student responses. Still, these aspects are important for comprehending how students commented on matters of context and environment, as we will see. Between the psychiatrist's explicit suggestions and school administrators' role in administering the questionnaires, students' responses were neither unmediated nor entirely unconstrained.

Student Responses

While all students ultimately answered the same questionnaire with the same questions, each did so in his own way, with his own understanding about what those questions were asking of him, his own motivations for responding, and his own concerns about what the potential consequences of his answers might be. Nevertheless, we can read their responses in ways that reveal the complex variety of meanings that may have emerged from such a coherent but fragmented set of voices.

One lens through which we can interpret the responses is in relation to what they suggest about medical practices in late colonial Nigeria. The history and anthropology of medicine in Africa has for decades concerned itself with studying vernacular healing ideas and practices. Janzen's (1978) study of communities of care in the lower Congo showed that kin were key in organizing the healing itineraries of afflicted relatives. His work began with an epistemological approach, continued by others, of studying healing as socially embedded, dynamic, and porous, thus central to the mixed and overlapping therapeutic landscapes found across the continent from well before the time that biomedicine arrived. Vernacular healing had long been recognized but was often characterized as religious, thus implying little efficacy. Vernacular healing has been a prime realm alongside biomedicine, a realm where African practices overlap with European ones and can be co-opted or explained in Western terms (Hunt 2013). In brain fag research, Prince was attempting to take vernacular speech about symptoms as articulated by "modern" students (who likely imagined themselves as separated from traditional or vernacular stances) and mold their words into a syndrome whose etiology could be understood in terms of European psychiatric knowledge. But a good number of their responses might be read as oblique references to common or popular ideas in southern Nigeria, and many of these did not necessarily lend themselves well to a psychiatric diagnosis or interpretation.

A few qualitative responses articulated symptoms in biomedical terms. A couple of respondents identified psychological symptoms in European terminology, such as "nervousness"[8] or "general depression"[9] and a good many more wrote about physical conditions in biomedical terms, such as "catarrh,"[10] "piles,"[11] or sensations in the "medulla oblongata."[12] And many of the described symptoms fit neatly into Prince's profile for brain fag syndrome. One student noted that he "fainted [in] 1955 and this was at the time that we were preparing for the school promotion examination" and that he had "declined right from that incidence."[13] A couple even wrote "brain fatigue"[14] in the qualitative symptom section.

Other responses seem more open to interpretation now. Let's return to the response found at the beginning of this chapter: "feeling of death at all times and thinking that this world is not the place for me."[15] While it might seem reasonable to interpret this response as a form of suicidal ideation, it

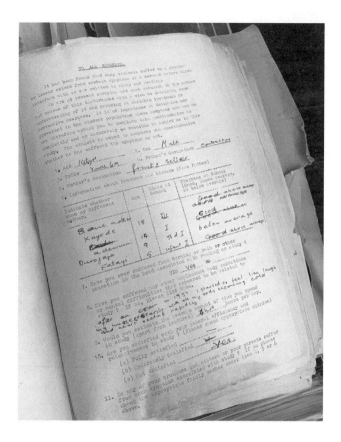

6.2 Response by fourteen-year-old with giddiness in Raymond Prince's 1959 survey of Nigerian students. (Prince Papers, Division of Social and Transcultural Psychiatry, McGill University. Photograph by Todd Meyers.)

could just as easily be a reference to southern Nigerian ideas about spirit children known as *abiku* (Yoruba) or *ogbanje* (Igbo), characterized by dying and being reborn by the same mother multiple times. Abiku children are believed to be denizens of the spirit world, continually drawn back to it even while living in the visible, human realm. They are often ambivalent about life and are often coddled as a means of convincing them to stay in this world. While abiku is associated with children who die before puberty, usually of an ambiguous illness, some abiku choose to remain in the world and live full lives. The response given by this student does not indicate whether he was considered an abiku child, but the characterization of "thinking that this world is not the place for me" lends itself as much to a vernacular as a psychiatric interpretation.

In a similar vein, the symptom—"a caterpillar . . . walking from one edge of my brain to the other"[16]—lends itself to being interpreted as a vernacular clue. The comment appears to be employing a simile to approximate a neurological sensation, as part of a biomedical framework. This comment seems to confirm Prince's primary symptoms of brain fag, which emphasized somatic complaints about itching and burning sensations in the body. However, complaints about "caterpillars" crawling in the body evoke widely held Yoruba ideas about illnesses caused by tiny creatures called *aràn*, a "worm, bug or relatively unformed organism" (Makanjuola 1987, 231). The consensus is that aràn are usually, but not always, the result of supernatural powers turned against a victim. When the aràn first enters the body through an orifice, it is extremely small but then migrates and grows inside the body to wreak havoc there. Several different types of aràn are thought to cause infertility in women, while others are associated with mental illness. For example, *odẹ orí* is a form of Yoruba madness believed to be caused by an *aràn*. Symptoms of ode orí include but are not limited to "a sensation of an organism crawling through the head and sometimes also other parts of the body, noises in the ears and palpitations" (Makanjuola 1987, 231). While the symptom profiles of brain fag and ode orí overlap, the idea of a caterpillar crawling across the brain works as a biomedical symptom only in metaphorical terms: it is intelligible in its literal form as a Yoruba cultural idiom. It would seem that either way, the student was expressing concerns about mental health in ways that the abiku example might not, but he was doing so in ways that might not translate as neatly into biomedical terms as it might appear at first blush. Interestingly, the Nigerian psychiatrist Roger Makanjuola found in his study from the 1980s that thirty patients easily diagnosed with ode orí by Yoruba healers had received ten different diagnoses from psychiatrists, and that those treated for ode orí saw much greater improvement than those receiving psychiatric treatment (Makanjuola 1987; Heaton 2013).

Such an analytical framework assumes pluralism within medical systems. The students likely had varying levels of knowledge about, or identifications with, such a range of therapeutic options. It is also possible that a relatively large number of students had little direct knowledge of any particular therapeutic system nor, relatedly, any interest in divulging personal information to an unidentified inquirer about their subjective psychological states. In addition to the declared assertions in the questionnaire responses, there is a good deal of "not knowing" suggested by the questionnaires. I take the concept of not knowing from Murray Last's influential essay on this subject. His purpose was to demonstrate the relatively unsystematic ways in which "traditional medicine" was practiced in northern Nigeria as a "non-system." Last's point was that such a medical culture does not require a coherent "system" of beliefs and practices openly shared and valued by practitioners and patients, since secrecy and hiding may also be important. For Last, medical "systems" of knowledge are found in biomedicine, in Islamic medicine, and within structural, political, economic, and social processes, as well as by the ontologies underlying them. I focus on the evidential basis that forms the foundation of this argument: Last's provocation that "every investigator has received the answer 'don't know' and has been unsure whether the answer was the truth or simply a snub" (Last 2007, 1). The prevalence of negative responses results in researchers privileging information gleaned from informants who claim to know and are willing to share it, bringing into focus elements of a "system" that might not be recognizable or meaningful to those engaging it.

To assess the brain fag questionnaires as examples of "not knowing" that open up interpretive categories, let us do a quick quantitative summary. Prince claimed in his publication of findings that the most common symptoms reported in the questionnaires were:

Head complaints alone: 138
Eye complaints alone: 31
Intellectual complaints alone: 41
Head and eye: 71
Head and intellect: 44
Other complaints: 133

These numbers gave Prince a grand total of 458 (of 844) students identifying symptoms. With this, he reached his conclusion that 54 percent of students complained of "symptoms associated with study" (Prince 1962, 201). If we remove the 133 "other complaints," only 38 percent identified symptoms that might fall under the rubric of brain fag syndrome as developed by Prince. Absent from his analysis was any recognition that the most common single response category was *no reported symptoms at all*, even though this category accounted for 46 percent of the returned questionnaires.

How are we to read the negatives? It is probable that many students did not find any relevant symptoms and that their responses were honest engagements with the exercise. There are, however, inklings of other possible interpretations. Some students did not identify specific symptoms, but still used the space provided to communicate. They wrote things like "No!"[17] and "Please, no,"[18] emphatically marking up the survey. Such marks could be benign, but could also indicate some level of resistance, fear, or discomfort with the nature of the question. Rather than consider the survey's implications, some students may have protested too much.

Some reported no symptoms but still struggled with how to answer the question. In a number of questionnaires, there are multiple marks, as though the student himself was unsure whether or not he had experienced these symptoms. In one survey, we can see that a student had crossed out both "yes" and "no" in response to the quantitative question before writing "No" in the box next to the negative response option.[19] In another, the student crossed out both "yes" and "no," then wrote both "yes" and "no" in the respective boxes next to the original, struck-through text, and later crossed out the handwritten responses before finally rewriting "no" as the apparent final response.[20] In these cases, students seem to have been communicating, perhaps unintentionally, that they really did not know if they had experienced the symptoms in question.

Finally, a number of students who answered positively may still have been expressing uncertainty or discomfort with how to characterize symptoms. One respondent, for example, noted that his only symptom was "just general bodily weakness especially in the morning, but I am not quite sure it's due to study."[21] Another claimed to have a condition whose symptoms he did not specify, but clarified that "the doctor calls it mental disorder."[22] The phrasing is intriguing. On the one hand, the student was confirming that he had symptoms classifiable as pathological within biomedicine. On the other hand, the ascription of the diagnosis by the doctor suggests the possibility that the student perhaps did not accept the diagnosis. The vagueness of calling it "mental disorder" suggests Last's language for "not knowing" beside an informant who did not know, did not want to know, or did not want to share.

The majority of survey responses seem to have been articulating something phenomenological, albeit with varying levels of certainty about how to categorize their experiences. Questions of what constitutes a symptom abound in the student responses. Part of the confusion may have lain in the phrasing of the question, which asked students if they had "ever suffered any other unpleasant body sensations or mental difficulties that appeared to be related to study."[23] The question was sufficiently vague to allow for a wide range of responses. The qualifier "ever" allowed respondents to reminisce about any instance of discomfort that might or might not have happened in indirect relation to their educational pursuits. Furthermore, the separation of mental and physical symptoms allowed respondents to identify a wide range of bodily pains and psychological responses. The relationship to studying was subjective, and it is unclear in many responses whether students actively considered their symptoms to be caused or exacerbated by study routines as opposed to preexisting symptoms that may or may not have affected their studies.

Take the single most commonly occurring symptom described by the students: eyestrain. According to Prince's computations, more than one hundred respondents complained of vision problems. Often, their complaints were associated with physical symptoms, such as head or body aches, or with mental concerns like an inability to concentrate or comprehend. But the context of the vision problems was usually absent, even when accompanied by other symptoms in the questionnaires. Usually, the respondent wrote something general like "eye strain" or "bad sight." It is difficult to know whether the vision problems were physical or psychological, whether they predated the student's educational pursuits, or whether the student experienced vision problems in everyday life outside his studies. It is clear that at least some of the respondents experienced eyestrain as a result of prolonged reading. "Eyes always red after study,"[24] declared one respondent, while another noted, "I always [have a] headache when I read for more than three hours."[25] While these symptoms were articulated as being related to study, they could be read as physiological responses to a task at hand: symptoms that most respondents likely experienced, but not all disclosed.

Students identified a variety of other symptoms—like eyestrain—that might be more appropriately identified as experiences that accompanied studying rather than symptoms of studying. One student noted that he became "hungry after reading for a long time,"[26] while another proclaimed that he occasionally felt dizzy "after break when I am hungry if I don't eat during break."[27] Others had medical conditions that they chose to disclose as symptoms, such as cough, piles, "dizziness occasionally after reading,"[28]

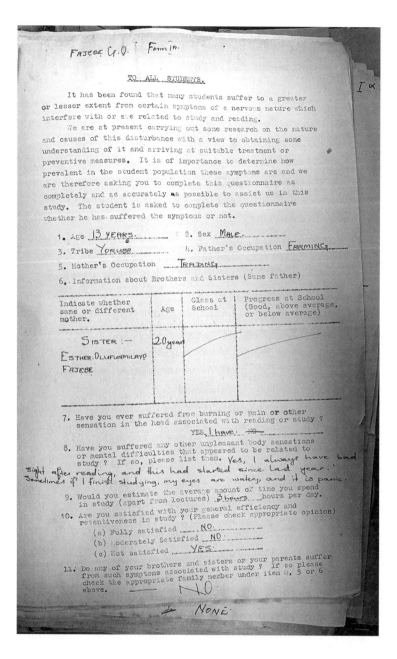

FAJEBE G.O. Form IA.

I ∝

TO ALL STUDENTS.

It has been found that many students suffer to a greater or lesser extent from certain symptoms of a nervous nature which interfere with or are related to study and reading.

We are at present carrying out some research on the nature and causes of this disturbance with a view to obtaining some understanding of it and arriving at suitable treatment or preventive measures. It is of importance to determine how prevalent in the student population these symptoms are and we are therefore asking you to complete this questionnaire as completely and as accurately as possible to assist us in this study. The student is asked to complete the questionnaire whether he has suffered the symptoms or not.

1. Age 13 YEARS.   2. Sex MALE.

3. Tribe YORUBA   4. Father's Occupation FARMING

5. Mother's Occupation TRADING

6. Information about Brothers and Sisters (Same father)

Indicate whether same or different mother.	Age	Class at School	Progress at School (Good, above average, or below average)
SISTER :— ESTHER.OLUFUNMILAYO FAJEBE	20years		

7. Have you ever suffered from burning or pain or other sensation in the head associated with reading or study ?
   YES, I have. ~~no~~

8. Have you suffered any other unpleasant body sensations or mental difficulties that appeared to be related to study ? If so, please list them. Yes, I always have bad sight after reading, and this had started since last year. Sometimes if I finish studying, my eyes are watery, and it is panic.

9. Would you estimate the average amount of time you spend in study (apart from lectures) 3 hours hours per day.

10. Are you satisfied with your general efficiency and retentiveness in study ? (Please check appropriate opinion)
    (a) Fully satisfied   NO.
    (b) Moderately Satisfied NO.
    (c) Not satisfied   YES.

11. Do any of your brothers and sisters or your parents suffer from such symptoms associated with study ? If so please check the appropriate family member under item 4, 5 or 6 above.   NO

    ⊥ NONE

6.3   "Bad sight" as a reported symptom in Raymond Prince's 1959 survey of Nigerian students. (Prince Papers, Division of Social and Transcultural Psychiatry, McGill University. Photograph by Todd Meyers.)

and a variety of other problems that caused discomfort. Yet the respondents did not offer any indication that these symptoms were linked with their studies. Some complained of bodily pains that affected their studying but were not caused by study. "Have a fractured knee which does not allow me to sit for long without pain," lamented one.[29] In these cases, it seems as if students' primary concerns lay with the ways that their physical and mental states affected their studies, rather than the other way around.

In keeping with the emphasis on academic performance, many expressed anxiety about their limited attention spans and intellectual capacities, and the effect they believed these aspects had on their overall performance. Respondents complained frequently of diminished cognition, claiming, "I sometimes read without knowing what I have read."[30] However, respondents offered some context for their comprehension failures, noting a lack of concentration and motivation. One student declared that his main symptom was that "after working problems for about 30 minutes I find that I can't work anymore,"[31] while another admitted that he "get[s] bored after a few hours reading" and had "difficulties in things dealing with figures."[32] One noted: "I can't concentrate well in the afternoon. But read well in the night."[33] Another confessed: "Very immoral things disturb my studies. These result in academic disturbances."[34]

These responses are a stark reminder that all who answered these questionnaires were adolescent youth navigating the physiological and psychological difficulties of that life stage. Only in rare instances did students connect their inability to focus with concerns about mental health. One student noted that he suffered from "general depression."[35] But many students with cognitive symptoms seem to have been concerned about their inability to study intensely and tirelessly.

Colonial Education and Nervousness

This chapter examines the limitations of the questionnaire as well as ways of interpreting student responses. Student efforts to grapple with the nature of their "symptoms" surely related to their environments, too. As Prince noted in his publication of findings, only 12 percent of the respondents indicated that they were "fully satisfied" with their academic performance, with 30 percent indicating that they were "not satisfied." The unanswerable question is whether their dissatisfaction had endogenous or exogenous roots.

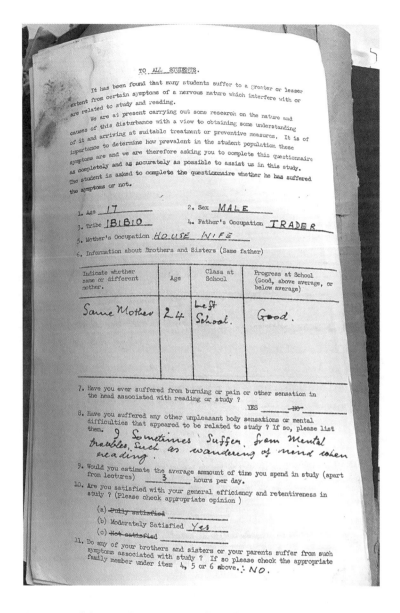

It has been found that many students suffer to a greater or lesser extent from certain symptoms of a nervous nature which interfere with or are related to study and reading.

We are at present carrying out some research on the nature and causes of this disturbance with a view to obtaining some understanding of it and arriving at suitable treatment or preventive measures. It is of importance to determine how prevalent in the student population these symptoms are and we are therefore asking you to complete this questionnaire as completely and as accurately as possible to assist us in this study. The student is asked to complete the questionnaire whether he has suffered the symptoms or not.

1. Age __17__   2. Sex __MALE__

3. Tribe __IBIBIO__   4. Father's Occupation __TRADER__

5. Mother's Occupation __HOUSE WIFE__

6. Information about Brothers and Sisters (Same father)

Indicate whether same or different mother.	Age	Class at School	Progress at School (Good, above average, or below average)
Same Mother	24	Left School.	Good.

7. Have you ever suffered from burning or pain or other sensation in the head associated with reading or study ?
   YES _____   NO _____

8. Have you suffered any other unpleasant body sensations or mental difficulties that appeared to be related to study ? If so, please list them. I Sometimes Suffer from Mental troubles, Such as wandering of mind when reading.

9. Would you estimate the average amount of time you spend in study (apart from lectures) __3__ hours per day.

10. Are you satisfied with your general efficiency and retentiveness in study ? (Please check appropriate opinion)
    (a) ~~Fully satisfied~~ _____
    (b) Moderately Satisfied __Yes__
    (c) ~~Not satisfied~~ _____

11. Do any of your brothers and sisters or your parents suffer from such symptoms associated with study ? If so please check the appropriate family member under item 4, 5 or 6 above. NO.

6.4   An Ibibio youth reporting on "wandering of mind when reading." Original response in Raymond Prince's 1959 survey of Nigerian students. (Division of Social and Transcultural Psychiatry, McGill University. Photograph by Todd Meyers.)

Were they unsatisfied with their performance in relationship to their surroundings, or their surroundings' performance?

Here I quote from the questionnaires in order to consider the context of late colonial education in Nigeria and the ways it provoked disquiet, doubt, and reservations, feelings implicit in many student responses to Prince's inquiry. Nancy Rose Hunt has urged for considering colonial milieus in relation to "nervousness." Distinct from anxiety as an embodied, clinical state, "nervousness" suggests a "kind of energy, taut and excitable," that semantically combines "vigor, force, and determination with excitation, weakness, timidity." It can be applied to "corporeal systems, historical epochs, nations, bodies, dispositions, and moods" (Hunt 2016, 5). To bring nervousness into this specific Nigerian milieu, it is helpful to turn to Chinua Achebe's classic novel *No Longer at Ease*, in which recent university graduate Obi Okonkwo struggles and fails to negotiate the inscrutable and bafflingly unscrupulous social environment of Nigeria, at almost exactly the time when Prince was sending out his questionnaires (Achebe 1960). Obi Okonkwo is intelligent, capable, upright (initially), and self-possessed, and yet he cannot maintain these traits while navigating the conditions of his life. In *No Longer at Ease*, Achebe illustrates the kind of "nervousness" described by Hunt: not embodied pathology, but a pervasive social mood of ambiguity. Achebe was a 1945 graduate of Government College, Umuahia, one of the schools to which Prince sent his brain fag questionnaire fourteen years later (Achebe 2009; Ochiagha 2015).

All of the secondary schools that Prince targeted with his questionnaire were extremely prestigious, among the oldest and best regarded in Nigeria, known for replicating the British education system and preparing students for success in the colonial system. Students from these schools could expect to have a reasonably good chance of going on to university in the United Kingdom or, after 1948, at the University of Ibadan, Nigeria's first degree-granting institution. The stakes were high for students at these schools. The pressure to succeed was real, and the stress that accompanied the expectations of family, friends, and entire communities was taxing for many students who felt the weight of the world on their shoulders, like their fictional archetype, Obi Okonkwo. Indeed, this stress was one of the primary factors that Lambo identified as contributing to Nigerian students' breakdowns in the United Kingdom in his government-commissioned report (Lambo 1958).

But beyond the educational pressures, much more was surely happening in these schools that could affect student well-being, not their studies

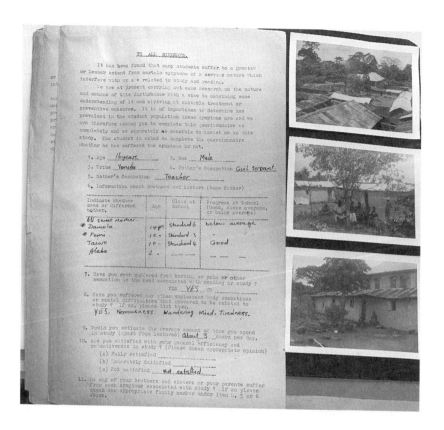

6.5 A rare survey mention of a symptom: "nervousness." Original response in Raymond Prince's 1959 survey of Nigerian students. (Division of Social and Transcultural Psychiatry, McGill University. Photograph by Todd Meyers.)

alone. All of the schools represented in the questionnaire responses were boarding schools. These adolescent male youth learned and lived on the campus. They stayed away from their families for long periods of time during the terms and were at the mercy of the school staff—not only for their education, but also for their personal development, well-being, and physical safety. The experiences that students had at the schools certainly affected them in positive and negative ways. But these experiences encompassed far more than classroom activities. They encompassed the entirety of adolescence. The everyday cultures and experiences of living in these educational environments should be considered in assessing how students interpreted "symptoms associated with study."

Achebe's alma mater provides a space to consider the contexts of "nervousness" navigated by these students. Government College, Umuahia achieved legendary status in postindependence Nigeria as the breeding ground for a disproportionate number of Nigeria's most renowned writers, artists, and public figures. In addition to Achebe, the school produced the novelists Elechi Amadi and Chukwuemeka Ike; the poet Christopher Okigbo; the painter Ben Enwonwu; and the writer, producer, governor, and political activist Ken Saro-Wiwa, among many others. Several prominent alumni wrote memoirs about their times at Umuahia. Even Achebe has written about his time at Umuahia (Achebe 2009). So too has Saburi Biobaku, one of the first Nigerians to join the faculty of the school in the late 1940s (Biobaku 1992). Chike Momah recounted his time at the school in a thinly veiled novelization from the same period (Momah 2003). While none of these memoirs specifically overlap with the time during which Prince distributed his questionnaire, they reveal manifold senses of the ambiguity of the colonial boarding school experience as well as the trauma it could produce.

All of the memoirs about Government College, Umuahia, emphasize the school's rigorous academics, the intense competition among students, and the strict discipline. The pressure that students and teachers felt in trying to succeed and maintain the school's high reputation is palpable. In some respects, these narratives reinforce Prince's notion that the educational experience might have been too much for many students to negotiate. However, they also demonstrate that there were other more personal, visceral, and relational issues that affected individuals in these close-knit but ultimately colonial environments. The school followed a Macaulayist curriculum, actively promoting all things British and denigrating the backgrounds and cultures of these students. Speaking in vernacular languages was forbidden on the campus, and British cultural norms, for everything from dress to dining, were strictly enforced. During the 1940s, the white faculty of the school actively sought to suppress anticolonial messages and forbid local newspapers, particularly Azikiwe's *West African Pilot*, from circulating on campus, ostensibly because the writing was poor and set a bad example for the students (Achebe 2009). Ultimately, the school taught Nigerian youth to reject their backgrounds and embrace the colonizer's worldview—a difficult path to navigate that had nothing necessarily to do with the rigorous education students were receiving.

The school's faculty sometimes failed the students, profoundly so. Momah discusses in his memoir the case of one of his classmates, who was overcome with anger and disillusionment after one of the white teachers at the school impregnated his relative's daughter and shortly thereafter left the school and returned to England, abandoning the woman and her unborn child. The student brought the situation to the attention of the principal, who claimed not to believe the account. "That's what the big man said," lamented the student after their palaver. "It seems he did not believe my story. But that's alright. I am learning to be patient" (Momah 2003, 60). It is not clear whether the school administration knew of the affair and removed the teacher as a result, or that the teacher had fled of his own accord. Either way, the colonial masters who preached responsibility and civilization had shown the hypocrisy of their racist paternalism to the students who knew about this scandal and demonstrated the extent to which their protectors were, in fact, also their assailants.

A different case from a few years later may have seemed less repugnant to the students, but it was powerfully enervating to several. In December 1948, one day before the Standard VI class was supposed to sit its Cambridge exam, Saburi Biobaku decided to take his class on a picnic as a reprieve from the rigors of cramming. He chose a spot near an estuary of the Imo River. In his memoir, Momah recalls Biobaku's reproachful reminders to the students not to swim in the river because of the strong undertow in the area. Most of the students disregarded his instructions and immediately waded into the water. Two students decided to have a race to the other side of the river: they were caught in the undertow and drowned. Their bodies were not immediately recovered, and the class returned to the school grounds in complete distress.

Both Momah and Biobaku recount this event in their autobiographies as a pivotal moment in their time at Umuahia. Both emphasize that the students in the class actually did quite well in their exams, but that the drowning incident had long-term consequences for all. Biobaku noted that "psychologically, things were not really the same after that experience" (Biobaku 1992, 143). He developed an amorphous illness, characterized by insomnia and weight loss. He ultimately took a leave of absence in Lagos before transferring into government service as an education officer.

The drowning incident was the climax of Momah's memoir. One of the main characters in this fictional account was Friday Stoneface, one of Momah's best friends throughout his time at Umuahia. Momah ends a key chapter with Friday Stoneface's drowning and the lamentations of another friend, "'Why did he have to go and die like that?' To which there was no answer. Only puzzlement. Puzzlement that life could be so unfair. And so screwed up" (Momah 2003, 310). He begins the next chapter with these words: "To this day, I cannot explain what came over me. I found, in January 1949, at the beginning of my second term of my last year in Umuahia, that I was suffering from a very serious academic malady. A malady I can only describe as a sudden diminished mental capacity for the sciences and mathematics. It was if an intellectual wall suddenly sprang up, from nowhere, cutting me off from those subjects" (Momah 2003, 311). Though he said that he does not know what came over him, the death of his friend clearly impacted him deeply. And while he did not describe the symptoms of brain fag as Prince described them, he did describe a sudden decline in his academic competence that was precipitated by an obviously traumatic event at school, which was less related to his studies than to the sudden, stark realization that the world was "so screwed up."

The unsettled and unsure quality to the responses received through Prince's questionnaires might reflect or tell of the students' "nervous" environments as much as anything else. When a student declares "this world is not the place for me," what world does he mean exactly? When a student worries that he does not retain enough of what he reads, to what is he comparing himself? When one complains of a fractured knee or a cricket ball to the nose, how much physical pain justifies the distraction it causes? How excellent does a student have to be to guarantee later success? Does he need to be an exemplary British subject? How much suffering, hunger, and humiliation should one be able to bear in pursuit of a particular future? These are some of the questions that the students seem to have been grappling with when describing their experienced "symptoms" in late colonial boarding schools.

Conclusion

And when you come to think of it, it was quite immoral of the headmaster to tell little children every morning that for every palm-kernel they picked they were buying a nail for Hitler's coffin.

So Obi Okonkwo reminisced as an adult in Chinua Achebe's (1960, 41) novel *No Longer at Ease*. Resentful of being corralled into forced labor, and uncomfortable with his role in the murder of a far-away cipher of an enemy, these experiences produced the opposite of the intended effect in Achebe's fictional character, Obi, who ended up kindling a sympathy for Hitler, even writing a letter to him. The headmaster intercepted the letter. He also publicly shamed Obi as a "disgrace to the British Empire" and guaranteed him that "if he had been older he surely would have been sent to jail for the rest of his miserable life." Obi was meant to feel grateful for getting off with only "six strokes of the cane to his buttocks" (Achebe 1960, 15). As an adult, Obi saw the situation for what it was: a confusing amalgam of signs, symbols, and expectations that no child could be expected to understand, but for which he had been held personally liable by the same authorities who influenced his behavior. The story serves as a metaphor for Obi's later arrest and conviction for taking a bribe under extreme duress. Though Obi did not suffer a psychological meltdown, his downfall suggests the precarity of navigating such a "nervous" colonial setting, very much like the one that the students in Prince's study negotiated daily, however they articulated it when replying to his queries about their "symptoms associated with study."

The notion that African students were vulnerable to mental distress dates back to those colonial fixations with "culture clash" and "detribalization" that Prince drew on when developing his brain fag etiology. The trope of the overwrought student struggling to cope with malaise remains common in African novels and other forms of storytelling up to the present day. Psychological distress and psychotic disorders frequently feature in fictional narratives, where they are often presented as an effect of marginalization and violence within milieus that neither value nor accommodate personality traits like compassion, idealism, individuality, and introspection (Dangaremba 1988; Bandele-Thomas 1993; Adichie 2003). Too often the emotional torment of African students has been interpreted through a narrow biomedical or psychological lens, emphasizing their symptoms as by-products of colonial or postcolonial pressures and fraught modernities. This chapter has suggested otherwise.

As this examination of Prince's 1959 brain fag questionnaires demonstrates, a medical model is by no means the only, the best, or even the most convincing lens by which to interpret the language of student responses. While some did articulate their symptoms through the terms of European medicine, the evidence suggests that other students may have been attempting to translate vernacular symptoms into the idioms of their English-only colonial educations. Still others seem to have been rejecting the assumptions

of the questionnaire altogether, choosing not to answer or distancing themselves from the exercise. Most commonly, the students seem to have been articulating deep uncertainties about their colonial conditions and environments,
which, they sensed, negatively affected their ability to feel confident about
whether they were effectively negotiating their way in the world.

The complexity of these student responses to such late colonial questionnaires defies all efforts to reach sole or all-encompassing readings. The archive offers up not definitive answers but multifarious possibilities. Several
interpretations have been elaborated here. The hermeneutic potential of
this singular archive is suggestive for all medical and psychiatric histories of
Africa, as the voices of patients, kin, and ordinary subjects vie with those of
hierarchical—often white colonial—figures like doctors, teachers, officials,
scholars, as well as an array of intermediaries. "The doctor calls it mental
disorder,"[36] offered up one student when naming his own condition. Yet the
same Nigerian youth likely had other terms for speaking about his condition
and health.

Notes

1   The answers cited refer to the original responses to a questionnaire that
    Dr. Raymond Prince sent out to five secondary schools in southern Nigeria in
    1959. I located the files in 2017 in the papers of Dr. Prince. At the time of pub-
    lication, they were housed in a filing cabinet in a storage room in the Division
    of Social and Transcultural Psychiatry at McGill University in Montreal, where
    Prince worked for his entire career and where they apparently have been
    stored since his death in 2012. My thanks to Dr. Laurence Kirmayer, Director
    of the Division of Social and Transcultural Psychiatry at McGill, for grant-
    ing me access to this collection. Almost none of the questionnaires contain
    names or dates for respondents; I have decided to anonymize those that do to
    protect the identity of the individual. The Prince Papers remain uncataloged.
    As such, my citations to specific documents can only be described in relation
    to the document, the school from which it came, and with a reference to their
    place within the larger collection of Prince's papers. For example, the "bad
    sight" quotation here is attributed to a document I cite as seventeen-year-
    old Ijaw male student from Government College, Umuahia, respondent of the
    "To All Students" questionnaire, Raymond Prince Papers, Division of Social

and Transcultural Psychiatry, McGill University, Montreal (hereafter Prince Papers).

2   Nineteen-year-old Yoruba male student from Government College, Umuahia, respondent of the "To All Students" questionnaire, Prince Papers.

3   E.A.O., seventeen-year-old Egba male student from Government College, Ibadan, respondent of the "To All Students" questionnaire, Prince Papers.

4   Fifteen-year-old Yoruba male student from Government College, Ibadan, respondent of the "To All Students" questionnaire, Prince Papers.

5   "To All Students" questionnaire, Prince Papers. This language is boilerplate and exists on every questionnaire.

6   "To All Students" questionnaire, Prince Papers. This language is boilerplate and exists on every questionnaire.

7   Raymond Prince to "Robin," December 5, 1961, Prince Papers.

8   Fifteen-year-old Yoruba male student from Government College, Ibadan, respondent of the "To All Students" questionnaire, Prince Papers.

9   Twenty-one-year-old Edo male student from King's College, Lagos, respondent of the "To All Students" questionnaire, Prince Papers.

10 Nineteen-year-old Qua male student from Hope Waddell Institute, Calabar, respondent of the "To All Students" questionnaire, Prince Papers.

11 Nineteen-year-old Bini male student from King's College, Lagos, respondent of the "To All Students" questionnaire, Prince Papers.

12 Twenty-one-year-old Yoruba male student from King's College, Lagos, respondent of the "To All Students" questionnaire, Prince Papers.

13 Eighteen-year-old Yoruba male student from Government College, Ibadan, respondent of the "To All Students" questionnaire, Prince Papers.

14 R.A., seventeen-year, seven-month-old Yoruba male student from Government College, Umuahia, respondent of the "To All Students" questionnaire, Prince Papers.

15 E.A.O., seventeen-year-old Egba male student from Government College, Ibadan, respondent of the "To All Students" questionnaire, Prince Papers.

16 Nineteen-year-old Yoruba male student from Government College, Umuahia, respondent of the "To All Students" questionnaire, Prince Papers.

17 Fifteen-year-old Yoruba male student from King's College, Lagos, respondent of the "To All Students" questionnaire, Prince Papers.

18 Nineteen-year, six-month-old Ibo male student from Government College, Umuahia, respondent of the "To All Students" questionnaire, Prince Papers.

19 Seventeen-year-old Ibo male student from Hope Waddell Institute, Calabar, respondent of the "To All Students" questionnaire, Prince Papers.

20 Fourteen-year-old Yoruba male student from Government College, Ibadan, respondent of the "To All Students" questionnaire, Prince Papers.

21 Twenty-year-old Itsekiri male student from King's College, Lagos, respondent of the "To All Students" questionnaire, Prince Papers.

22 Twenty-two-year-old Yoruba male student from King's College, Lagos, respondent of the "To All Students" questionnaire, Prince Papers.

23 "To All Students" questionnaire, Prince Papers. This language was boilerplate, in the sense that it existed on every questionnaire provided.

24 Fourteen-year-old Yoruba male student from King's College, Lagos, respondent of the "To All Students" questionnaire, Prince Papers.

25 Sixteen-year, six-month-old Yoruba male student from King's College, Lagos, respondent of the "To All Students" questionnaire, Prince Papers.

26 Twenty-year-old Yoruba male student from King's College, Lagos, respondent of the "To All Students" questionnaire, Prince Papers.

27 Thirteen-year-old Ibo male student from King's College, Lagos, respondent of the "To All Students" questionnaire, Prince Papers.

28 Nineteen-year-old Bini male student from King's College, Lagos, respondent of the "To All Students" questionnaire, Prince Papers.

29 E.A.O., seventeen-year-old Egba male student from Government College, Ibadan, respondent of the "To All Students" questionnaire, Prince Papers.

30 Seventeen-year-old Yoruba male student from King's College, Lagos, respondent of the "To All Students" questionnaire, Prince Papers.

31 Seventeen-year-old Yoruba male student from King's College, Lagos, respondent of the "To All Students" questionnaire, Prince Papers.

32 Twenty-year-old Ijaw male student from King's College, Lagos, respondent of the "To All Students" questionnaire, Prince Papers.

33 Eighteen-year-old Urhobo male student from Government College, Umuahia, respondent of the "To All Students" questionnaire, Prince Papers.

34 Sixteen-year, six-month-old Yoruba male student from King's College, Lagos, respondent of the "To All Students" questionnaire, Prince Papers.

35 Twenty-one-year-old Edo male student from King's College, Lagos, respondent of the "To All Students" questionnaire, Prince Papers.

36 Twenty-two-year-old Yoruba male student from King's College, Lagos, respondent of the "To All Students" questionnaire, Prince Papers.

Sources

Archival Material

Raymond Prince Papers, Division of Social and Transcultural Psychiatry, McGill University, Montreal, uncataloged.

Literature

Achebe, Chinua. 1960. *No Longer at Ease*. London: Heinemann.

Achebe, Chinua. 2009. *The Education of a British-Protected Child*. New York: Alfred A. Knopf.

Adichie, Chimamanda Ngozi. 2003. *Purple Hibiscus*. New York: Workman.

American Psychiatric Association. 1994. *Diagnostic and Statistical Manual of Mental Disorders*. 4th ed. Washington, DC: American Psychiatric Association.

Anumonye, Amechi. 1973. "Emotional Illness among Students of Developing Countries." *Papua New Guinea Medical Journal* 16:183–88.

Ayonrinde, Oyedeji A., Chiedu Obuaya, and Solomon Olusola Adeyemi. 2015. "Brain Fag Syndrome: A Culture-Bound Syndrome That May Be Approaching Extinction." *British Journal of Psychiatry Bulletin* 39, no. 4: 156–61.

Bandele-Thomas, Biyi. 1993. *The Sympathetic Undertaker and Other Dreams*. London: Heinemann.

Berkenkotter, Carol. 2008. *Patient Tales: Case Histories and the Uses of Narrative in Psychiatry*. Columbia: University of South Carolina Press.

Biobaku, Saburi O. 1992. *When We Were Young*. Ibadan, Nigeria: University of Ibadan Press.

Carothers, John Colin. 1953. *The African Mind in Health and Disease: A Study in Ethnopsychiatry*. Geneva: World Health Organization.

Dangarembga, Tsitsi. 1988. *Nervous Conditions*. London: The Women's Press.

Falola, Toyin, and Matthew M. Heaton. 2008. *A History of Nigeria*. Cambridge: Cambridge University Press.

Field, Margaret J. 1960. *Search for Security: An Ethno-Psychiatric Study of Rural Ghana*. Evanston, IL: Northwestern University Press.

Gilman, Sander. 1985. *Difference and Pathology: Stereotypes of Sexuality, Race, and Madness*. Ithaca, NY: Cornell University Press.

Heaton, Matthew M. 2013. *Black Skin, White Coats: Nigerian Psychiatrists, Decolonization, and the Globalization of Psychiatry*. Athens: Ohio University Press.

Hornstein, Gail. 2017. *Agnes's Jacket: A Psychologist's Search for the Meanings of Madness*. New York: Routledge.

Hunt, Nancy Rose. 2013. "Health and Medicine." In *The Oxford Handbook of Modern African History*, edited by John Parker and Richard Reid, 378–95. Oxford: Oxford University Press.

Hunt, Nancy Rose. 2016. *A Nervous State: Violence, Remedies, and Reverie in Co-lonial Congo*. Durham, NC: Duke University Press.

Janzen, John. 1978. *The Quest for Therapy in Lower Zaire*. Berkeley: University of California Press.

Jegede, R. Olukayode. 1983. "Psychiatric Illness in African Students: 'Brain Fag' Syndrome Revisited." *Canadian Journal of Psychiatry* 28:188–92.

Jones, Edgar, Shahina Rahman, and Brian Everitt. 2012. "Psychiatric Case Notes: Symptoms of Mental Illness and Their Attribution at the Maudsley Hospital, 1924–35." *History of Psychiatry* 23, no. 2: 156–68.

Lambo, Thomas Adeoye. 1958. *A Study of Social and Health Problems of Nigerian Students in Great Britain and Ireland*. Ibadan, Nigeria: Government Printer.

Last, Murray. 2007. "The Importance of Knowing about Not Knowing." In *On Know-ing and Not Knowing in the Anthropology of Medicine*, edited by Roland Little-wood, 1–17. London: Routledge.

Makanjuola, Roger O. A. 1987. "'Ode Ori': A Culture-Bound Disorder with Promi-nent Somatic Features in Yoruba Nigerian Patients." *Acta Psychiatrica Scandi-navia* 75:231–36.

McCulloch, Jock. 1995. *Colonial Psychiatry and "the African Mind."* Cambridge: Cambridge University Press.

Momah, Chike. 2003. *The Shining Ones: The Umuahia School Days of Obinna Okoye*. Ibadan, Nigeria: Ibadan University Press.

Morakinyo, Olufemi. 1980. "A Psychophysiological Theory of a Psychiatric Illness (the Brain Fag Syndrome) Associated with Study among Africans." *Journal of Nervous and Mental Disease* 168, no. 2: 84–89.

Ochiagha, Terri. 2015. *Achebe and Friends at Umuahia: The Making of a Literary Elite*. Woodbridge, UK: Boydell and Brewer.

Prince, Raymond. 1960. "The 'Brain Fag' Syndrome in Nigerian Students." *Journal of Mental Science* 106:559–70.

Prince, Raymond. 1962. "Functional Symptoms Associated with Study in Nigerian Students." *West African Medical Journal* 11:198–206.

Prince, Raymond. 2010. *Why This Ecstasy? Reflections on My Life with Madmen*. Montreal: Amvor Art and Cultural Foundation.

Sadowsky, Jonathan. 1996. "The Confinement of Isaac O.: A Case of 'Acute Mania' in Colonial Nigeria." *History of Psychiatry* 7, no. 25: 91–112.

Schöhl, Stephanie, and Volker Hess. 2019. "War Imprisonment and Clinical Narra-tives of Psychiatric Illness, Psychiatric Hospital Charité, Berlin, 1948–56." *Jour-nal of the History of Medicine and Allied Sciences* 74, no. 2: 145–66.

Swartz, Sally. 2018. "Asylum Case Records: Fact and Fiction." *Rethinking History* 22, no. 3: 289–301.

PART III

PRACTICES
AND LONG DURATIONS

Sloan Mahone 7

Casting out Anger

Stress, Possession, and
the Everyday in Taita, Kenya

For a brief period in the 1950s, the isolated Taita Hills in Kenya attracted the interests of the British colonial government, two anthropologists from Cambridge and a Canadian psychiatrist who doubled as an amateur photographer. The cross section of competing claims about Taita stress that emerges gives us an opportunity to read into everyday Taita life amid a surge of new economic and political pressures, external interference, and strategies of coping and self-reliance. Government observations of insanity cases with related outbursts of violence were growing out of control, prompting a call to experts, and an analytical turn toward local and colonial articulations regarding the pressures of modern life. In considering Taita, in Kenya's Coast Province (now Taita-Taveta County), as a case study, this chapter presents a unique snapshot of a complicated colonial encounter.[1] Madness and patients may be in short supply here, but the angst associated with the threat of forms of madness, oftentimes expressed as an angry or dangerous heart, shows itself in vernacular practices that confounded outsiders to these hills. *KidaBida*, the language and philosophy of "being Taita," organized local life with a zeal for predicting chaos and protecting order.

Histories of interactions between psychiatrists and colonized communities are increasingly well documented for Africa and elsewhere throughout former colonial empires. Often, the reports from both doctors and administrators showcase an array of outmoded theories (even for their time), recast as new ways to assert that indigenous people crumbled as "modernity" threatened their presumed traditional ways of seeing the world. Doctors' reports, branded by the government in the metropole as authoritative, often incorporated ethnographic writing about weaning practices, marriage and kinship, witchcraft belief, and various interpretations of African custom and cosmology. Anthropologists, frequently funded by the Colonial Office, were not necessarily immersed in imperial politics, and many produced important ethnographies that today serve as foundational texts and eloquent pieces of writing. This volume highlights, when possible, vernacular expressions and practice, eschewing overarching representations of colonial thought and bias and illuminating the everyday where the colonial could be both ever-present and ignored. This chapter turns its attention to spirit possession among that Taita, or rather the colonial fixation on possession practices as a screen by which to diagnose mental states, frenzy, breakdown, and "hysteria." The assumption is not that these colonial readings of a ubiquitous vernacular healing form were wrong—though a fearful primitivist colonial lens could distort. Rather this density of European expert knowledge tells us much about colonial panic and nervousness and reminds us of the paucity of ways of entering into this dialogue about mental instability from Taita perspectives from the time.

The Taita in Kenya

In the 1950s, the scrutiny of Taita by outsiders marked a curious endeavor, considering the government's necessary preoccupation with higher Kenyan politics and the increasing turmoil of the Mau Mau war. With the state of emergency declared in 1952, the war in the forests escalated rapidly, and tens of thousands of mostly Kikuyu men and women were either incarcerated in detention camps situated throughout the country or displaced and relocated as the government sought to "rehabilitate" oath-taking terrorists.

The Taita seemed far removed from this, although both the MacKinnon Road and Manyani detention camps were broadly in their midst. Nonetheless, a province that had been seen as a sleepy backwater began to stand out, curiously, as a region in flux. Government reports and missionary testimonies suggesting that urgent assistance may be required, depict the growing concerns within the district. From 1950 to 1952, two young anthropologists, Alfred and Grace Harris, conducted fieldwork in Taita for their Cambridge PhD theses, but they also provided the government with quasi-official reports to explain Taita life and behavior in anthropological terms. Finally, in 1956, the newly appointed psychiatrist in charge of Mathari Mental Hospital in Nairobi, Edward Margetts, was summoned to Taita to give expert medical opinion on the extremely high levels of insanity said to be occurring in the region and to suggest possible remedies for it.

With serious unrest brewing closer to Nairobi, Taita was quietly navigating pressures of its own. Emerging industries such as asbestos and graphite mines, factories producing cement pipes, and most notably sisal plantations drew young men in as wage laborers, shifting the norms of self-sufficiency, ownership, and adulthood. Witchcraft was a significant player in the area—sometimes handled internally, but in serious cases, witch cleansers from outside (such as Tanzania) were brought in to diagnose and expel sinister activity. Traditional healers, diviners, and seers of different specializations abounded in the Taita Hills, and heritage and lineage were revered, most notably in the keeping of shrines (*Ngomenyi*) where the skulls of the departed were kept in the caves dotting the rocky landscape. In short, the Taita were religious and reverent, with a strong sense of Taita-ness, while particularly noting the differences between the people of the hills and the people of the plains. The sense that the Taita were breaking down psychologically stood in stark contrast to the government's previous assertion that the Taita were generally happy and quite at peace with the world.

A Note on Source Material

The voluminous paper trail left by these various outsiders, including a series of photographs taken by Edward Margetts, portray a dynamic picture of 1950s Kenya in the isolated Taita Hills. These documents present a fascinatingly precise point of contact as they converge, with their varying motivations and approaches, within a tight time frame of a few years. The anthropologist, the psychiatrist, and the colonial administrator all brought to the table the tropes of their respective disciplines. We can add to this the doctor's alter ego as photographer and documentarian—a contribution we shall discuss separately. For the purposes of this story, we see the utility of engaging not with one colonial archive but with several, with the benefit of witnessing how they intersected during this brief explosion of interest in the region. While the overarching identity of these self-appointed observers was deeply entangled with colonialism, they still engaged with Taita resistances (or sometimes indifference) in unique ways.

Is it here that we might discover vernacular forms? Taita engagement with the various reports on their customs and behaviors reveals cooperation, rebuttals, exasperation, and at times an impatience to get on with things. Western preoccupations with finding "madness" or "hysteria," in individuals and the collective, point to a familiar tale of colonial angst and a patronizing distrust. With not only one outsider agenda but three to contend with, it is possible to glean from this raw data a Taita engagement with a dynamic and sometimes tense social space where words and actions were well documented, but perhaps poorly understood. There is ample evidence that these outsiders were observing *something*, but one is left with the feeling that, unsurprisingly, the questions were wrong, and a good deal of energy was spent searching for something not lost.

The archival material related specifically to the question of Taita psychiatric instability comes in the form of regional reports and correspondence from doctors, government and missionary accounts and letters, published ethnography, medical case notes, diary entries, and Edward Margetts's photographs—often with accompanying explanations or captions. The most extensive early relationship with the region, however, is presented by anthropologist Grace Gredys Harris.

Casting out Anger

At the heart of the analysis of Taita life are the PhD thesis and published ethnography authored by Grace Harris, as well as her influential article on "possession hysteria," published in the journal *American Anthropologist*. Although her fieldwork, government reports, and article all appeared in the 1950s, she would not publish her ethnographic study of Taita religion until 1978. Thus, her encounters with the government, the traveling psychiatrist, and the Taita themselves did not fully incorporate the analyses she employed in her later years as an anthropology professor in the United States. However, Harris makes clear in her preface what she revised from her thesis, and we can consider her fieldwork notes to be largely frozen in time. Ultimately, Harris became a faculty member at the University of Rochester in New York, initially as a part-time spousal hire. She remained at Rochester until her retirement, when she became emeritus professor. She died in December 2011 at the age of eighty-five. Harris's written corpus remains sparse, but she embarked on new research mid-career, publishing on aspects of stress and decision-making among hospital patients in the United States (Harris 1989, 3–21).

We consider first the place of Harris's ethnography, *Casting out Anger*, which concerns itself with Taita religion and the centrality of the ritual *kutasa*: the spraying of liquid out of the mouth while uttering phrases or exhortations to "cast out anger" from the heart. Kutasa was not merely a symbolic act, but a way of altering a wrong path, provided that the performer was indeed sincere with a "clean" and "cool" heart (Harris 1978, 26). This means of stabilizing harmony in the heart within individuals, families, and the community was intrinsic to KidaBida: the "Taita way," or the "way of the Hills." Today, *Casting out Anger* is a critical text for any historical grounding in the region, particularly when speaking of the locality of the Taita Hills. Ethnographies of surrounding regions present similar themes and practices in a very extensive literature on healing, possession, and ritual along the East African Swahili coast, but much of the work on Taita touches on the quite reflective identity politics in a region marked by migration and mixing for many years. Bill Bravman's longue durée approach to Taita, in his monograph *Making Ethnic Ways* (1998), makes use of oral history to illustrate dynamism and change across and within generations. Bravman's interviews reveal, for instance, the Ngomenyi skull shrines, representing a profound symbol of Taita ancestry, reverence, and security. These were, by the 1950s, contested or neglected as competing concerns about education, economic independence, and Christianity began to hold sway (Bravman 1998, 202). Bravman shows that, while the strains of colonial-era life may have fractured some communities, what came to be a staunch Taita ethnicity coalesced (Bravman 1998, 139). Like Harris, Bravman recounts that this notional sense of being Taita or KidaBida was a central expression within daily life.

James Howard Smith's *Bewitching Development* (2008) also makes use of Grace Harris's foundational work to provide an illuminating account of modern development practice and aspirations in Taita as filtered through the language of witchcraft. Struggles during Smith's fieldwork in the 1990s depict familiar generational, gendered, and economic stresses in the Taita Hills. These tensions may seem removed from economic and labor conflicts under colonialism but are echoed in recent decades by the legacy of heavy-handed structural adjustment policies. Like Harris's ethnographic accounts of "being Taita" and Bravman's memoirs from the mid- to late colonial period, the Taita are seen to be a people who have continually memorialized, reinvented, and reengaged their history, as even the most potent Taita symbols required new responses, or sometimes abandonment, with successive generations.

When *Casting out Anger* finally appeared in print, Harris acknowledged that she was not writing in the then fashionable "ethnographic present," but suggested that her work was a "picture" of Taita religion as observed in the middle of the twentieth century (Harris 1978, vii). The time lag between fieldwork and publication allowed Harris to come to conclusions about anthropology's turn to what she saw as an "overuse of semiotically-inclined searches for meaning" and a troubling "view of symbolism as representing what somehow 'really' exists outside the rituals" (Harris 1978, viii). Harris differentiated her own approach as showing "the forms making up rituals as *presenting* realities that are lived in ritual itself" (Harris 1978, viii).

Casting out Anger was widely reviewed, albeit with a range of contrasting opinions about what it had truly accomplished. Paul Spencer, the British social anthropologist of the Samburu and the Maasai, was perhaps the most critical in his disappointment that such an important subject, with fieldwork carried out during "a vintage era for anthropological field work on African indigenous religions," fell short in terms of intellectual depth and theoretical purpose (Spencer 1979, 587). Meyer Fortes, as one of Grace Harris's mentors at Cambridge, found the ethnography a "treatise of fundamental general and theoretical import" and "written with admirable economy of language and conceptual clarity" (Fortes 1979, 569). Fortes's cogent and generous summary of the book praised the sidestepping of the usual thick description for an analysis of the core cosmological and ritual significance of casting out anger or kutasa. In Taita, kinship obligations and entitlements were interwoven with the dangerous anger that lived in the heart and threatened the harmony and stability of the community. Lucy Mair differentiated anthropology's familiar interpretations of witchcraft's embodiment as the enmity or envy of neighbors with a more unique Taita perspective that eschewed a "special category of witches whose anger can do harm" with the ubiquitous seeking out of "angry hearts" that could be found everywhere and in everybody (Mair 1979, 571).

Harris stressed that central to the act of "casting out anger" was not the ritual performance, but the inner state of the performer. Anger from the heart could only be expelled when the participant was without "inner reservations" (Harris 1978, 46). In fact, insincerity when practicing kutasa could result in not only the ritual's failure, but the faker's "words hidden in the heart" might also lead to sorcery and a counter-effect to what was intended (Harris 1978, 47). The practice of kutasa was integral to managing the danger inherent in the "angry hearts" of individuals, particularly toward their close family members. Harris likened this to a more universal human concern with what she called the "potentially dangerous psychobiological individual 'inside' the social person" (Harris 1978, 175). However, it was not this potential for hidden anger that made it most visible to outsider observations and interest.

Watching Taita

In the mid-1950s, various district and medical officers, missionaries, and local politicians weighed in on the alarming rise of insanity and associated violence in Taita. The district commissioner, R. A. Wilkinson, sent a memorandum to the provincial commissioner to insist that the incidence of insanity in Teita District was "incomparably greater" than in any other district he had seen during the last twenty years of his service. He buttressed this claim by consulting "responsible African opinion," which concurred that insanity was "definitely increasing."[2] The provincial commissioner wrote to the secretary for African affairs to highlight concerns about "mental instability among the Teita," suggesting that the new psychiatrist in charge of Mathari Mental Hospital might shed light on whether the rate of mental instability was higher in the Taita Hills than elsewhere in Kenya, whether madness was indeed on the increase, what the causes might be, and what steps might be taken to reduce the rate of insanity.[3]

The local Catholic mission also weighed in on "lunacy in Teita." Father Madigan wrote to the district medical officer, situating the crises within the context of the worsening social problems that accompanied a rapidly modernizing population:

Drink: The old Teita law in this matter must be restored if we are to avoid serious social upheavals. The old custom forbade young men to drink until they got married. Then they were initiated by the drinkers, and were only allowed to imbibe through a reed, until they were accustomed to restraint in the matter. . . . Now with the advent of the public beer shops and partially fermented brews and tilting bottles as long as one can pay, [this] is really responsible for mental disorders. . . . Drunk tonight, incapable of work to-morrow, further quenching of the thirst to-morrow night . . . denying the wife and family money for household expenses—hunger, rags, disease—stealing from the wife's shamba and selling to get more money; robbing others; unpaid debts . . . worry, worry, worry, and the mind snaps. [4]

Father Madigan commented further on the rising tensions caused by "materialism" among the Taita—a tendency that appeared to be supplanting traditional religious values and practices in the region: "The African caught up in this individualism is not capable of adjusting himself, becomes a super-materialist, a living lie to what is traditional in him. Then, when the material world withdraws its support (in times of poverty or family trouble) the mind snaps." [5]

Despite frequent descriptions of bhang and alcohol use on the rise as well as the violence of young men, contrasting reports referred to the Taita as "pleasant drunks" who, unlike some regions, had an abhorrence of violence. According to one district officer, "any dispute which leads to physical violence is looked on with amazement and horror, and the assailant is rapidly hauled before the African court." [6] Witchcraft was implicated for specific forms of derangement and for a unique act of violence called *kuloga* or *kuroga*, which involved hiring a sorcerer to administer a slow poison that caused both derangement and a decline of general health to the point of death. Lastly, medical officers felt compelled to document the seemingly absurd political aspirations of the Taita, noting: "It would appear that [the Taita] have taken to the slogan of 'Self-Government by 1960.'" [7] Despite such sentiments making their way into annual reports, Taita grievances about land, the most traditional form of wealth, seem not to have been taken very seriously, and the population was seen as not particularly adept at organizing itself. Grace Harris recalled that the Taita land use system was poorly understood by the British government, "some of whom thought that the Taita made an unduly large amount of fuss over the alienation of relatively small pieces of land" (Harris 1978, 179n24).

While district officers might have been instrumental in procuring anthropological and psychological reports regarding what they saw as rampant mental illness in Taita, there is evidence that Kenyans from neighboring communities also wanted the madness in Taita to stop. Prominent Kenyan politician Ronald Ngala wrote to the medical officer in charge of Wesu, Taita, on behalf of his worried constituents in Kigombo, suggesting that the government conduct a "special investigation" into the matter.[8] What stands out from the Taita district records is the insistence that high rates of insanity and chaotic behavior were not only new to the area but that it was a far greater problem than existed anywhere else in the colony. This was an extraordinary claim as far as the colonial government was concerned as Kenya was full of not only the Mau Mau in this period but widespread antigovernment sentiment, rebellious prophets, charismatic diviners, bewitchers, and nomadic witch cleansers. Taita's mild reputation was becoming more unstable, and the presumed severe spike in lunacy and hysteria was pulling it out of the shadows.

A Psychiatrist Comes to Taita

In November 1955, a Canadian psychiatrist arrived in Kenya from McGill University in Montreal to take up the post of chief psychiatrist and medical superintendent of Mathari Mental Hospital in Nairobi. In what proved to be a decade-long habit, Edward Margetts began a personal diary—recording his travels, notes about colleagues and contacts, and impressions of his new environment including any customs, rituals, healing practices, and local stories he might collect. The diaries are full of both insight and the mundane, but they are wonderfully meticulous in recording names of places, people, and terminologies that the doctor encountered. It was not long after his arrival that Margetts was invited most urgently to the Coast Province to deal with reports from district officers who insisted that they had never seen such high levels of hysteria anywhere in Kenya as they had in Taita. In advance of his first trip to the region in 1956, Margetts had at his disposal all available district administrative and medical reports, correspondence with local officials, a list of people to interview, and the reports to the Colonial Office written by Grace and Alfred Harris. The doctor sometimes recreated these conversations or excerpts from reports in hand-written notes in his diary—amending official observations with skeptical comments or questions of his own. Local observations noted the seasonality of some of the hysteria hitting the Hills between June and September—roughly corresponding to higher incidences of malaria, as well as the use of easily obtained antimalarial drugs, which were associated with psychosis. Bhang and alcohol consumption were also said to be worryingly on the rise as traditional values about drinking (by whom and how much) were under assault. Inbreeding was said to be common due to Taita's isolation and preferred sense of separateness. But, most significantly, there was a feeling of foreboding in the Hills and a presumed weakening of Taita moral codes as economic pressures increased.

Pepo Ngoma

In reading this correspondence, it becomes apparent that the psychiatrist soon developed an agenda of his own. His letters indicated that he would forgo tours of the hospital, showing little interest in the actual diagnoses of medical cases. Instead, he asked to tour the district for general impressions and to be present at some of the rituals and ceremonies for which the WaTaita were well known. In particular, he asked to observe a ritual dance called *pepo*. He also came armed with a camera.

In the first instance, Margetts noted that there might be difficulty in differentiating pepo in Taita from true psychosis, meaning that the ubiquitous reports of an increase in hysteria might represent either a "manifestation of an unstable, hysteria prone population," or might be an "acceptable form of tribal behaviour."[9] He often couched his reports in the language of anthropology, but he also momentarily considered a quasi-experimental approach, suggesting that finding another nearby "tribe" to act as a control group might prove clinically interesting. In total, Margetts made three medical trips to Taita, accompanied by his translator and senior medical assistant, Henry Mwariri. He wrote up his findings after each visit and titled his investigations as "anthropological–psychological notes" on the Taita. He situated his own findings alongside the anthropological reports of Grace and Alfred Harris, as well as previous work on the region, such as the ethnographic survey of Dutch anthropologist A. H. J. Prins (1952), whose work Grace Harris criticized as "inaccurate" due to the short nature of his visits to Taita (Harris 1978, 179n15). Published accounts by the Reverend Peter Geoffrey Bostock (1950) from the Church Missionary Society in Kenya from 1935 to 1958, and Charles William Hobley's early accounts of traveling through Tsavo and the Taita highlands (1895), rounded out his background on the region. He indicated in his notes that he intended to correspond with the Harrises, and he commented on the "very good work" in their government reports. However, he added the caveat that he wished the anthropological reports had contained more information about "witchcraft, poisons, *pepo*, and other subjects which tie in with the problem at hand."[10] Finally, Margetts interviewed district officials and four WaTaita employees of the district hospital in Wesu. He recounted the impressions of others who described the Taita to him as "very emotional, rather unpredictable, theatrical in behaviour, friendly and polite." He rejected previous characterizations of Taita men as "effeminate."[11] The report summarized the key problem as defined by the district: the rise in violence and, particularly, cases of murder. The possibility of associating such violence with an increase in mental illness needed differentiation, he wrote, noting that relevant categories for analysis might be the general functional psychoses (such as mania or schizophrenia), toxic-infective states (such as advanced neurosyphilis or malaria), and, finally, "emotional or neurotic illness," which he classed as "particularly hysteria—the 'PEPO' of the Wataita."[12]

Margetts reported the descriptions of pepo as given by his informants: "hysterical outbursts and dances and rituals involving hysterical mechanisms are said to be unusually common amongst the Wataita." The fact that cases of pepo might be mistaken for psychosis seemed likely to falsify the contention that psychotic behavior was a unique and increasing problem in the region. He surmised that pepo should not in itself be considered a psychiatric problem. Margetts concluded his report with the suggestion that if it can be shown that mental illness (and related violence) was on the increase, it was likely due to factors such as significant increases in alcohol and bhang consumption, the "in-breeding" known to occur in the Hills, and endemic diseases such as malaria. The doctor also gave his broad impressions of the increasingly unstable religious life among the Taita, and questioned whether the long-standing missionary efforts to Christianize the already religious Taita was the right thing to do: "there are some things which the missions brought which were of universal appeal, such as help in time of need and of bright clothing etc. Whether they brought the spiritual conversion they wanted is another story, certainly not a universal one."[13]

Margetts took no photographs of the hospitals in Wesu, Voi, or any other towns in the district, but there are myriad photos of pepo as performed both in Taita and the surrounding areas of the Kamba people. He curated these photographs together but did differentiate the unique practices of distinct groups. He interviewed and photographed dance leaders (*vilongozi*) and local healers, and documented key terminologies, including the mistakes made by previous observers such as Prins. He wrote descriptions in his diaries of the ceremony, dress, the types of props employed in pepo dances, the skill and the drunkenness of the drummers, and the reactions of the crowds. He took special interest in the actions of women dancers, who he described as convulsing rapidly before falling into a trance state, if not completely unconscious. These were attacks of *saka*—the pepo spirit that made demands of the women it visited, or, more to the point, made demands of the husbands of the afflicted women. Margetts noted the "attention-seeking motive" of pepo and thought it often "based on sexual conflicts which may be quite subconscious."[14]

Ultimately, Margetts wrote up his findings, clearly differentiating between hysteria in individuals who might be viewed as hysterical personalities, and group hysteria as witnessed in the ceremonial dances, seen as socially sanctioned and populated by "quite normal people." Traumatic events triggered some hysterical reactions, he noted, such as one woman who went into "hysterics" at the scene of a suicide. The doctor was clearly intrigued by the props on display during the dances, including whistles, staffs, the ubiquitous red fez, and one woman "who was seen dancing with a whisky bottle balanced on her head—no mean feat considering the activity of her movements. This was obviously a pure show-off."[15] Both Margetts as an amateur anthropologist and Harris as a psychologically minded ethnographer reified the everyday, but notably foreign, objects on display as culturally telling but also absurdist performance that suggested instability rather than purposeful meaning. Fritz Kramer places such "arbitrary collections" from possessing spirits in opposition to the equally arbitrary curiosities of nineteenth-century travelers and anthropologists who collected objects, customs, and manners of their human objects of study (Kramer 1993, 241). In Taita, the primacy of such object use was noted for its peculiarity, but also as a common local response to the stresses of modern life.

Photographing Pepo

Margetts's photographs appear in multiple forms. They were often repurposed within correspondence and district reports (with strict demands for their return), in publications (chiefly medical journals or textbooks, but also newspaper or magazine articles), on display in exhibits at international psychiatric conferences, in teaching slides, and in his personal photograph albums. In all these cases, the photographs are accompanied by captions that he altered to suit his intended audience. Margetts often commented on the process of taking photographs, including when he met hostility or indifference, what he gifted or paid people who agreed to pose, and where technical matters of light and exposure made a difference to the outcome. He requested to attend pepo dances (or have them organized for him) early in the day when the light was best, although Grace Harris noted that dances were generally held around 9:00 p.m. and continued late into the night. In some cases, Margetts took film footage. His intent early on was to publish, and he made references to articles he was writing about Taita in his correspondence, which often included clarifying questions about things he had witnessed. In some cases, he differentiated the pepo dances from *cases* of pepo (as illness), including with one woman he photographed at Mgangi Dawida who "was feeling pretty ill with malaise and headache, and readily accepted an offer to be taken to hospital where malaria was diagnosed. She is one of a family in which *pepo* is prevalent. Rag around forehead and medicine cuts above eyebrows had been administered for headache."[16]

Margetts's report included a lengthy description of pepo as experienced through a form of possession characterized by "shaking, or shivering, or shrugging, rhythmic chatter, whistling in an isolated and irregular manner or in a tune. The afflicted one generally expresses a desire to have something (which may be very peculiar) to eat or drink." The report gave some examples, too: "Sugar cane juice, sea water, sweet smelling soap, kerosene or may ask for a shirt, a buckle, or some other article." He added that the dance (or *ngoma*) centered around the afflicted but that among the drummers and other onlookers and participants it became "quite a party."[17] The rest of the report engages with vernacular notions of mental illness, with terms differentiating types of anxiety states (and their causes), other illnesses, and pathological actions, including suicide and murder.

Pepo dances became a key interest, with photographs taken along the route through the province. One report takes the form of an article he hoped

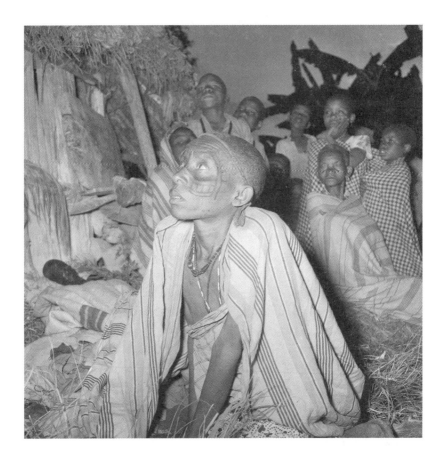

7.1   Original caption reads: "Pepo. Mtaita. C. 35. M. Also Pepo. Rag around
       head, medicine cuts above eyebrows, for headache (she had malaria)."
       Mgangi Dawida, 1957.

to publish, "Pepo Ngoma of the Wataita," which he hoped to illustrate with
his photographs. The draft incorporates existing anthropological literature
on the Taita from Harris and others, but also includes grander references to
Aldous Huxley's *The Devils of Loudun* (1952) and Harrer's *Seven Years in
Tibet* (1953), as well as snake-handling "cults" of the southern United States
and European dancing manias—a tendency of Margetts to reference the
universality of human behaviors, particularly those that could be considered
ancient.[18] He then prompted the district medical officer, Robert McKnight,
to rewrite his previous medical report in article form entitled "Hysterical
Behaviour (Pepo) amongst the Wataita," to be submitted at the same time.

Margetts suggested that McKnight could focus on the general medical impressions of hysteria he witnessed as a medical officer in Wesu and that he should include a "detailed description of the individual case of pepo at the suicide [observed] at Upper Mbale."[19] There is no indication that either Margetts or McKnight succeeded in publishing their articles in the ensuing years, although Margetts did continue to display his photographs in exhibits at various international psychiatric conferences. His visual representation of his encounters in Taita is included in the Proceedings of the 1983 World Congress of Psychiatry meeting in Vienna, where he described pepo as a "highly ritualized dance (ngoma) in order to encourage the manifestations of spirit possession (saka, Sw[ahili], pepo) usually trance, fit or automatic running" (Margetts 1985, 701). So engaged was Margetts with Taita possession states and pepo dances that he shot several reels of film in the late 1950s. His personal notes reflect a rejection of terminology such as "hysterical," suggesting instead that such cases ought to be seen as dissociative, "until we know more about them."

"Possession Hysteria" (the Saka Complex)

While this Canadian psychiatrist engaged with a form of self-styled anthropology in assessing Taita ways of dealing with anxiety, the anthropologist, from her vantage point two decades later, indicated that she would like to have paid more attention to the "psychological formations" surrounding saka possession (Harris 1978, 178n2). Grace Harris first described pepo (or saka) in her article "Possession 'Hysteria' in a Kenya Tribe," published in *American Anthropologist* in 1957. She differentiated saka or pepo dances from "saka attacks," which happened most frequently to married women as part of everyday life in the community. The dance and the "illness" (which saka was considered to be) were linked, as the dance was intended to relieve the visitation of the spirit that makes its demands known through the trance and speech of afflicted women. Harris referred to this entanglement of pepo, the afflicted, the family, the community, and relief as the "saka complex," comprising "the set of symptoms to which people give the name saka; the distribution in the population of susceptibility to attacks; the immediate causes of the attacks; the form of treatment; and Taita notions about saka" (Harris 1957, 1047).

Harris remarked that women who were susceptible to saka would show signs of "generalized restlessness and anxiety," and she described a typical

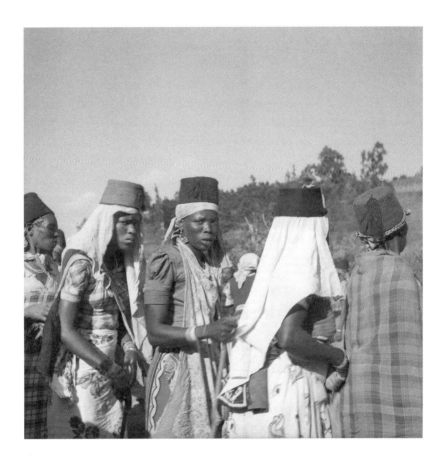

7.2 Original caption reads: "Possession—Taita; Saka (pepo) possession, Mgangi, Taita Hills, 2nd February 1958; women with Fez hats." This photograph was reproduced in Margetts's personal photo album with the caption: "THE FEZ."

case: "Sometimes without any obvious warning a woman begins the characteristic convulsive movements. The upper part of the body trembles but often the head and shoulders are more affected so that, while the shoulders shake rapidly, the head is moved rhythmically from side to side. As the attack continues the eyes may close and the face become expressionless. Some women perform certain simple acts in monotonous repetition, or they repeat strange sounds which are supposed to be foreign words" (Harris 1957, 1048).

The remoteness of the Taita Hills in the early 1950s meant that some accoutrements of European life sometimes acted as a trigger for individual

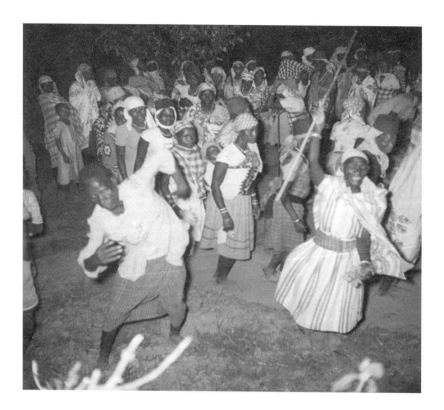

7.3   Original caption reads: "Possession—Taita; Saka (pepo) possession, Mgangi, Taita Hills, 2nd February 1958." This photograph, reproduced in Margetts's personal photograph album, carried the caption: "By 7:00 P.M., most of the men and a few of the women are intoxicated. Women are jovial enough, men inclined to be a little hostile, so we move out."

women performing expressions of a saka attack at "the sight of a motor car, the sound of a train whistle, the sight or smell of a cigarette, the sound of a match being struck, the sight of a bright piece of cloth, the smell, sight, or taste of bananas" (Harris 1957, 1048). This last trigger was not European as such; however, it represented a male cash crop rather than a food staple and clearly delineated the distinct realms of men and women. Harris gave examples of saka attacks, describing a remote part of the Taita Hills where the rare sighting of a European might trigger saka (although she herself did not seem to trigger attacks). Observing a Taita woman who came upon a parked car, Harris noted that she "went into convulsions. She began to dance back and forth, apparently trying to make herself go around the car and continue on her way. Trembling and with her head shaking in the saka fashion, she danced toward the car and then away from it, seeming to find it impossible to approach slowly and go around. Eventually someone else held her arm and helped her to get by" (Harris 1957, 1048).

The strike of a match sent another woman into a convulsion, whereupon a child was sent to bring her a toy concertina. The woman strolled about "playing the concertina's two notes over and over and making sounds which were supposed to be English words. The only intelligible ones were 'sit down' and 'thank you.' These she repeated in monotonous tone, interrupting herself only to assure the two Europeans present, in Kiswahili, that 'nothing was wrong.' When we left the village an hour or so later she was still walking about, jerkily playing the concertina and intoning the same words" (Harris 1957, 1048).

Like Margetts, Harris noted the centrality of objects in expressing saka. Pepo spirits speaking through women demanded material objects from husbands or household needs like sugar, but pepo might even demand a husband's blood. Symptoms were relieved when demands were met. Harris grouped such objects of demand into three categories: items that are normally forbidden to women (such as cigarettes); items of clothing that women do not normally wear; and men's "skills," such as playing the concertina. A second category included purchased items such as sugar or cloth. And, lastly, foreign objects like cars, train whistles, foreign words, and the fez were highlighted (Harris 1957, 1051). Everyday objects, which those of "foreign" extraction soon *became*, were dynamically employed in both shared and individual expressions of saka. Harris's accounts echo early twentieth-century reportage from colonial administrators (often dealing with potentially subversive prophet movements), travelers, and ethnographers. Similarly, there is a wealth of literature on the Swahili coast (and elsewhere) about the incorporation of symbols like the fez and other foreign objects into rituals. These could act, as Harris described, as a "trigger" for emotive expressions of possession. Katherine Luongo's article on prophet and possession movements in the neighboring Kamba region describes the frequency with which British observers recorded the alarming reactions of the Kamba to foreign objects, or items of clothing such as the fez or the pith helmet (Luongo 2012, 191–216). Anthropologist Gerhard Lindblom described these "psychical disturbances" in terms of "epidemics" that spread throughout the Kamba country (Lindblom 1920, 238–39).

These early twentieth-century colonial encounters documented swaths of madness, not in a clinical sense but at least psychologically, and suggested evidence for the dangerous excitability of Africans, particularly when under the influence of "fanatical" leaders (Mahone 2006, 241–58). However, within the context of the everyday, what these demands, symptoms, objects, and relief had at their core, according to Harris, was differences between men and women. "Wage-labour, inheritance, ownership, and land rights sit outside the purview of women in Taita. Even access to towns is largely forbidden as the male presumption is that women who go to the towns succumb to prostitution," she wrote, and Taita women "have far less experience of the world outside the Native Land Unit. . . . Their familiarity with European machines and equipment is slight, and to many of them a camera is still an exceedingly sinister object" (Harris 1957, 1052).

Harris's diagnosis of women—and her thinking was in part diagnostic—within the context of saka recognized women as "uncontrollable consumers; as persons without experience of the outside world. . . . In short, they are shown as contrasting in every way with men, and the contrast is symbolized as a personal malady" (Harris 1957, 1060).

Harris also noted a crucial difference between the "attack" on the individual and the dance in a community of women: "the saka dance turns the saka attack on its head" (Harris 1957, 1060). Comportment in dance is far more composed and dignified. Male garments are worn proudly, community drummers are present to support the dance and are paid for by husbands, onlookers are respectful and attentive. If the saka attack is a form of illness demand, the saka dance is an expression of women's rights to make such demands in a dependency relationship—an expression that speaks to the imbalance of property ownership and access to the outside world. Attack and dance, according to Harris, are "two manifestations of a single situation." So interwoven are these expressions that women engaging in a saka dance might *also* experience the uncontrollable convulsions of a saka attack, as "attack and dance can be translated into one another" (Harris 1957, 1061). Despite Harris's contention that women could be viewed as intellectually isolated and left to only extreme and symbolic ways of making themselves seen and heard, they are nonetheless shown to be central to Taita expressions of well-being and entitlements. The stereotyping of women as "flighty, foolish and irresponsible, in need of masculine guidance and control" was in fact manipulated through religious doctrine to subvert "the mutterings of the everyday battle of the sexes" (Harris 1978, 176). A broader gendered "battle" could be seen in generational terms as well, with Harris reporting that some young men considered saka to be "all pretense," and laughed at anyone taking part. Others in the community, including converted Christians, considered saka attacks to be either the "work of the devil," or a "product of foreign sorcery" sent to ruin the Taita (Harris 1957, 1050). District officials cited memories of imported witchcraft and foreign charms as a source of stress, and reported that the "great war" of 1939 was thought by locals to be the point when witchcraft (previously thought to be hereditary) entered the Hills. It was said that this helped to explain why there were now so many "funny lunatics" in the region.[20] Madness was accepted as present within the region, and there were distinct categories of such illnesses. However, true insanity was associated with violence and such cases could be dealt with harshly, if not fatally. As such, the Taita were far more careful in their use of such terms and accusations of insanity than were contemporary British medical officers (Harris 1978, 49).

Furthermore, Harris remarked on the interpretation of women as "deprived persons," whose behaviors could be seen as arising from the psychological tensions associated with envying men (Harris 1957, 1054). She gives little space to this, however, although such an interpretation would fit squarely within the eventual dominance of I. M. Lewis's theorization of women's cult activities as a response to their peripheral status (Lewis 1971), though a view that has since been challenged by a broad scholarship. Harris briefly noted the Freudian symbolism of certain objects, but her overall contention was that the saka complex must be viewed along a continuous scale of ritual life and whose specific form can be said to "symbolize and expound the social order" (Harris 1957, 1055).

As the saka complex was, in part, about individual expression (the attack), Harris addressed the suggestion and the obvious imagery of a psychiatric disturbance or condition. She recounted the diversity of women she personally knew who suffered saka attacks, stressing a range of personality types, from "mousy shyness" to "sardonic cantankerousness" (Harris 1957, 1062). In this instance, Harris had the distinct advantage over other outsider observers in knowing the individuals involved and gauging their levels of control over their actions or, in some cases, the possibility that they *might have* genuinely neurotic personalities. She also posited that understanding susceptibility to saka attacks would make for a useful psychiatric study, particularly as it might shed light on the "self-induced hypnotic states" of some attacks, as well as the value of saka dances as a form of psychotherapy (Harris 1957, 1062). Harris concluded by remaining open to the suggestion that a psychological interpretation of saka would have value, although she stressed the vital contribution of social anthropology in understanding this Taita idiom: "if they are neurotic; it is in the Taita fashion" (Harris 1957, 1065).

Discussion

With this snapshot of the Taita Hills at a critical decade in late colonial history, I have brought together competing (and sometimes complimentary) claims, observations, and interests of the district government, alongside their engagement with anthropologists and psychiatrists. All were present in this terrain at the same time. What do such encounters and forms of knowledge production tell us about the everyday in this region as decolonization neared? The reportage of such a range of non-Taita witnesses depicts a common zeal for documenting behaviors viewed as exceptional amid conditions that all agreed seemed to be worsening. There is evidence that neighboring communities also witnessed a growing turmoil with rising cases of "insanity" threatening to destabilize the region. Colonial concerns about the Taita also generated one of the first ethnographies of the area, albeit one written with the benefit of hindsight and a revisiting of decades-old fieldnotes. As such, *Casting out Anger* (1978) represents a transformation of anthropological fieldwork into a form of colonial-produced memory. In parallel to this frenetic production of reports, ethnographies, and photographic displays, the Taita simply got on with life through KidaBida—the Taita way.

In her early article on possession hysteria, Harris situated the saka complex within similar possession activities in neighboring groups along Kenya's coast (chiefly the Giriama) as well as further afield, among the Zulu (Junod 1927), the Somali (Ross 1956), and the Songhay (Rouch 1954). The reliance on foreign symbols as a means of expressing anxiety, desire, and seeking out consumable things and experiences was related, according to Harris, to the world of wage labor that surrounded but excluded women. Worried colonial officials used the word *hysteria* nonclinically, but often. The term spoke to the emotive powers of saka possession as a form of communal expression and as an individuated malady that looped back and through all women's concerns. The psychiatrist Margetts rejected the presence of explicit mental illness, hysteria, or madness. He allowed for the possibility of feminine deception in the zeal to acquire material objects or forms of wealth not normally associated with women. He saw the ubiquity of pepo as evidence of mystical thinking common to Africa, but he also meticulously documented and compared key differences in concepts, language, and practice among neighboring groups. Consistently, the colonial government was the most insistent that the Taita were going increasingly mad yet still seeing the area's turmoil as largely unrelated to politics and livelihoods. Most disturbing was the realization that this once placid region could suddenly turn to anger. An older Taita generation might have experienced a similar anxiety, but such vernacular perceptions are difficult to locate.

We may reread these fraught moments of witnessing alongside more recent ethnographic work on the region. James Smith's work portrays a similar period of crisis, expressed in part by an "alarming increase in uncontrollable and deadly forms of witchcraft," handled internally by a few sublocations in the Taita Hills, alongside the help of a prominent witchfinder from Tanzania. According to Smith, the witchfinder's public activities over the course of six months brought controversy and conflict, but also "drew attention to local concerns about the erosion of local social and moral boundaries under conditions defined, at least in part, by recent economic and political liberalization" (Smith 2005, 141–58). This movement, he writes, was articulated as "global in that it was seen as emanating from beyond Taita and also highly local, in that it seized on and transformed localized conflicts and histories as well as people's emotions, which were perceived as increasingly vulnerable because of a diversity of contemporary hardships" (Smith 2005, 143). Smith's interlocutors cited the unease felt in Taita in the 1990s, with clear echoes of the anxious colonial past of the 1950s, including "the rapid increase in violent crime and death, social facts that seemed to directly contravene the image of their region as a place of serenity and cool heartedness in a troubled nation" (Smith 2005, 145–46). The ineffective police response in both periods resulted, in some cases, in violent vigilantism—adding to the sense of chaos and disorder. Under the exigencies and precarities of postcolonial structural adjustment, the Taita today are experiencing pressures and witnessing stresses reminiscent of a time decades earlier when vernacular practices and values were eroding and anxieties surfaced due to the relentless pressure to pay taxes, perform wage labor, and consume commodities.

Notes

1 Taita refers to the region but may also refer to the people. Alternatively, "Wa-Taita" may be used. The region is sometimes written in colonial documents as "Teita" as the official administrative district of the government.

2 Mental Disease—Teita, April 21, 1956, Kenya National Archives (hereafter KNA), BY/9/335.

3 Annual Medical and Sanitary Reports, February 9, 1955, Wesu, KNA, BY/9/335.

4 Catholic Mission Bura, Lunacy in Teita, July 22, 1956, KNA, BY/9/335.

5 Catholic Mission Bura.

6 Annual Medical and Sanitary Reports.

7 Annual Medical and Sanitary Reports.

8 Increase of Number of Mad People Taita: Disturbing Inhabitents [sic], October 29, 1959, KNA, DC/TT/3/9/5.

9 Re: Alleged Higher Incidence of Mental Illness in the Wateita, August 13, 1956, KNA, BY/9/335.

10 E. Margetts to R. A. Wilkinson, DC Taita, August 15, 1956, KNA, BY/9/335.

11 E. Margetts to R. F. McKnight, Re: "PEPO," May 12, 1958, KNA, BY/9/335.

12 Alleged Higher Incidence.

13 Alleged Higher Incidence.

14 Alleged Higher Incidence.

15 Re: The Pepo Ngoma of the Wataita, June 27, 1958, KNA, BY/9/335.

16 Anthropological–Psychological Notes on the Wataita, November 21, 1957, KNA, BY/9/335.

17 Anthropological–Psychological Notes.

18 Pepo Ngoma of the Wataita.

19 E. Margetts to R. F. McKnight.

20 "Witchcraft in Teita District," October 23, 1956, KNA, DC/TTA/3/9/44.

Sources

Archival Material

Kenya National Archives (KNA), Nairobi, Kenya.

Literature

Bostock, Peter Geoffrey. 1950. *The Peoples of Kenya: The Taita*. London: Macmillan.

Bravman, Bill. 1998. *Making Ethnic Ways: Communities and Their Transformations in Taita, Kenya, 1800–1950*. Oxford, UK: James Currey.

Fortes, Meyer. 1979. "Review: *Casting out Anger: Religion among the Taita of Kenya.*" *Man* 14, no. 3: 569–71.

Harris, Grace. 1957. "Possession 'Hysteria' in a Kenya Tribe." *American Anthropologist* 59, no. 6: 1046–66.

Harris, Grace. 1978. *Casting out Anger: Religion among the Taita of Kenya*. Cambridge: Cambridge University Press.

Harris, Grace. 1989. "Mechanism and Morality in Patients' Views of Illness and Injury." *Medical Anthropology Quarterly* 3, no. 1: 3–21.

Hobley, Charles William. 1895. "Upon a Visit to Tsavo and the Taita Highlands." *Geographical Journal* 5, no. 6: 545–61.

Junod, Henri-Alexandre. 1927. *The Life of a South African Tribe*. London: Macmillan.

Kramer, Fritz. 1993. *The Red Fez: Art and Spirit Possession in Africa*. London: Verso.

Lewis, Ioan Myrddin. 1971. *Ecstatic Religion: An Anthropological Study of Spirit Possession and Shamanism*. Harmondsworth, UK: Penguin.

Lindblom, Gerhard. 1920. *The Akamba in British East Africa*. Uppsala, Sweden: Appelbergs Boktryckeri.

Luongo, Katherine. 2012. "Prophecy, Possession, and Politics: Negotiating the Supernatural in 20th Century Machakos, Kenya." *International Journal of African Historical Studies* 45, no. 2: 191–216.

Mahone, Sloan. 2006. "The Psychology of Rebellion: Colonial Medical Responses to Dissent in British East Africa." *Journal of African History* 47, no. 2: 241–58.

Mair, Lucy. 1979. "Review: *Casting out Anger: Religion among the Taita of Kenya.*" *African Affairs* 78, no. 313: 570–71.

Margetts, Edward Lambert. 1985. "The Medicine Man—and Woman—East Africa." In *History of Psychiatry, National Schools, Education, and Transcultural Psychiatry*, edited by Pierre Pichot, Peter Berner, Rainer Wolf, and Kenneth Thau, 697–701. Vol. 8 of *Psychiatry: The State of the Art*. New York: Plenum.

Prins, Adriaan Hendrik Johan. 1952. *The Coastal Tribes of the North-Eastern Bantu*. London: African International Institute.

Ross, A. D. 1956. "Epileptiform Attacks Provoked by Music (Clinical Note)." *British Journal of Delinquency* 7, no. 1: 60–63.

Rouch, Jean. 1954. *Les Songhay*. Paris: Presses Universitaires de France.

Smith, James Howard. 2005. "Buying a Better Witch Doctor: Witch-Finding, Neoliberalism, and the Development Imagination in the Taita Hills, Kenya." *American Ethnologist* 32, no. 1: 141–58.

Smith, James Howard. 2008. *Bewitching Development: Witchcraft and the Reinvention of Development in Neoliberal Kenya*. Chicago: University of Chicago Press.

Spencer, Paul. 1979. "Review: *Casting out Anger: Religion among the Taita of Kenya*." *Bulletin of the School of Oriental and African Studies* 42, no. 3: 586–87.

Richard C. Keller

8

The Universal, the Particular, and Vernacular Resistance in Colonial Algeria

When I published *Colonial Madness* (Keller 2007a) in spring 2007, developments in French politics underscored some of the book's major arguments. Just two years earlier, the National Assembly had passed the Law of 23 February 2005, mandating that teachers in French *lycées* (secondary schools) impress upon their students the positive aspects of France's colonial past, with specific attention to French colonialism in North Africa. Meanwhile, the struggle to determine who would succeed President Jacques Chirac in the republic's highest office involved a bitter fight over immigration, with a close focus on what France's political Right labeled a tight link between immigration from France's former African colonies and crime in peri-urban Paris. Already in 2002, the Center Left had been eliminated in the first round of the presidential elections due to the rapid rise of the radical right-wing Front *National* (FN) (since 2018, the Rassemblement National, RN) on the issue of immigration. In the 2007 election, the Union pour un

Mouvement Populaire candidate, Nicolas Sarkozy, running from the position of interior minister, ran his campaign directly from the FN playbook, using his powerful position within the government to deploy police powers in a mission to cast himself as unrelenting on crime. In the process, he labeled the descendants of migrants from North and West Africa in Paris's suburbs "scum" who needed to be "power-washed" off the streets, a move that helped to set off intense protests in October and November 2005. One of the main arguments of *Colonial Madness*—about the effort by colonial scientists and physicians to cast Islam as a pathogenic force and North African Muslims as inherently different behaviorally from Europeans—had a powerful legacy in the French present (Keller 2007a). This argument appeared relevant in a moment when prominent French politicians and academics made proclamations blaming Islam and polygamy for producing criminal behavior in the *banlieues* (*Le Monde* 2005; Sciolino 2005).

Contemporary developments indicate that these issues have, if anything, intensified in the years since the book's publication, prompting a revisiting of some of the book's arguments. Questions of race and France's legacy of African colonialism have brought politics to a fever pitch. In July 2020, French president Emmanuel Macron commissioned the historian Benjamin Stora to produce a report on France's colonial history in Algeria in particular. The report, published in January 2021, led to the establishment of a memories and truth commission, and made a series of recommendations for how to mend the relationship between France and Algeria. Yet the report skirted the issue of French torture of Algerians during the war for independence and stopped short of recommending any kind of apology or reparations. Beginning in 2020, the government also implemented tight restrictions on access to archives relating to the military during the Algerian War, making them essentially off limits to scholars. And in December 2020, the National Assembly introduced a *projet de loi* (or a bill) in defense of the principles of the republic. Ostensibly targeting foreign funding of radical Islamist groups in France, many accused the law of stigmatizing Islam in general. In a debate on the law hosted on the French political talk show *Vous avez la parole* on February 11, 2021, Macron's interior minister accused the radical Right RN leader Marine Le Pen of being "too soft on Islam."

Meanwhile, as COVID-19 continued to batter France in the winter of 2020–21, amid a botched state response and with a presidential election approaching, a curious debate raged among politicians and academics. In something of a reversal of his 2017 invitation to American scholars to pursue academic freedom in France, Macron decried the American academy as a toxic force bent on destroying the republic. Historians, sociologists, and literary scholars in US universities had deployed theories about race, ethnicity, and identity to expose France's failure to come to terms with its colonial past. In so doing, Macron argued, they engaged in an "ethnicization of the social question" with the goal of "breaking the republic in two" (Onishi 2021). A number of prominent senior humanists and social scientists quickly came to Macron's defense, with a hundred of them signing an open letter in *Le Monde* asserting that "racialist and anticolonial ideologies (imported from North American campuses) are widely present" in French universities, where they were "feeding a hatred of 'whites' and of France" (*Le Monde* 2020). By contrast, younger scholars, and particularly scholars of color, contended that France willfully cultivated racial blind spots in the name of preserving an illusory universalism, and that such theories and concepts were essential for the nation to address the legacy of colonialism and the persistence of racism in French society.

Plus ça change: tensions over the universalist aspirations of republican citizenship and the particular lived experiences of those in France have marked the nation since 1789. France's model of citizenship, articulated in the course of the revolution and a constantly debated part of republican rhetoric since, relies on the abstraction of the individual into the figure of the citizen, who is then capable of representing an equally abstracted nation through a willful disregard of particular differences. In the ideal model, individual particularities are private: factors such as wealth, religion, and race may privately distinguish people from one another, but they have no bearing on public life. Jews, initially excluded from citizenship during the revolution, became citizens by declaring their primary allegiance to the republic rather than to religion. Yet some differences remained as impossible barriers to abstraction: sex, for example, excluded women from active citizenship until the 1940s (and arguably until the turn of the twenty-first century). Islam has been another hotly contested particularity that many have argued is incompatible with the republican model. The veil has remained an important symbol of difference as a public attestation of religion rather than a privately held belief, generating fierce controversy in a republic asserting the importance of universal abstractability (Scott 2004, 2007; Robcis 2013). Likewise, defenders of this model consider any assertions about the importance of allegedly private distinctions for public life—as in claims of a specifically Black experience in France—to be

American-style multiculturalist identity politics, something they claim is a rejection of universalism.

Passionate debates over the capacity of universalism to erase the particular have been especially acute in discussions about mental health and its treatment, in ways that reveal the persistence of psychiatry's challenges in navigating the political landscapes of republicanism and colonialism. This chapter puts the debate over universalism and particularism in a historical context by reexploring the implications of colonial psychiatry for the question of citizenship. It frames that narrative in a longer history of psychiatry's struggles with universalism, racial or ethnic difference, and the contest over citizenship in the mid-twentieth century. It argues that, despite a scientific need to advance the idea of a universal subjectivity—a need dating back to the origins of the profession—French colonial psychiatrists in Algeria insisted on an ineradicable psychological difference between European settlers and the colonized. Yet a particular form of vernacular resistance emerged among a small number of ethnographically sensitive practitioners, who recognized the essential humanity of their patients while respecting the ways in which language, culture, and the politics of colonial rule marked a particular experience that challenged typical French approaches to psychiatric practice.

Work by some of the psychiatric profession's first luminaries often reveals their profound concerns about ethnicity and culture in nascent theories about health and illness, at the same time as they sought to develop a universalizing theory of mind. The writings of Philippe Pinel—widely considered the founder of the modern psychiatric discipline—reveal his immersion in French revolutionary discourse on universality and citizenship. In 1795, as the almost certainly apocryphal story goes, Pinel ordered the unchaining of the inmates at Paris's Bicêtre hospice for the insane, and later at the Salpêtrière, Bicêtre's counterpart for women. The supposedly monstrous insane behaved uncontrollably only because they had been imprisoned and treated as monsters. Willing patients to tranquility by treating them as human, Pinel "elevated the madman to the dignity of the patient" (Keller 2005). In so doing, he launched a half-century-long project of reform in which the state-run, medically organized asylum—one that protected both patients' rights and society—came to be an ideal that marked European care for the insane (Goldstein 1987).

Most accounts of this story position Pinel as embodying the revolutionary ideals of liberty, equality, and fraternity. While these may have been an influence, it is critical to recognize that other factors were probably more important motives. As a French country doctor who had long been excluded from the inner circle of Parisian academic medicine, Pinel took advantage of the deregulation of medical practice in the 1790s to fill a vacuum in the treatment of mental illness. He then dedicated much of his life's work to bringing psychiatry into parity with other medical specializations. Crucial to this effort was grounding psychiatric theories in a universalist philosophical tradition.

As a product of European enlightenment thought, Pinel closely hewed to Jean-Jacques Rousseau's philosophy on the origins of mental instability. Rousseau had argued that insanity marched in step with the progress of civilization; the true nobility of reason existed in man's natural state, and social progress brought with it only a corruption of mind and spirit. Insanity resulted principally from "a reversal of the laws of nature" (Pinel 1813, III, 5; also Jacob 1994). Pinel thus rejected the colloquial term "*folie*," or madness, to designate mental illness, and instead posited the idea of "*aliénation mentale*," or mental alienation, to highlight the process by which one literally lost one's true nature, one's psychic self. *Aliénation* was the price Europeans paid for living in civilization; by implication, psychological well-being was the privilege of the so-called primitive.

What was at stake here was not merely bringing a new science of mental illness and health into line with a philosophical grounding. Much more important was to underscore the universal applicability of a theory of mind in order to establish psychiatry as a legitimate science. With the advent of the anatomopathological clinic, Paris was emerging as the global center of a new biomedical science. By observing symptoms in clinical settings and then immediately analyzing the affected tissues postmortem, French physicians were establishing what they considered objective with broadly applicable laws of the body and its potential failings. As with the *Description de l'Egypte* and the *Encyclopédie*, the body was subject to minute description through its close observation, whereby generalized conclusions established its dominion by science (Ackerknecht 1967; Waddington 1973; Foucault 1994; Warner 1994).

The human mind, in this view, is no different from the body. Rather, a universal mind is compatible with a similar model of citizenship and is analogous to the body in its subjugation to scientific scrutiny. Pinel's theory of mind argues that the materiality of consciousness and intelligence is a substance universally shared. In drawing on Rousseau to articulate a conception of mental estrangement from a true nature, he is explicit that this nature is the province of all men. Rather than cast an irremediable gulf between and among human races and ethnicities—which his polygenist contemporaries had been doing for the past half century—he argues that it is a deviation from our natural roots, a sort of deracination that steers us onto the path of madness. Social and cultural factors—chiefly the malevolent influence of civilization—pull us away from our nature and into madness. Just as the 1789 Declaration of the Rights of Man and Citizen notes that "men are born and remain free and equal in rights," and that "social distinctions may be founded only upon the general good," with the state the guarantor of sovereignty to protect against inequalities, an emergent psychiatry established itself as the guarantor of mental sovereignty over the unrooting of mind under the pressures of modern civilization.

Pinel was vague about who exactly constituted man in his natural state. His successors made such suggestions explicit. Writing in 1839, Alexandre Brierre de Boismont echoed Pinel and Pinel's student Jean-Étienne-Dominique Esquirol, arguing that "mental illness is far more frequent, and in more diverse forms, where peoples are more civilized, while it becomes far rarer where they are less enlightened" (Brierre de Boismont 1839, 293). Yet he drew on field research conducted among specific populations in order to support his claim. He traced a pattern of increasing awareness and incidence of mental illness in Europe from antiquity to the nineteenth century, which he then compared to an apparently lower prevalence in Asia, Latin America, and, most specifically, in Africa. Borrowing from population surveys conducted by British and French explorers, Brierre argued that there was effectively no incidence of mental illness in Egypt or Abyssinia. While his sources identified a number of cases that presented forms of religious madness among Muslim pilgrims, they also asserted that most of these cases were likely faked, either to intimidate strangers or as a kind of religious performance. This left merely a handful of cases that presented forms of alienation linked to what Brierre and his colleagues called moral causes. And "to give this proposition a deeper degree of evidence," he pointed to the numbers of cases of mental illness in relation to their populations. Whereas London showed one case per 200 residents, and Paris one case per 222 residents, Cairo showed one case per 30,000 residents (Brierre de Boismont 1839, 287).

These are, of course, extremely problematic data, with little consistency in what constitutes a diagnosable case of mental illness across both time and place, as well as no accounting for over- or underreporting of cases. What is far more important is that Brierre took them as fact and used them to argue the general principle that madness was fundamentally a moral corruption of mind caused by an alienation from a more natural or "primitive" state—the purest form of which he conveniently found in a North Africa over which France was struggling to exercise hegemony. By drawing on these data, Brierre plotted a continuum that both supported the dominant theory on the causes of insanity and demonstrated the condition's universality along that continuum.

As French annexation expanded in North Africa, however, psychiatrists' position on the uniformity of the psyche began to fray in tandem with their increased experience in the region. Just four years after Brierre published his essay on the relationship between madness and civilization, Esquirol's former student Jacques-Joseph Moreau de Tours published his "Recherches sur les aliénés en Orient" in the premier issue of France's flagship psychiatric journal, the *Annales médico-psychologiques*, which detailed his observations of mental illness and its treatment in Malta, Istanbul, Smyrna, and Cairo. Unable to secure a position after completing his medical degree, Moreau undertook an extensive trip through the Mediterranean. He spent most of his time in Cairo, where he conducted research on the influence of hashish as both a cause of and a treatment for mental illness and worked in a number of hospitals, making a range of observations on insanity as part of his duties (Moreau de Tours 1845; Guba 2020).

Moreau is an important transitional figure. His experience on the ground in Cairo led him to conclude that Brierre and others' conclusions about the rarity of mental illness in North Africa was in part due to undercounting of cases. "Arabs," he argued, "only consider the confinement of one class of the insane, those for whom their *idées fixes*, their disturbances, make them dangerous or intolerable." In other words, only those few among the mentally ill who presented a danger to public safety found themselves in custody, resulting in extremely low case numbers. By contrast, Moreau asserted, "among the peoples of the Orient, madness is generally seen as a holy illness," so most patients remained with their families (Moreau de Tours 1843, 13). Nevertheless, he remained convinced that there were still far fewer afflicted with mental illness in North Africa than there were in Europe. Yet Moreau's strongest differences with his peers were on the causes of this distinction. Unlike Brierre and Esquirol, Moreau was an ardent physicalist, as David Guba (2020) has indicated. Where Brierre, Esquirol, and Pinel agreed that the roots of mental illness were moral, Moreau argued that they were physical, that "madness was a disorder of cerebral functions." Islam and its fatalistic influences, a concern for material satisfactions rather than intellectual activity and the pleasure of the mind (*"les jouissances de l'esprit"*), marked the North African subject; where the European "lives more through the mind than through the body," the "Oriental" is the opposite (Moreau de Tours 1843, 20). The Egyptian, through the influences of Islam and a lack of intellectual stimulation, never experienced the kinds of intellectual development that could lead to the sophisticated complication of mental illness.

This subtle change in Moreau's model—the advancement of a concept of the physical origins of mental illness—coincided with the advancement of French interests in North Africa. While the conquest of Algiers began in 1830, the struggle to annex Algeria unfolded over eighteen years; it was not until 1848 that France seized the colony and began to settle it as a part of the French nation. Moreau's work indicates a kind of sea change in French psychiatric perspectives toward Islam and North Africans. Where metropolitan psychiatrists often hewed to a universalist model, those who practiced in North Africa tended to emphasize an inherent difference between the mentalities of North African Muslims and Europeans—and, increasingly, European settlers in Algeria.

The Crémieux Decree of 1870 represents another important turning point in the intersection of French colonial interests and the production of psychiatric knowledge about North Africans. The decree granted French citizenship to Algeria's European and Jewish populations, despite the fact that few of them had any connection to France. Although a number of French migrated to Algeria amid the disruption of the 1848 revolution, the bulk of Europeans in the colony had arrived from Spain, Malta, and Italy, and the Sephardic Jewish population had little recent connection to Europe. Meanwhile, the decree also explicitly excluded Arabs and Berbers, thereby subjecting them to a separate legal and criminal code.

Whereas before 1870 there were a handful of articles and theses expressing curiosity about mental illness in North Africa, the period after the Crémieux Decree witnessed a dramatic uptick in such work. As settlement increased in Algeria after 1870, and with the establishment of the Tunisian protectorate in 1881, French psychiatrists recreated Moreau's sojourn, touring local facilities for the confinement of the insane and advocating for the establishment of European-style asylums on grounds of public safety. They decried the contemporary practice of transporting mentally ill Algerians to asylums in the south of France as inhumane and impractical. They also further developed theories that highlighted psychic differences between Europeans and Muslims. Whereas anthropologists and other social scientists were focused on careful and often nuanced distinctions among populations within these new colonial spaces—focusing in particular on the differences between Arabs and Kabyles in Algeria—psychiatrists increasingly eschewed these subtleties and developed hardened lines marking a distinct difference between Europeans and Muslims.

As I have argued elsewhere, by the late nineteenth century, psychiatrists produced a discourse suggesting that not only were North African Muslims inherently different from Europeans psychically, but they were also dangerously so. In 1884, Adolphe Kocher studied records from the criminal court in Algiers to conclude that Algerian Muslims were far likelier to commit violent crimes than Europeans (Kocher 1884). A decade later, his colleague Abel-Joseph Meilhon agreed, and argued that such tendencies were biologically determined: the Muslim's "instinctive" nature was a result of "cerebral inferiority" (Meilhon 1896, 17–18). By the early twentieth century, the psychiatrist Auguste Marie, who had traveled extensively in the Middle East and North Africa, had developed what he considered a Darwinian biological theory, one which accounted for the differences in an Arab mentality based in "anatomical characteristics."

These ideas culminated in the work of the so-called Algiers school of French psychiatry, which emerged in the aftermath of World War I. Founded by Professor Antoine Porot—who had trained in Lyon and worked for years in Tunis before moving to Algiers's military Hôpital Maillot during the war—the group comprised Porot's students from the University of Algiers, who trained under his direction at the Hôpital Mustapha in the interwar period. Porot and his students conducted extensive research, beginning with Porot's "Notes de psychiatrie musulmane," which appeared in the *Annales médico-psychologiques* in 1918, and which established him as the empire's leading expert on psychiatry in the colonies. Unlike psychiatrists in other colonial settings, the Algiers school's members published prolifically in top journals, giving them wide exposure and elevating them to the top of their field. Porot also drew French psychiatry's most prestigious conference, the Congrès des médecins aliénistes et neurologistes de France et des pays de langue française, to the Maghreb three times in his career—to Tunis in 1912, Rabat in 1933, and Algiers in 1938.

It was not just their prominence within the French psychiatric profession that distinguished the Algiers school's members from earlier researchers on psychiatry in North Africa. Porot and his counterparts in Morocco and Tunisia built an extensive network of psychiatric hospitals and clinics across the Maghreb, which opened in the 1930s. At their opening, these were modern facilities that were unrivaled in France or the empire, where institutions, if they existed, were often a century or more old. These clinics gave them unparalleled access to colonial subjects to conduct study after study on psychopathology among North African Muslims. And their work reached highly specific conclusions. It asserted that North African Muslims remained unassimilable into French culture due to a pathological cortical structure in their brains that rendered them criminally impulsive and irremediably primitive (Porot and Sutter 1939; Bardenat 1948; Porot and Bardenat 1960). Therefore, any attempt to assimilate them into French society and culture was bound to fail, resulting in either an outburst of violence or, in some cases, the subject's suicide (Donnadieu 1939). Instead of investing in schools, museums, or radio programs designed to facilitate Muslim integration into French culture, the Algerian government should put its resources into a streamlined penal system and an expanded psychiatric hospital network for the protection of settler communities (Porot and Arrii 1932).

These conclusions are significant because they came to light in the context of passionate debates over Algerian citizenship in the interwar period. As with the upticks in psychiatric interest in North African mentality at the moment of initial French expansion and after the Crémieux Decree, intensifying discussions about citizenship for Algerian men in the interwar period met with a surge of research on Algerian psychopathology. Although abolition of slavery in France's so-called old colonies in the Caribbean and the Atlantic had resulted in citizenship for formerly enslaved people after 1848, since 1865, the French government had classified Algerian Muslims as "*indigènes*" (natives), granting them French nationality but denying them citizenship. They could appeal for citizenship, but only by effectively renouncing Islam, which few were willing to do. The Crémieux Decree had done nothing to change this, and most efforts after 1870 came to nothing. This situation changed in 1919, when Jonnart Law outlined a pathway to citizenship for certain categories of Algerian Muslims: those who had completed military service, rural property owners, or those who had demonstrated an affinity for French civilization. The move sparked outrage in Algeria, and represented little improvement over the status quo for Algerians, as the

Algerian governor general retained the capacity to deny citizenship in any case. A much more serious effort unfolded with the Blum-Viollette proposal of 1936. It was ushered in as part of the Popular Front's governing platform, along with expanded educational and cultural programming aimed at France's working class—the same types of programs Porot and his colleagues described as useless for Algerians. The proposal promised to enfranchise Algerian Muslims into similar categories as the Jonnart Law: those with service records, those who had completed French secondary education, and those who were elected representatives serving the Algerian population. As with the Jonnart Law, the Blum-Viollette proposal was met with outrage from both groups of stakeholders in Algeria: settlers became radicalized in their rejection of the very notion of Muslim equality, however limited in scope; and Algerian Muslims became equally resolute, seeing independence as the only path forward (Blévis 2012; see also Ageron 1968; Cole 2019).

It is critical to note that precisely at the moments when the French National Assembly was considering the expansion of citizenship to Algerian Muslims, a scientific discipline was marshaling evidence for why it should be rejected. I am not arguing here that psychiatrists disproportionately influenced the debate over citizenship, nor that they ultimately determined the failure of the Blum-Viollette proposal. Rather, their explicitly political advocacy in works published in the 1930s underscores their vested interests in preserving settler domination in Algeria. This body of work determined with increasing specificity the highly particular psychic makeup of Algerian Muslims in such a way that made them incompatible with enfranchisement in a republic that depended on their capacity for abstraction into the role of universal citizens, and thus it constitutes a critical artifact reflecting the sensibilities of this moment.

It is important to signal another rhetorical component of the Algiers school's work in the context of debates on Algerian citizenship. The constitutional committee that devised the concept of citizenship in 1789 also divided the French population into two overarching categories: those of active and passive citizens. Active citizens had the rights and responsibilities of political citizenship, and consisted of men who paid the equivalent of three days' wages in taxes per year. Passive citizens included virtually everyone else in France. Specific categories of passive citizens were women, children, criminals, and the insane. By using the tools of psychiatric science to label Algerian Muslims as highly—and physiologically—predisposed to violent criminal insanity, Porot and his students not only signaled the particular difference of that population, but they also associated that group with two readily accepted categories of those who could only belong to a second tier of citizenship at best.

Porot's students—and eventually his son Maurice—generally presented a united front. The group's position on issues such as psychopathological predisposition, citizenship, appropriate methods of care, and hard and fast differences between Europeans and North African Muslims were of a piece. There was a notable exception, however, whose story deserves close attention. Suzanne Taïeb, one of the very few women practitioners and very few Arabic speakers who worked in Algerian psychiatric institutions in the period, departed from her *maître* (mentor) in important ways. Her work is significant in its own right for the insights into the experiences of women Muslim patients—she is one of the few colonial psychiatrists to have worked closely with them and to have published about them. But it is also crucial because it shows a kind of vernacular resistance to some of the dominant themes in the Algiers school's work. It indicates that there was a way to draw on knowledge gleaned through clinical contact with Muslim patients to recognize the cultural differences between Europeans and Muslims in Algeria, while still acknowledging the universality of the psyche and, by extension, Algerian Muslims' full humanity.

Born in Béja, Tunisia, in 1907, Taïeb was the eldest child in a large Jewish family. Her father was a wheat merchant and the family was relatively well off. In the 1930s, Taïeb enrolled at the University of Algiers, where Porot encouraged her to pursue her studies at the Faculté de Médecine. She spent three years as an intern at the Hôpital Psychiatrique de Blida-Joinville, Algeria's premier psychiatric facility (Faranda 2012; Studer 2015). Her sex and her language skills allowed her to work more closely with women Algerian patients than anyone had before. Historians have focused on this aspect of her work as the most important (Bégué 1989; Berthelier 1994). Her thesis also includes some of the most detailed case histories of any produced by members of the Algiers school. Yet perhaps what is most significant about her work is that, in part due to her status as a relative outsider when compared with her peers, she provides a significantly different perspective on North African Muslim subjectivity from that of her colleagues.

In some ways, Taïeb's work is of a piece with that of her colleagues. She begins by reciting a litany of tropes about North African Muslims and their psychology. She adheres closely to her colleagues' pronouncements about the so-called fatalism and primitivism of North Africans, as well as their intellectual inferiority. Yet, for Taïeb, the causes of these phenomena were external ones rather than inherent and biologically fixed differences. Where there were higher rates of mental debility among North African Muslims, she argued that these were a function of high syphilis rates and prevalent encephalitis infections among children (Taïeb 1939).

Taïeb also paid close attention to the idioms of madness in settler versus Muslim patients. Where the content of Europeans' delusions included figures from daily life, including priests, neighbors, and doctors, among North Africans, the influences of sorcery were more pronounced. Vernacular experiences, then, rather than innate physiological difference, shaped local psychological distress and outcomes. This perspective constituted a form of intellectual resistance: in describing psychological phenomena in this way, Taïeb granted her patients a kind of psychic malleability and adaptability that her colleagues rejected. Perhaps most telling is her concluding observation: "What is curious to note is the progressive transformation of these themes of influence among natives who have begun to enter our civilization. Among those whose education or social life has called them to live our lives and take on our habits, one sees a critical attitude begin to develop" (Taïeb 1939, 148–49).

Taïeb's recognition of assimilability comes at the end of a thesis that, for the most part, reiterates the principal themes of her colleagues' work. Yet her fluency in Arabic language and colloquial practices, which she gained by growing up with Muslim Arab women in Tunisia—she wrote that she drew on her "childhood memories, because I had the good fortune to live among [Muslim women] in the little town in Tunisia where I was born"— provided her the opportunity to learn more from her patients about their experiences than her exclusively francophone colleagues. According to Taïeb's biographer, Laura Faranda (2012), Taïeb took photographs of her patients so that she could more easily recognize them and remember their names, a practice her colleagues failed to do. And as I argued in *Colonial Madness* (Keller 2007a, 116), as a result of these factors, her case histories go into detail about the ways in which colonial biases and violence informed her patients' illness experiences. She alone among members of the Algiers school was able to navigate mistranslations and crossings, and to identify the ways in which racialized structures of rule manifested in her patients' suffering, where they surfaced as deliria of persecution by settlers, with regular abuse by Europeans as the foundation of their illnesses.

In the early 1940s, with the arrival of German forces and Vichy policies in Algeria, Taïeb lost her position at Blida due to her Jewish status. She never practiced in Algeria again, although she moved to the outskirts of Paris, where she opened a clinic in Gennevilliers, serving primarily the North African migrant community in the *bidonvilles* in the area until her death in 1979. She never published again after her thesis, so it remains unclear how her perspective developed, although she did remain in touch with her former colleagues for the rest of her life. Two psychiatrists who arrived at Blida more than a decade after Taïeb's ouster, however, read her work and built on it extensively. Frantz Fanon is, of course, the face of French anticolonial resistance in Algeria; but he was also a committed psychiatric reformer who saw in his profession the possibility of psychic liberation (Robcis 2021; Keller 2007b). His intern Jacques Azoulay was no less engaged in this endeavor.

Like Taïeb, Fanon saw the ways in which the colonial situation produced psychopathology in his patients. Also like Taïeb, it was his experience as an outsider that informed his clinical perspective on colonial pathogenesis. Yet in contrast with not only Taïeb but the entirety of French psychiatric discourse about North African Islam and the personality of the colonized, Fanon was not so naive as to focus on simplistic formulations like the universal and the particular. As his *Black Skin, White Masks* makes patently clear, Fanon recognized the fiction of French universalism on his arrival in France from Martinique. Although he was a citizen by birth, based on his lineage in one of France's so-called old colonies, his reception in Lyon continually reminded him of his perpetual status as an outsider. This was among the reasons Fanon sought a post in Algeria from the outset: disillusionment with his experiences of racism in the course of his medical education as well as his first residency in France led him to seek a professional outlet whereby he might both find greater acceptance and accomplish his goals of developing a liberatory psychiatric practice (Cherki 2000; Macey 2000).

Where their predecessors saw either a universal spectrum from the primitive to the civilized that placed the North African on one end and the European on the other, or a particular and ineradicable physical difference that prevented the Muslim from having any capacity for assimilation, Fanon and his intern Azoulay saw something far more complex. Azoulay's thesis provided the basis for several coauthored papers that highlight a novel perspective on normal and abnormal Muslim psychology in Algeria. The thesis involved an experiment that Azoulay and Fanon conducted in two separate wards at Blida: a European women's ward and a Muslim men's ward. Drawing on Fanon's experience at the Saint Alban hospital in France, they implemented a kind of sociotherapy in the wards, engaging the patients in the running of a cinema series, the production of a newspaper, among other activities. The experiment was a great success in the European women's ward, but a complete failure among the Muslim men as it adopted elements of an everyday register that only comported with the expectations of one of these patient populations. For Muslim men, there was a complete disconnect— they took no interest in the activities, and if anything the attempt provoked disturbances in the ward (Fanon and Azoulay 2015a). A second experiment proved more promising, however. Recognizing that film and print media played only a minor role in the lives of Algerian patients outside the hospital, Azoulay and Fanon took a different tack. They engaged the patients in the operation of a traditional Algerian café and gardening work, and even cleared a field to create a football pitch on the hospital grounds. These referents aligned more closely with patients' expectations of colloquial practice and drew their enthusiastic response. Within a year, Fanon and Azoulay reported positive results.

The difficulties that Fanon and Azoulay had encountered prompted them to dig further into an understanding of Algerian Muslims from a cultural perspective. They noted quite literally vernacular tensions in the clinic: the violence of attempting to practice across a language barrier. Even with an interpreter the effort was bound to fail: most Algerians' experiences with interpreters were "administrative or judicial," preconditioning mistrust in their presence (Fanon and Azoulay 2015a, 310). They also concluded that cultural determinants played such a significant role in shaping both the illness experience and the efficacy of psychiatric methodology that any notion of a universal psyche was misguided. Yet difference did not need to be physical, or by its nature pathological. Of course, it was impossible to achieve good results by implementing "a western-inspired socio-therapy in a ward for mentally ill Muslims"—their mistake as psychiatrists was "to reflexively adopt the politics of assimilation" (Fanon and Azoulay 2015a, 305). Recognizing that their patients' psychic touchstones were organized through religion, agricultural practice, and the political economy of a colonial fracturing in their society, Fanon and Azoulay understood the failure in their initial experimental design and redoubled their efforts to understand patients' vernacular frames. After Fanon's death, Azoulay reported that Fanon had immersed himself in learning about Muslims' understandings and expectations of mental illness and its treatment, attending traditional healing ceremonies. He also visited *douars*, or small agrarian villages, where he sought to learn about everyday material practices in rural Algerian spaces that most of his patients called home (Murard 2008). What he found was a population destined to strike Europeans as other, but also that alterity was a result of European prejudice rather than racial difference. In an unpublished paper, Fanon and Azoulay argued that "certain behaviors, certain reactions could appear to us to be 'primitive,' but that is only a value judgment, arguably dependent on poorly defined characteristics, and that offers little insight into an understanding of the Algerian Muslim man" (Fanon and Azoulay 2015b).

Fanon and Azoulay were unique in their framing of Algerian subjectivity. Early nineteenth-century psychiatrists could only account for difference in a civilizational framework, seeing North Africans as people living in a natural state, uncorrupted by society, and therefore protected from the ravages of mental illness (albeit cut off from intellectual sophistication as well). This frame supported the notion of a universal psyche, which was subject to moral influence that could lead to pathology, but also to healing. In so doing, they drew on an episteme of universalism that informed both the novel experiment in republican citizenship, but also a nascent science of the mind that sought to align itself with other medical specializations that cast themselves as universally applicable. By contrast, with the expansion of colonial settlement in North Africa, and in the context of furious debates over the question of citizenship, psychiatrists in the colonies broke with this epistemic imperative and insisted on particular differences inherent in the Algerian psyche that made the Muslim incompatible with assimilation. Although Suzanne Taïeb never engaged specifically with the question of citizenship, she pierced this logic, arguing by way of her linguistic facility and direct knowledge of her patients that a cultural adaptation of Algerians could set them on the pathway to assimilability.

By contrast, Fanon and Azoulay's research led them to see the psychological differences between Europeans and North Africans as profound. They were cultural differences rather than biological ones, to be sure, but they remained significant. The critical distinction is that Fanon and Azoulay saw the discourse of assimilation as threatening to Muslim Algerians' identity and to the effectiveness of therapeutic practice. They found that Muslim Algerians differed from Europeans in their fundamental frames of reference, yet colonial psychiatrists insisted that "the native does not need to be understood in his cultural originality"; instead, "the effort should be made by the 'native' and he has every interest in becoming in his type the model of man that is proposed." Fanon and Azoulay were forced to struggle against this perspective:

"Indeed, a revolutionary attitude was essential, as we need to move from a position in which the supremacy of western culture was self-evident to a cultural relativism" (Fanon and Azoulay 2015a, 305).

In the postcolonial era, colonial knowledge about Muslims of North African descent has retained its relevance. Waves of immigration in the 1960s and 1970s brought renewed attention to Porot and his students' work on the supposedly innate criminality of the Algerian, which had by then made its way into prominent psychiatric textbooks. In the summer of 1973, a mentally ill Algerian living in Marseille inexplicably attacked and killed a bus driver, an incident that prompted a furious outburst of racialized violence in and around the city and fed a resurgent right-wing view on the mental instability of Arab migrants (Gastaut 1993). As Abdelmalek Sayad argued in 1977, the migrant body was subject to fear and policing as the function of a colonial discourse in a postcolonial moment: there was no difference that was not also threatening to the fabric of the republic (Sayad [1977] 1999). Such debates have only intensified since, with the increasing electoral presence of the Front National—now renamed the Rassemblement National in an effort to underscore its broad appeal. Meanwhile, straying (at least rhetorically) from its strongly Catholic roots, the party has adopted a policy of strictly endorsing *laïcité* (secularism) condemning radicalism but insisting that, in private practice, Islam is a religion like any other.

This is the context in which Fanon's insistence on the importance of vernacular difference remains not only relevant, but critical. As I write this conclusion, France is torn over the place of race in contemporary society and its legacy of African colonialism. As younger scholars increasingly investigate racial tensions in France, they are invariably poking at a wound with its roots in Africa and most specifically in North Africa. (It is notable that so much of this discourse is centered on the role of colonialism in Africa and the Caribbean, in comparison to, for example, Southeast Asia.)

In early February 2021, a press interview with the sociologist Rachida Brahim centered on the question of race and how it fits into the republic's fictions of the universal and the particular. France is suffering from structural racism, she argues, as a function of "particularization and universalization, racialization and deracialization," which both "creates race and denies it at the same time." While a post-1945 discourse denies the biological reality of race, French administrative practices have reinforced it at every turn. In the 1960s, immigration officials established a record of stigmatizing "African migrants as a group of unassimilable and potentially deviant individuals," effectively racializing migration while simultaneously denying the existence of race as a concept. Brahim insists that the university itself is implicated in the continued preservation of this status quo. When she was writing her dissertation on racial violence in France, her own doctoral adviser, she recounts, insisted that she could not see that her subject was really class, rather than race, as "the fact that I am of Algerian descent prevented me from distancing myself from the subject." In rejecting race as a concept, the adviser signaled the ways in which her racial difference threatened her scholarly objectivity. The university—the institution at the heart of contemporary debates over race and France's colonial legacy—"is primarily a statist institution in the same sense as the police or justice system. It does what the State expects it to do. Its goal is not to produce knowledge to radically improve society, but to maintain the dominant thought that benefits from the established order" (Brahim 2021).

Brahim's work is thus at the center of France's moral panic over critical race theory and intersectionality. Moreover, it points to the inextricability of this crisis from France's inability to come to terms with its colonial past in Africa. A continued insistence on the universality of the citizen is based on the rejection—or rather, the ignoring—of particular differences and, above all, particular interests. Yet for many French citizens, that difference and that interest define their interaction with state and society—they are inseparable from their identity as constructed through their experience. Just as the political economy and structural violence of the Algeria of Fanon's era produced a specific and ineluctable experience for those subject to its rule, similar phenomena organize the frame of reference for a growing population in France. At the same time, the cultural relativism that Fanon insisted held the key to resolving the tensions of France's colonial legacy remains institutionally unacceptable, and instead, in Macron's words, threatens to "break the republic in two."

Sources

Ackerknecht, Erwin. 1967. *Medicine at the Paris Hospital, 1794–1848*. Baltimore, MD: Johns Hopkins University Press.

Ageron, Charles-Robert. 1968. *Les Algériens musulmans et la France, 1870–1919*. Paris: Presses Universitaires de France.

Bardenat, Charles. 1948. "Criminalité et délinquance dans l'aliénations mentale chez les indigènes algériens," parts 1 and 2. *Annales médico-psychologiques* 106, no. 2: 317–33, 468–80.

Bégué, Jean. 1989. "Un siècle de psychiatrie française en Algérie, 1830–1939." Mémoire de these, Université Pierre et Marie Curie.

Berthelier, Robert. 1994. *L'Homme maghrébin dans la littérature psychiatrique*. Paris: L'Harmattan.

Blévis, Laure. 2012. "Quelle citoyenneté pour les Algériens?" In *Histoire de l'Algérie à la période coloniale (1830–1962)*, edited by Abderrahmane Bouchène, Jean-Pierre Peyroulou, Ouanassa Siari Tengour, and Sylvie Thénault, 352–58. Paris: La Découverte.

Brahim, Rachida. 2021. "Mettre en lumière les crimes racistes, c'est nettoyer nos maisons." *Ballast*, February 5, 2021. https://www.revue-ballast.fr/rachida-brahim-mettre-en-lumiere-les-crimes-racistes-cest-nettoyer-nos-maisons/.

Brierre de Boismont, Alexandre. 1839. "De l'influence de la civilisation sur le développement de la folie." *Annales d'hygiène publique et de médecine légale* 21:241–95.

Cherki, Alice. 2000. *Frantz Fanon: Portrait*. Paris: Éditions du Seuil.

Cole, Joshua. 2019. *Lethal Provocation: The Constantine Murders and the Politics of French Algeria*. Ithaca, NY: Cornell University Press.

Donnadieu, André. 1939. "Psychose de civilization." *Annales médico-psychologiques* 97, no. 1: 30–37.

Fanon, Frantz, and Jacques Azoulay. 2015a. "La socialthérapie dans un service d'hommes musulmanes: Difficultés méthodologiques." In *Frantz Fanon: Écrits sur l'aliénation et la liberté*, edited by Jean Khalfa and Robert Young, 297–313. Paris: Découverte.

Fanon, Frantz, and Jacques Azoulay. 2015b. "La vie quotidienne dans les douars." In *Frantz Fanon: Écrits sur l'aliénation et la liberté*, edited by Jean Khalfa and Robert Young, 314–24. Paris: Découverte.

Faranda, Laura. 2012. *La signora di blida: Suzanne Taïeb e il presagio dell'etnopsichiatria*. Rome: Armando.

Foucault, Michel. 1994. *The Birth of the Clinic*. Translated by Alan Sheridan. New York: Vintage.

Gastaut, Yves. 1993. "La flambée raciste de 1973 en France." *Revue européenne de migrations internationales* 9, no 2: 61–75.

Goldstein, Jan. 1987. *Console and Classify: The French Psychiatric Profession in the Nineteenth Century*. New York: Cambridge University Press.

Guba, David. 2020. *Taming Cannabis: Drugs and Empire in Nineteenth-Century France*. Montreal: McGill–Queens University Press.

Jacob, Françoise. 1994. "La psychiatrie française face au monde colonial au XIXe siècle." In *Découvertes et explorateurs: Actes du colloque international, Bordeaux 12–14 juin 1992. VIIe Colloque d'Histoire au Présent*. Paris: L'Harmattan.

Keller, Richard C. 2005. "Pinel in the Maghreb: Liberation, Confinement, and Psychiatric Reform in French North Africa." *Bulletin of the History of Medicine* 79, no. 3: 459–99.

Keller, Richard C. 2007a. *Colonial Madness: Psychiatry in French North Africa.* Chicago: University of Chicago Press.

Keller, Richard C. 2007b. "Clinician and Revolutionary: Frantz Fanon, Biography, and the History of Colonial Medicine." *Bulletin of the History of Medicine* 81, no. 4: 823–41.

Kocher, Adolphe. 1884. *De la criminalité chez les Arabes au point de vue de la pratique médico-judiciaire en Algérie.* Paris: J. B. Baillière et fils.

Le Monde. 2005. "Le ministre de l'emploi fait de la polygamie une 'cause possible' des violences urbaines." November 16, 2005. https://www.lemonde.fr/societe /article/2005/11/16/le-ministre-de-l-emploi-stigmatise-la-polygamie_710615 _3224.html.

Le Monde. 2020. "Enseignement supérieur: 'Sur l'islamisme, ce qui nous menace, c'est la persistance du déni.'" November 1–2, 2020.

Macey, David. 2000. *Frantz Fanon: A Biography.* London: Picador.

Meilhon, Abel-Joseph. 1896. "L'aliénation mentale chez les Arabes: Etude de nosologie comparée." Parts 1–6, *Annales médico-psychologiques* 54, no. 1: 17–32, 177–207, 364–77; and no. 2: 26–40, 204–20, 344–63.

Moreau de Tours, Jacques-Joseph. 1843. "Recherches sur les aliénés en Orient." *Annales médico-psychologiques* 1, no. 1: 1–30.

Moreau de Tours, Jacques-Joseph. 1845. *Du haschish et de l'aliénation mentale.* Paris: Esquirol.

Murard, Numa. 2008. "Psychotherapie institutionelle à Blida." *Tumultes* 31:31–45.

Onishi, Norimitsu. 2021. "Will American Ideas Tear France Apart? Some of Its Leaders Think So." *New York Times*, February 9, 2021. https://www.nytimes.com /2021/02/09/world/europe/france-threat-american-universities.html.

Pinel, Philippe. 1813. *Nosographie philosophique ou méthode de l'analyse appliquée à la médecine.* Paris: Brosson.

Porot, Antoine. 1918. "Notes de psychiatrie musulmane." *Annales médico-psychologiques* 76:377–84.

Porot, Antoine, and Don Côme Arrii. 1932. "L'impulsivité criminelle chez l'indigène algérien—ses facteurs." *Annales médico-psychologiques* 90, no. 2: 588–611.

Porot, Antoine, and Charles Bardenat. 1960. *Anormaux et malades mentaux devant la justice pénale.* Paris: Maloine.

Porot, Antoine, and Jean Sutter. 1939. "Le 'primitivisme' des indigènes Nord-Africains: Ses incidences en pathologie mentale." *Sud médical et chirurgical*, April 15, 226–41.

Robcis, Camille. 2013. *The Law of Kinship: Anthropology, Psychoanalysis, and the Family in France.* Ithaca, NY: Cornell University Press.

Robcis, Camille. 2021. *Disalienation: Politics, Philosophy, and Radical Psychiatry in Postwar France*. Chicago: University of Chicago Press.

Sayad, Abdelmalek. (1977) 1999. *La double absence: Des illusions de l'émigré aux souffrances de l'immigré*. Paris: Seuil.

Sciolino, Elaine. 2005. "Immigrant Polygamy Is a Factor in French Unrest, a Gaullist Says." *New York Times*, November 18, 2005. https://www.nytimes.com /2005/11/18/international/europe/immigrant-polygamy-is-a-factor-in-french -unrest-a.html.

Scott, Joan. 2004. "French Universalism in the Nineties." *differences* 15, no. 2: 32–53.

Scott, Joan. 2007. *The Politics of the Veil*. Princeton, NJ: Princeton University Press.

Studer, Nina. 2015. *The Hidden Patients: North African Women in French Colonial Psychiatry*. Zurich: Bohlau.

Taïeb, Suzanne. 1939. *Les idées d'influence dans la pathologie mentale de l'indigène nord-africain: Le rôle des superstitions*. Algiers: Ancienne imp. Heintz.

Waddington, Ivan. 1973. "The Role of the Hospital in the Development of Modern Medicine: A Sociological Analysis." *Sociology* 7, no. 2: 211–24.

Warner, John. 1994. *Against the Spirit of System: The French Impulse in Nineteenth-Century American Medicine*. Baltimore, MD: Johns Hopkins University Press.

PART IV

UNEXPECTED ARCHIVES AND ETHNOGRAPHIC INVESTIGATIONS

Romain Tiquet

9

Precarious Families, "Danger," and Psychiatric Internment in 1960s Dakar

An Archive of Kin Letters

On January 8, 1968, a woman we shall call A.N.[1] sent a petition to Governor Pape Malick M'Bengue of Cape Verde Peninsula (Cap-Vert, a region of Dakar, Senegal) in "hopes" of arranging psychiatric internment for her daughter, A.T., then residing in her mother's home. A.N. wrote: "I have the honor to ask for your great benevolence in the internment at Fann Hospital of my child A.T. who has been suffering from mental disorders for some time. She is becoming very angry and is picking on the inhabitants of the house."[2] The reply was not long in coming. On the same day, the governor sent a letter to the director of the Fann psychiatric clinic, requesting A.T. be admitted in order to decide "whether in her actual state she is a danger to public order."[3]

This chapter sheds light on a collection of such previously unexplored letters, written to the governor of Cap-Vert in the 1960s asking to commit a relative to a psychiatric unit. In 1960s Senegal, only two neuropsychiatric services existed: the psychiatric clinic of Fann and the hospital of Thiaroye. Thiaroye, opened in 1960, was an annex of Fann psychiatric clinic, and was meant for chronic patients (Ozouf, Collignon, and Sylla 1977). The neuropsychiatric service at Fann hospital opened in 1956, late in the colonial period. It was to serve all of colonial French West Africa, and it became a psychiatric clinic in 1958, after Senegal was declared a republic. The Fann clinic was deeply influenced by Henri Collomb, who directed the service from 1959 to 1978, and Moussa Diop, the first Senegalese psychiatrist (Collignon 1978; Arnaut 2009; Kilroy-Marac 2019).

The Fann clinic became a cradle of transcultural psychiatry and intense reflections on African psychopathologies (Bullard 2022). Collomb and his team surrounded themselves with ethnologists, sociologists, and anthropologists to think about the social, economic, and cultural aspects of mental illness. *L'École de Fann* developed a mixed practice, with technical aspects of Western psychiatry combined with a local theoretical basis inspired by the experiences of Senegal's traditional therapists (Thiam and Moro 2014; Bullard 2022). Such a "psychiatry without borders" sought to break down asylum walls and open up a health-care institution to local definitions and representations of mental disorders. It influenced many institutions in West Africa (Kilroy-Marac 2019).

This historiographic reflection lies at the crossroads of two themes. By examining letters requesting to intern relatives, I investigate what happened before any "entry into psychiatry," thereby expanding the history of psychiatry, which thus far has focused mainly on colonial psychiatric wards (Vaughan 1983; Collignon 2010; Quarshie 2011). In histories of mental health care, hospitalization was but one treatment practice among others, often presumed to be the last therapeutic option chosen by West African families. I also add a historical dimension to the literature on relationships between family care and mental illness in Africa (Gruénais 1990; Hunt 1999; Kilroy-Marac 2014; Parle 2014; Aït Mehdi 2018; Diagne and Lovell 2020). Some scholars have focused on relationships between family solidarity and community-based approaches to treating mental illness, often idealizing the African family as the primary source of care (Janzen 1978; Collignon 1983; Read 2012). Another strand, from the field of medical anthropology, has focused on elements leading to forms of family exclusion or "social abandonment" (Biehl 2005; Povinelli 2013). The psychiatric hospital often reveals the limits of family care (Whyte 2012; de-Graft Aikins 2015; Petit 2020). Yet the notion of abandonment has been criticized for producing an overdetermined, passive image of the family, denying forms of autonomy (Dracchio 2020).

Fann clinical teams were interested in their patients' family ties, organizing long interviews with immediate kin (mainly parents) and even traveling to villages to gain a better understanding of the social and cultural environments of patients (Fann 1968). Did this comprehensive approach, unlike the repressiveness of "classic" colonial asylums, have an influence on families' willingness to commit a relative to Fann? Henri Collomb suggested something different in an interview with Hubert Fichte in the mid-1970s, recalling how he "came to the pessimistic conclusion that in the end, a stay at Fann only accelerates and reinforces the alienation of our patients. The patient is a member of society as long as he or she has not left traditional healing processes. . . . [Yet if these do not work] . . . or if society excludes him or her . . . the family considers him mentally ill [*aliené*]. Only then does the family send him to Fann, wanting us to keep him here forever" (Fichte 1990, 38).

A close exploration of kin letters allows for a more complex analysis and reveals the agency of families. Forms of care for the mentally ill were dependent on multiple factors, which must be taken into account in analyzing how moral—but also social and economic—ideals of family care were challenged on a daily basis, according to a range of parameters: access to resources for care and healing, the nature of severe mental illness, the strength of family solidarity, and the like (Quinn 2007; Read and Nyame 2019).

The letters examined here come from regional archives in Dakar and are composed of two types: first, letters, usually handwritten, from family members asking the governor of Cap-Vert for a psychiatric commitment of a relative; and second, the governor's requests to the director of Fann hospital for a diagnosis of the individual, to determine whether they should be committed.

The family-authored letters assembled here include nearly sixty in all, written after Senegal's decolonization. I use the term "family" in a broad sense: not as a stable category but to suggest networks of shifting relations among immediate and extended family members. The letters were written between 1961 and 1969, although it is conceivable that others may have been received before and after these dates without being processed or kept by the authorities. A variety of family members—mothers, fathers, cousins, uncles, brothers, and close neighbors—wrote them. People of all ages were the ill subjects of these letters—children, adolescents, and people over sixty years old. Nearly 25 percent of the corpus requests the internment of women relatives.

What else makes these letters special? First, petitions have rarely been investigated within the frame of Africa's histories of madness or in the continent's social history (Sifou 2004; Lawrance 2006; Rodet and Tiquet 2018). Attention has heretofore been devoted to petitions asking for the psychiatric release of kin (Edington 2019, 122), but never to petitions asking to commit a relative to a psychiatric ward. In *Imperial Bedlam*, Jonathan Sadowsky (1999) mentions that the majority of letters he found were release requests, while requests for internment were few. Many of the petitions discussed here were found outside the psychiatric ward, within Dakar's regional archives. We need a multisited exploration of such a source to assemble histories of madness that are not limited by psychiatric archives. By looking at letters written after the country gained independence, their analysis opens up new avenues for the history of madness in Senegal and West Africa, and beyond much current scholarship that still focuses too narrowly on colonial psychiatry (McCulloch 1995; Mahone and Vaughan 2007; Akyeampong, Hill, and Kleinman 2015).

The requests sent by the governor to the Fann clinic's director were template letters: only the name of the individual ever changed. The template was in keeping with Article 5 of the General Order of June 28, 1938, stipulating that either the governor or the security services could order that a subject deemed dangerous be presented to a qualified alienist for examination or internment.[4] This 1938 colonial decree also established psychiatric assistance in French West Africa (including Senegal). The same decree remained in place in postcolonial Senegal. Not until 1975 did Senegal pass a national law reorganizing its psychiatric services.[5]

The families who wrote the letters were mainly from Dakar, the capital city, and a key focus of attention for Senegalese authorities during those early postindependence years of shaping the country into a nation. Dakar remains the site of daily repression of urban marginality—of vagrants, lepers, prostitutes, and "lunatics"—by police seeking to "clean up the city" and make it attractive for foreign investors (Ndiaye 1979; Collignon 1984; Faye and Thioub 2003). In this vexed context, interning a "mentally ill" individual as "dangerous" remains a way to remove and erase them from "public space."

The historical literature on madness in Africa tends to focus on psychiatric knowledge under colonial rule. Relevant studies of British African colonies—pioneers in this field of research and care—have pointed out the wide range of ideological tools used by colonial authorities to control, usually unsuccessfully, the bodies and minds of the colonized (Vaughan 1983; McCulloch 1995; Sadowsky 1999; Quarshie 2011; Heaton 2013; Linstrum 2016). In contrast, historiography on colonial psychiatry in French colonies in Africa has lagged behind (D'Almeida 1997; Collignon 1999, 2010), at the same time that the francophone anthropological literature on madness has in many senses been more innovative.

I am aware of the risk of overinterpreting individual situations when grappling with this corpus of letters, especially since insights provided by letters arise from relatively succinct texts (in letters that rarely exceed a few paragraphs). Still, it remains possible to suggest several lines of thought through a fine-grained analysis. In the first section, I analyze how letters describe, name, and suggest a diagnosis for a mental disorder, and some-times beyond psychiatric words. This step sideways enables interrogating the development of relationships between family care and mental disorder, and the emergence of an imported psychiatry from Europe alongside the opening of the Fann psychiatric clinic just a few years before independence.

The second section focuses on a persistent question arising from this corpus of letters: what caused families to seek hospitalization for a relative who they perceived as mentally ill? Was it because the person seemed to pose a threat to themselves, their families, or their surroundings? Strikingly, the speedy answers of the governor underline quite a different concern: public order, and the need for Senegalese authorities to repress urban marginal-ity and "dangerous lunatics" in this decolonizing context of developing a strong, clean nation in the 1960s.

Finally, monetary deficiency played an important role in the limitations of family care. Economic precarity drove many families to ask for relatives to be admitted to a psychiatric service because the moral—but also financial—costs seemed too heavy to bear. This socioeconomic aspect opens up matters of how families tried to meet the ethical and practical demands of care.

Before Entering the Psychiatric Unit

On November 18, 1968, S.S., a young man of twenty-eight years, seemed affected by "mental dementia and suffering from various diseases."[6] Al-though some letters feature the common categories of medical staff or the political authorities, like "mental dementia," "mental alienation," or "mental troubles," different expressions also announced to the authorities that a relative was mentally ill. These terms highlight a constant negotiation over what was understood as "madness" by a variety of actors: medical staff, family members, the authorities, and the like (Parle 2014).

In January 1965, the daughter of M.J.P. explained that her mother was "affected by THE madness," using capital letters in her text.[7] Similar language appeared in a letter from February 1966, when S.B.S. requested assistance for his niece, O.H.D., "affected by the Madness" (with the "M" capitalized).[8] Some letters expressed that mental disorder was the result of an outside intervention. In September 1965, the cousin of M.D. explained that his relative "had a furious insanity attack"[9] (or a *crise de folie*, a crisis of madness). In December 1964, a daughter described M.A. as "invaded by the madness."[10] In these petitions, madness was sometimes personified as a distinct entity, and sometimes seen as the result of an outside attack, underlying local, vernacular forms of understanding madness.

Such expressions aligned with representations of madness, observed in Senegal and West Africa. Indeed, as studies by several scholars have shown, three main explanations of the cause of mental disorders are common in the region: first, possession by spirits, manifest in trance phenomena; second, attacks by "witches," manifested by terrible anguish and feelings of losing one's body; and third, *maraboutage*, which lies at the crossroads of religion and magic (Zempleni 1968; Sow 1978; Fassin 1984). Nevertheless, this tripartite categorization deserves a critical eye due to some overinterpreting objects, words, or practices as madness or mental disorder (Olivier de Sardan 1994).

My corpus of letters illustrates how family members linked an unusual behavior with mental disorder. Shouting, insults, incoherent language, physical threats, and nudity were alleged in the petitions as signs of insanity. On August 13, 1964, I.D., the landlord of F.F., wrote that his female tenant was "not enjoying her mental faculties, crazy in the true sense of the word, [she] constantly comes to my home, night and day, makes a lot of noise, shouts, insults, and threatens to harm my family members and in particular attacks the children."[11] Sometimes, letter writers explained a mental disorder in the form of a diagnosis. For instance, A.D. mentioned that his brother M.D. "has been drinking too much, which leads him to make these monstrous brutalities."[12] A.D. suggested that alcoholism explained his brother's mental disorder.

Finally, these letters are a testament to the long duration of troubles affecting the individuals involved and to the various forms of care put in place by families. M.N. explained in September 1965: "My mother has been severely mentally ill for several years now and her condition is getting worse every day."[13] The long endurance of some disorders raises questions about the care provided by the family before they requested the internment of a relative in the Fann psychiatric clinic or Thiaroye hospital.

The first form of family care tended to be "traditional" healers or religious figures like marabouts. To avoid overinterpreting the evidence, it is important to note that "traditional" healers and religious figures were never explicitly mentioned in the letters, only suggested. Nevertheless, the literature does show that "traditional" medicine still appears as one of the first forms of care provided by a family to a relative affected by a mental disorder (Ouango et al. 1998; Read 2012; Lovell and Diagne 2019). Thus, when the daughter of M.A. explained that "our family has been trying everything for a long time to heal [my] mother," it is likely that she was including the use of "traditional" healers.[14] Traditional treatments were also at the core of reflections made at Fann by Collomb and his team (Bullard 2022).

A common form of family treatment was to chain the person undergoing a severe crisis. In September 1965, the cousin of M.D. mentioned that M. was "getting very dangerous, that is why he is currently chained to a tree in my house."[15] I found only two similar cases in the corpus of letters, yet this form of treatment was not uncommon and is often mentioned in the literature (Ae-Ngibise et al. 2010; Petit 2018). The use of such a coercive and violent treatment enables introducing nuance into the idea that the family environment was always benevolent and tolerant of a relative with a mental disorder. Indeed, the family remains a place of physical—with chaining and confinement—and also of stigmatizing, symbolic violence.

The written requests offer critical insights into ways of understanding madness beyond medical vocabulary and diagnostics.[16] It is important to interrogate the multiplicity of uses and interpretations of madness, along with the various representations of and treatments for madness within the family sphere. The archival corpus shared here highlights a vital component of the history of mental illness in Senegal: the first space of care for those affected by a mental disorder tended to be the family. Given this fact, additional questions arise. What were the consequences of the way that European psychiatry, imported into Senegal, emerged? And how did relationships between families, madness, and institutions of psychiatric care develop within Senegalese society?

The letters suggest that placement in a psychiatric unit was a matter of last resort for the vast majority of families. Yet this does not mean that medical care and hospitals were never used. Hospitals became important in the colonial period and have been a consistent form of therapeutic resort for African families, even if only a late or last resort.[17] Some letters reveal that families were in contact with the Fann neuropsychiatric service for a consultation or medical treatment request before officially asking to place their relative in the unit. On June 17, 1963, a worried father explained to the governor that his twin children "do not enjoy their mental faculty as attested by the [past] visit and treatment reports from the Fann hospital center."[18] However, previous medical visits to the Fann psychiatric unit seem to have failed to heal many patients. The father of C.C., a twenty-seven-year-old man, explained that his son was "suffering from very dangerous and incurable crises despite the repeated efforts of the Fann hospital center. . . . He is becoming more and more dangerous; it is in a way complete madness [*folie complète*]."[19] The same language recurred in a letter from the city councilor of Cap-Vert regarding his brother, thirty-one years old: "My young brother S.M. doesn't enjoy his full mental abilities and despite having been admitted twice to Fann, he has relapsed since Tuesday."[20]

All the letters arrived from individuals living in the Cap-Vert region, mainly Dakar, the capital and largest city in the country. This geographical aspect raises a broader question of upheavals brought about by the emergence of imported psychiatry in the form of an asylum and within the rapidly changing—urbanizing—Senegalese society a few years after independence. Broader relationships among city families, mental illness, and psychiatric practice need to be taken into account. Increasing urbanization, itself part of the aftermath of World War II, intensified along with national development plans following independence (O'Brien, Diouf, and Diop 2002; Colin 2007).

Senegalese society underwent a whole range of lifestyle changes, including consumption, employment, education, and access to services. For many, an urban lifestyle was a sign of modernity, and opposed to communal ways of life found in rural areas (Gary-Tounkara 2003; Tiquet 2018, 2019). City life changed balances within families, and also changed tolerant attitudes toward mental illness. Senegalese urban society became as if a "cultural in-between," to quote the former head of psychiatry at the Fann clinic, poised in between increasing urbanization and disintegrating family solidarity, between greater use of psychiatric placement and unraveling family care (Guèye 2013, 35). When a mother wrote to the Cap-Vert governor in

January 1968, explaining that her son showed "signs of dementia," she spoke to an important kind of fragmentation: "The people who help me prevent him from doing harm to himself and others cannot devote themselves any longer" to such labors of care, "due to other obligations."[21] Although not stated explicitly, one can imagine that after devoting time and energy without success, care no longer remained the same priority within this family. As a result, the mother asked for help from the governor in having her son committed to the Fann clinic. Her request recalls the hypothesis of Henri Collomb (1973) that familial forms of rejecting the mentally ill—especially, as we will see, when the person seemed dangerous—and committing them, tended to increase in urban areas due to lifestyle changes in the years immediately following independence.

Danielle Storper-Perez worked for a long time at the Fann clinic with Collomb. In *La Folie Colonisée* (1975, 120), she suggested that due to this pervasive "cultural in-between," the mentally ill were no longer "accepted by a social and cultural consensus," and instead found themselves sent to a former colonial psychiatric hospital for treatment, or "locked up, guarded, relegated." Although my corpus of letters bears witness to these increased demands of the 1960s for psychiatric placement, it was not only such a "cultural in-between" that threatened family care at home. Indeed, family care was usually provided for long periods of time before a family member was placed in a psychiatric unit, suggesting that the moral force of family care seems to have often remained. Following the analysis of Ursula Read and Solomon Nyame (2019, 22) on precarity, social change, and family care for those with mental illness in contemporary Ghana, what was at stake was the ability of families to meet "the practical and moral demands of care" for relatives affected by mental disorder.

This aspect can be explored through two strands: the sense of danger provoked by the mental illness of a relative, and the economic precarity of the family.

Family Care or Public Order?

The grandfather of A.N., a man of twenty-four years, wrote in 1963 that his grandson's condition "predisposed him to acts of violence that constituted a danger to himself and his family."[22] In another case, the father of B.B. requested to intern his son in April 1966 because he was suffering from "furious madness," and "presents a permanent danger to the entire population of the district."[23] A similar formulation was in use for A.S., whose brother stated in a letter of June 1969, that A.S. "attacks the people of the house" and appears to be "a permanent danger to his relatives."[24] The letters followed a similar format. The risk of violence associated with mental disorder reinforced requests for a psychiatric placement. In August 1964, I.D. mentioned in reference to F.F., a woman for whom he provided housing, "I have the honor to ask your high benevolence to capture this patient so that my safety is maintained because her presence in my home is a danger to me and my family."[25]

By associating potential—or real—violence with mental disorder, a boundary came to be progressively drawn between an "acceptable" mentally ill person, tolerated by family and society, and a "dangerous" individual whose behavior was judged to be a risk, and who required confinement and isolation far from family within a psychiatric unit. C.C.'s father described his son in June 1965 as "becoming more and more dangerous. It is kind of a complete madness."[26] This father indicated that the gravity of his son's danger had reached total madness, so difficult he was to manage on a daily basis. By associating the word *complete* with the degree of danger, the father suggested that it was not only his son's mental disorder but also his potential for violence that necessitated his commitment at a psychiatric unit.

Another letter told of Y.D., "suddenly mentally ill" and "angry and dangerous."[27] Perhaps Y.D. had been suffering from a mental disorder for some time, though he had been relatively acceptable to his family because he did not behave violently. However, a crisis of violence induced his brother to write that Y.D. had "suddenly" gone mad. This example raises the question of differentiated perceptions of families before mental disorder, according to the level of risk or to the danger to the patient and others around.

As some Senegalese psychiatrists (Sylla et al. 2011, 69–71) note in an article on contact and connections between families and mental illness in contemporary Senegal, patients experiencing intense psychological suffering (with depression, inhibition, and the like), but remaining calm, tend to be accepted or at least do not unduly alarm their families. Their behavior is "more consistent with those social values of *kersa* (modesty, timidity, deference) and *sutura* (discretion, respect for intimate life) appreciated by the family group." In contrast, displays of delirium, agitation, aggressiveness, and exhibitionism in the streets, such symptoms break with accepted social codes, producing shame (*rus*) and jeopardizing a family's honor (*jom*).[28] Similar criteria and codes—increasing distance between a patient and relatives—likely drove families to request psychiatric placements.

The father, C.C., who we met above, described his son in 1965: "When he has a crisis, he threatens people with a knife and if I don't intervene, it will be fatal. . . . I am not in a position to face the consequences for his actions."[29] Were the son to commit a crime, the consequences might not be a legal issue alone but also a moral one, since C.C.'s misconduct would stain the honor of the entire family. To avoid such harmful consequences, C.C.'s father requested an internment for his son. Another father wrote in December 1965 that his son, D.D., "no longer enjoys his mental faculties and might commit unforgivable crimes in the vicinity."[30] The term "unforgivable" is important. It suggests the seriousness of acts his son might commit, and, in a literal sense, points to potential moral consequences of a future crime. D.D.'s crime would not be forgivable, due to the dishonor and shame posed to the entire family. Again, to avoid such a result, the father proposed having his son placed in the hospital.

Such cases of the potentially "dangerous" mentally ill were taken very seriously by the authorities in 1960s Senegal, at a time when they were repressing all forms of public disorder. After they received one such letter, the authorities quickly responded through the voice of the Cap-Vert governor. According to the dates on the letterhead, usually only a few days—sometimes a few hours—passed between receiving a family letter and the reply of the governor. He always sent a standardized letter to the Fann director, requesting a medical examination "to determine whether the person is dangerous to the public order and the safety of persons" and whether the person "must be hospitalized in a special unit," one that keeps such persons "away from harm inflicted on themselves or others."[31]

Maintaining public order was central to official replies, and family letters sometimes underlined the issue as well. A letter of May 1963 explained that F.C. "is dangerous, because he threatens our neighbors with sharp tools. I would be very grateful if you could help the family, me, and the public through his internment."[32] The same term—dangerous—was part of a letter written by N.T.'s brother in September 1963, describing N.T. as "very dangerous to public space [*espace public*]."[33] For Senegalese authorities, public order is related to the risks of physical danger and transgression of social norms, like forms of public nudity. The mayor of Dakar's third arrondissement explained in June 1963 that twins, A.S. and O.S., "constitute a danger to the public because they walk naked in the street. They must be urgently interned."[34]

The governor and, more broadly, Senegalese authorities made it their priority not so much to care for the mentally ill, but to isolate them by locking them up in a psychiatric unit in the interest of public order. The rapidity with which the authorities reacted to these letters was related to stigmatization and the suppression of urban marginality in Dakar and Senegal. The figure of the "lunatic," if dangerous and transgressive of social codes, was seen as disruptive to social order within the city in the newly decolonized nation. In the aftermath of independence, the government—led by President Léopold Sédar Senghor and Mamadou Dia, *président du conseil* before his 1962 ouster—wanted the capital city to showcase the country's emergence and to attract tourists and international business. The authorities publicly displayed a will to "cleanse" Dakar of an entire section of the population—so-called deviants—considered obstacles to this national flourishing because their presence disturbed social and economic order. Such alleged deviants included the unemployed, youth, prostitutes, alcoholics, lepers, vagrants, hawkers, and the mentally ill (Ndiaye 1979; Faye and Thioub 2003).

All such social categories occupied public space, that is, the streets. Senegal's postcolonial authorities stigmatized them through forms of control, suppressing those they alternately defined as part of a "social plague" (*fléaux sociaux*) or later as "human clutter" (*encombrements humains*) (Collignon 1984). Police roundups and forms of confinement and isolation were the means contributing to the erasure and invisibility of these persons and categories in urban space.

My corpus of letters between families and the governor also allows for an analysis at a different scale. Each letter expresses individualized pain within a private or intimate story. These letters also spoke to social issues, with collective concerns about the care of the "dangerous" mentally ill and of the public order. The governor's letters suggest an administrative process with three stages: (1) the moment of receiving letters of suffering, with the family's inability to manage a mentally ill relative or the related risk of danger; (2) the moment when the administration, in the governor's voice, viewed such persons and private stories from a social level, and when he questioned the wider implications of such situations for public safety and order; and (3) the moment when Senegalese authorities consolidated "common sense," involving the stigmatization and suppression of those mentally ill individuals deemed dangerous, and seeking to render them invisible in the public sphere. In sum, assistance to mentally ill individuals was not on offer by the authorities, but rather assistance to society at large *against* the potentially dangerous repercussions of violent, mentally ill individuals.

Precarity and Family Care

Scholars have shown that an increase in precarity in contemporary Africa represents an important barrier for families caring for relatives suffering from mental disorders, including their difficulties in accessing treatment and in the disintegration of family solidarity (de-Graft Aikins and Ofori-Atta 2007; Diagne 2016; Read and Nyame 2019; Diagne and Lovell 2020). Indeed, it is possible to trace the impact of difficult economic situations on everyday family care, usually before a family asks to have a relative committed at an institution like the Fann clinic or Thiaroye hospital. Although a dangerous individual was the main reason families requested to place a relative in the Fann clinic, the precarious economic condition of a family appears to have been critical in the decision to ask for help from the authorities.

Mental illness has moral and financial costs for families caring for a sick relative. It is a daily financial burden that involves seeking and administering treatment, and often organizing a daily schedule to keep up with routine expenses. Moreover, for poor families, a mentally ill individual was usually unable to carry out any income-generating activity, making them dependent on family members without bringing in any income to offset the costs of their care. For many poor families, the financial burden became complicated or impossible, leading to abandonment, as several letters suggest.

In September 1965, A.D.'s son explained that his "unemployed" father was living under extremely precarious conditions. His mother, A.D.'s wife, "has been seriously mentally ill for several years . . . hangs around the city, goes anywhere and she is becoming dangerous." At the end of the letter, A.D.'s son added about his mother: "My efforts are exhausted, that's why I appeal to your spirit of kindness to confine her at Fann or Thiaroye."[35] This letter suggests a son's distress and fatigue at no longer being able to care for his mother, as well as the great precarity that led him to abandon her, with her left wandering around the city.

In a similar letter from March 1965, we learn that M.D. was mentally ill, but his brother, A.D. (who wrote the letter), was not financially able to care for him: "I am not solvent, so you will help me with an indulgence for him [*sic*], since if I tell you that I can provide for him, it would be a big lie." About his brother, A.D. added: "His name is M.D., he speaks five foreign languages: American, English, German, Norwegian and French. If only he could be readapted [*réadapté*] to normal life, he would be of great use as an interpreter, which is why I don't leave him rotting in the city."[36] This second part of the letter shows that M.D. risked being left on his own in the city because of a lack of family care caused by financial precarity. This letter also shows that the brother positively addressed the need for the psychiatric internment for his brother, who he said would be a "useful" individual—"he speaks five languages"—to society if "rehabilitated."

We see here how a discourse on the social utility of an individual could aim at justifying psychiatric internment. The vocabulary of "rehabilitation" is reminiscent of Collomb's (1973, 349) comments on the relationship in the 1960s between Senegalese society and European psychiatric hospitals. The use of a psychiatric hospital leads to an attitude toward madness that is "resolutely medical in the biological sense of the word," Collomb wrote, adding: "Madness is reduced to mental illness; the patient is no longer a carrier of meaning and cannot be listened to. He can only be treated, handled as an object who must be restored to his proper working condition."

For families living in poverty, psychiatric internment appeared as a solution to "relieve" the financial costs caused by the sickness of a loved one: food, accommodation, daily care, and the like. At the same time, internment was an admission of failure, since relatives viewed the hospital as a better option than care at home. By taking account of the precarious situation of families who wrote letters, it becomes possible to interpret with nuance the idealized vision according to which family care was *the* alternative to institutional treatment. In fact, poor households experiencing increasing precarity were, in many cases, unable to take care of a close mentally ill relative. Although danger was the main reason families gave when requesting to commit a relative, precarity played a determining role in their decisions to seek help from the authorities.

Psychiatric commitment was not without costs. According to the 1938 general decree on psychiatric assistance (which still applied in 1960s Senegal), "all patients are admitted after payment of fees."[37] Thus, the question of financial responsibility for hospitalization arises, as does that of the difficulties posed for poor families.

Many families wishing to place relatives in hospital indicated their socioprofessional situation adjacent to their letterhead. It is possible to trace the socioeconomic background of some families requesting psychiatric hospitalization of a relative. Not all families writing to the governor were in a situation of economic insecurity. Many minor civil servants, traders, and even politicians—one letter is from a Dakar City Hall councilor—wrote to the governor. This urban middle class could afford to pay for psychiatric hospitalization.

In contrast, less fortunate families suffering from deep economic deprivation were unable to provide the monies needed to pay for a relative's placement at Fann. The daughter of M.A. mentioned in her letter from December 1964 that she was "a woman without support," with "no resources to meet the obligations stipulated by the administration."[38] Note the similar language of the father of O.D., who wrote regarding his son in November 1962: "My son has been mentally ill for several years . . . thus making life difficult for us. His behavior constitutes a serious threat to the safety of our neighbors and myself. . . . I don't know what to do at the moment because I find myself unable to bear the costs of his admission to an asylum. I am retired from administrative services and only receive a small pension."[39]

In addition to requesting internment, it was not uncommon for letters to request a certificate of indigence in order to be relieved of hospitalization costs. This measure was governed by the same 1938 law, which stated that "the indigent shall be treated at the expense of their community of origin (colony and possibly commune)."[40] The sister of S.S. asked in July 1963 for a certificate of indigence for her brother because she was a "woman without any resources, unable to bear the costs of placement" for her brother.[41] A similar request was made by the father of D.D. in 1965; he requested a certificate of indigence for his son to "allow him to be admitted to Fann hospital" at no cost.[42]

Mental illness entailed heavy daily costs for families, but so did psychiatric internment. Precarity was a determining factor in whether a mentally ill person was placed in hospital or not. In many cases, precarity was a significant challenge for families trying to care for relatives with a mental illness. Focusing on the economic aspects of the care provided by families reveals that the viability of family care was profoundly vulnerable to poverty. This analysis of the relationship between precarity and care underlines how poor families found it difficult to meet the practical and moral demands of care.

Conclusion

This analysis of an archival corpus of petitions seeking psychiatric internment for kin in 1960s Senegal raises two important points. First, the letters allow us to look at vernacular dimensions of madness beyond a psychiatric framework. By exploring in a fine-grained manner the multiple representations, understandings, and meanings of mental disorder as expressed by families, these letters show that madness was—and remains—a labile and plastic category. Second, the letters highlight the complexities that led families to seek to intern relatives. Be it the physical danger posed by a mentally ill relative or the social and economic situation of a family, many parameters came into play, challenging daily family care and also home-based solidarities related to mental illness.

The corpus lends itself to analysis at different levels. The family level suggests relationships between families, mental illness, and psychiatry. At the level of the Senegalese authorities, the governor's requests highlighted how psychiatric internment of "dangerous lunatics" aligned with the state's prioritization of public order. I have shown that studying madness well means not analyzing it as a rigid or fixed phenomenon, but rather as a *label* sometimes applied to individuals or groups due to particular behaviors or language (Aït Mehdi and Tiquet 2020). Madness must be understood first and foremost as a category within which beliefs, practices, and political and clinical knowledge are assembled and combined, giving rise to many patterns, including social control.

The question remains: what happened to individuals whose families requested internment? In these letters, the ill person remains more an object than subject of their own history. They began as the subjects of a family complaint and commitment request, and they became the objects of an administrative process undertaken by Senegalese authorities (known as confinement for the sake of public order). In order to overcome the biases inherent in these letters and avoid framing the mentally ill as passive or insane, it is important to do further research on certain individuals mentioned in the letters through examining the patient case files held at Fann. By focusing on those considered to be "mad," and how they were treated by a variety of actors and institutions (with therapeutic treatments or punitive measures), it may be possible to analyze how individuals resisted or challenged a diagnosis, and the ways in which madness came to be deployed or understood on a daily basis. These aspects will be explored in future publications.

It is clear from patient files that a family who requested a relative's commitment usually continued to play an important role in the life of this relative-turned-patient. Fann's staff took into account the social and family environments of patients and, in the 1970s, made the presence of a family member during a hospital stay a central tool in the therapeutic process—*parcours*—of patients (Gbikpi and Auguin 1978; Kilroy-Marac 2014; Koundoul 2015). Some families asked for the release of their sick relative after a few weeks to care for them at home once more. It is likely that some families behaved otherwise, though their relative inaction or abandonment went unrecorded.

There is still much to explore regarding the history of madness in Senegal and West Africa. Patient files enable reconstructing person-centered histories of mental disorder, focusing on ordinary experiences of madness (Aït Mehdi and Tiquet 2020), and the complex relations among patients, families, and psychiatric institutions. Such a case-based archive facilitates leaving behind that limited approach still widely used in historical writing on psychiatry in Africa, which sheds light only on psychiatric discourse, medical staffing, and state authorities. Treating patient case files in relation to "minuscule lives" (Revel 1996, 12) offers an unassuming, intimate, and textured version of history, revealing the social and political realities that patients, kin, and doctors were navigating during this time of decolonization. With a focus on families, as well as on a key decade, the 1960s, such a social and cultural history pushes beyond a historiography that, with some profound anthropological exceptions (Kilroy-Marac 2019; Diagne and Lovell 2020; Bullard 2022), has for Senegal, at least so far, mainly focused on administrative and colonial histories of psychiatry.

In exploring "minuscule" dimensions, a partial foundation may be created for a multisited history of madness during Africa's years of decolonization. This chapter is a call for ethnographic histories that explore peculiar relations among madness and its production in relation to postcolonial governmentality, the decades immediately after independence, and everyday families. Such multisited histories stand to contribute to writing social and political histories of the continent since decolonization, a subject worthy of further exploration (Nugent 2004; White 2015).

Indeed, historians would do well to not only investigate discourses on and practices of madness in Africa as produced out of politics and societies, but also question what madness says about politics and society on the continent.

Notes

This chapter is based on research that received funding from the European Research Council under the European Union's Horizon 2020 research and innovation programme (grant agreement number 852448: "A History of Madness in West Africa: Governing Mental Disorder during Decolonisation").

1   All the names are anonymized in order to protect the privacy of the persons quoted in the letters, some of whom may still be alive.

2   Lettre concernant A.T., Archives Régionales de Dakar, January 8, 1968, B172. Correspondances diverses avec le centre hospitaliser de Fann, 1962–1970 (hereafter ARS, B172). All translations from French to English are mine.

3   Lettre du Gouverneur de la région Cap-Vert au directeur de l'hôpital de Fann, January 8, 1968, ARS, B172.

4   "Arrêté général du 28 juin 1938 créant un service d'assistance psychiatrique," *Journal Officiel de l'AOF*, no. 1783, July 9, 1938.

5   "Loi n° 75–80 relative au traitement des maladies mentales et au régime d'internement de certaines catégories d'aliénés," *Journal Officiel de la République du Sénégal*, no. 4436, July 21, 1975.

6   Lettre concernant S.S., November 18, 1968, ARS, B172.

7   Lettre concernant M.J.P., January 12, 1965, ARS, B172.

8   Lettre concernant O.H.D., February 1966, ARS, B172.

9   Lettre concernant M.D., September 1965, ARS, B172.

10 Lettre concernant M.A., December 1964, ARS, B172.

11 Lettre concernant F.F., August 13, 1964, ARS, B172.

12 Lettre concernant M.D., March 29, 1965, ARS, B172.

13 Lettre concernant A.D., September 1965, ARS, B172.

14 Lettre concernant M.A., December 1964, ARS, B172.

15 Lettre concernant M.D., September 1965, ARS, B172.

16 It is also possible that a relative perceived as mentally ill by their family was, in fact, not.

17 See, for instance, record cases from the late nineteenth century of family members asking for help from the central hospital of Saint-Louis. Archives Nationales du Sénégal, Série Santé Sénégal H, Aliénés 1888.

18 Lettre concernant A.S. et O.S., June 17, 1963, ARS, B172.

19 Lettre concernant C.C., June 22, 1965, ARS, B172.

20 Lettre concernant M.S., August 1963, ARS, B172.

21 Lettre concernant le fils de F.A., January 19, 1968, ARS, B172.

22 Lettre concernant A.N., April 23, 1963, ARS, B172.

23 PV de A. B. père de B.B., April 19, 1966, ARS, B172.

24 Lettre concernant A.S., June 19, 1969, ARS, B172.

25 Lettre concernant F.F., August 13, 1964, ARS, B172.

26 Lettre concernant C.C., June 22, 1965, ARS, B172.

27 Lettre concernant Y.D., December 24, 1965, ARS, B172.

28 Terms in Wolof.

29 Lettre concernant C.C., June 22, 1965, ARS, B172.

30 Lettre concernant D.D., December 31, 1965, ARS, B172.

31 See all the letters from the governor, using this formulation: ARS, B172.

32 Lettre concernant F.C., May 18, 1963, ARS, B172.

33 Lettre concernant N.T., September 25, 1963, ARS, B172.

34 Lettre concernant A.S. et O.S., June 17, 1963, ARS, B172.

35 Lettre concernant A.D., September 1965, ARS, B172.

36 Lettre concernant M.D., March 1965, ARS, B172.

37 "Arrêté général du 28 juin 1938."

38 Lettre concernant M.A., December 1964, ARS, B172.

39 PV de police du père de O.D., November 20, 1962, ARS, B172.

40 "Arrêté général du 28 juin 1938."

41 Lettre concernant S.S., July 18, 1963, ARS, B172.

42 Lettre concernant D.D., December 31, 1965, ARS, B172.

Sources

Archival Material

Archives Régionales de Dakar (ARS), Senegal.

Literature

Ae-Ngibise, Kenneth, Sarah Cooper, Edward Adiibokah, Bright Akpalu, Crick Lund, and Victor Doku. 2010. "'Whether You Like It or Not People with Mental Problems Are Going to Go to Them': A Qualitative Exploration into the Widespread

Use of Traditional and Faith Healers in the Provision of Mental Health Care in Ghana." *International Review of Psychiatry* 22, no. 6: 558–67.

Aït Mehdi, Gina. 2018. "La mère, le fils et la folie: Expériences partagées d'une maladie chronique à Niamey." *Tsantsa*, no. 23: 154–62.

Aït Mehdi, Gina, and Romain Tiquet. 2020. "Considering the Everyday of Madness." *Politique Africaine* 157, no. 1: 17–38.

Akyeampong, Emmanuel, Allan G. Hill, and Arthur Kleinman, eds. 2015. *The Culture of Mental Illness and Psychiatric Practice in Africa*. Bloomington: Indiana University Press.

Arnaut, Robert. 2009. *La folie apprivoisée: L'approche unique du Professeur Collomb pour traiter la folie*. Paris: De Vecchi.

Biehl, João. 2005. *Vita: Life in a Zone of Social Abandonment*. Berkeley: University of California Press.

Bullard, Alice. 2022. *Spiritual and Mental Health Crisis in Globalizing Senegal: A History of Transcultural Psychiatry*. New York: Routledge.

Colin, Roland. 2007. *Sénégal notre pirogue: Au soleil la liberté*. Paris: Présence Africaine.

Collignon, René. 1978. *Vingt ans de travaux à la clinique psychiatrique de Fann-Dakar: [1958–1978]*. Dakar: Société de psychopathologie et d'hygiène mentale.

Collignon, René. 1983. "À Propos de la psychiatrie communautaire en Afrique noire: Les dispositifs villageois d'assistance: Éléments pour un dossier." *Psychopathologie Africaine* 19, no. 3: 287–328.

Collignon, René. 1984. "La Lutte des pouvoir publics contre les encombrements humains à Dakar." *Canadian Journal of African Studies* 18, no. 3: 573–82.

Collignon, René. 1999. "Le traitement de la question de la folie au Sénégal à l'époque coloniale." In *Enfermement, prison et châtiments en Afrique: Du 19e siècle à nos jours*, edited by Florence Bernault, 227–57. Paris: Karthala.

Collignon, René. 2010. "La psychiatrie coloniale française en Algérie et au Sénégal: Esquisse d'une historisation comparative." *Revue Tiers Monde* 187:527–46.

Collomb, Henri. 1973. "L'avenir de la psychiatrie en Afrique." *Psychopathologie Africaine* 9, no. 3: 343–70.

D'Almeida, Ludovic. 1997. *La folie au Sénégal*. Dakar: Association des chercheurs sénégalais.

De-Graft Aikins, Ama. 2015. "Mental Illness and Destitution in Ghana: A Social-Psychological Perspective." In *The Culture of Mental Illness and Psychiatric Practice in Africa*, edited by Emmanuel Akyeampong, Allan G. Hill, and Arthur Kleinman, 112–43. Bloomington: Indiana University Press.

De-Graft Aikins, Ama, and Angela L. Ofori-Atta. 2007. "Homelessness and Mental Health in Ghana: Everyday Experiences of Accra's Migrant Squatters." *Journal of Health Psychology* 12, no. 5: 761–78.

Diagne, Papa Mamadou. 2016. "Soigner les malades mentaux errants dans l'agglomération dakaroise." *Anthropologie et Santé. Revue internationale francophone d'anthropologie de la santé* 13. https://doi.org/10.4000/anthropologiesante .2171.

Diagne, Papa Mamadou, and Anne Lovell. 2020. "Vivre avec la folie dans le Sénégal mondialisé: Contraintes économiques, *care* et reconfiguration des solidarités dans des zones péri-urbaines." *Politique Africaine* 157, no. 1: 143–54.

Dracchio, Cecilia. 2020. "(Extra)ordinary Collaborations in Zones of Social Abandonment? Mental Health Care between Psychiatry and Prayer Camps in Rural Ghana." *Politique Africaine* 157, no. 1: 165–82.

Edington, Claire. 2019. *Beyond the Asylum: Mental Illness in French Colonial Vietnam*. Ithaca, NY: Cornell University Press.

Fann (Centre hospitalier de). 1968. "Psychopathologie et environnement familial en Afrique." *Psychopathologie Africaine* 4, no. 2: 297–311.

Fassin, Didier. 1984. "Anthropologie et folie." *Cahiers Internationaux de Sociologie* 77:237–71.

Faye, Oussenou, and Ibrahima Thioub. 2003. "Les marginaux et l'État à Dakar." *Le Mouvement Social* 204:93–108.

Fichte, Hubert. 1990. *Psyché: L'histoire de la sensibilité (Extraits)*. Paris: L'Harmattan.

Gary-Tounkara, Daouda. 2003. "Quand les migrants demandent la route, Modibo Keïta Rétorque: 'Retournez à la terre!' Les Baragnini et la désertion du 'chantier national' (1958–1968)." *Mande Studies* 4:49–64.

Gbikpi, Paul A., and Roselyne Auguin. 1978. "Évaluation d'une pratique institutionnelle à Fann, l'admission d'un accompagnant du malade à l'hôpital." *Psychopathologie Africaine* 14, no. 1: 5–68.

Gruénais, Marc-Éric. 1990. "Le malade et sa famille: Une étude de cas à Brazzaville." In *Sociétés, développement et santé*, edited by Didier Fassin and Yves Jaffré, 227–42. Paris: Ellipses.

Guèye, Momar. 2013. "La psychiatrie après Collomb." In *L'Afrique symptôme*, 25–44. Paris: L'Harmattan.

Heaton, Matthew M. 2013. *Black Skin, White Coats: Nigerian Psychiatrists, Decolonization, and the Globalization of Psychiatry*. Athens: Ohio University Press.

Hunt, Nancy Rose. 1999. *A Colonial Lexicon: Of Birth Ritual, Medicalization, and Mobility in the Congo*. Durham, NC: Duke University Press.

Janzen, John M. 1978. *The Quest for Therapy in Lower Zaire*. Berkeley: University of California Press.

Kilroy-Marac, Katie. 2014. "Of Shifting Economies and Making Ends Meet: The Changing Role of the Accompagnant at the Fann Psychiatric Clinic in Dakar, Senegal." *Culture, Medicine, and Psychiatry* 38, no. 3: 427–47.

Kilroy-Marac, Katie. 2019. *An Impossible Inheritance: Postcolonial Psychiatry and the Work of Memory in a West African Clinic*. Berkeley: University of California Press.

Koundoul, Adama. 2015. "La professionnalisation de l'accompagnement des malades en milieu psychiatrique au Sénégal." *Le journal des psychologues* 332, no. 10: 42–51.

Lawrance, Benjamin N. 2006. "Petitioners, 'Bush Lawyers' and Letter Writers: Court Access in British-Occupied Lomé, 1914–1920." In *Intermediaries, Interpreters and Clerks: African Employees in the Making of Colonial Africa*, edited by Benjamin N. Lawrance, Emily L. Osborn, and Richard L. Roberts, 94–114. Madison: University of Wisconsin Press.

Linstrum, Eric. 2016. *Ruling Minds: Psychology in the British Empire*. Cambridge, MA: Harvard University Press.

Lovell, Anne, and Papa Mamadou Diagne. 2019. "Falling, Dying Sheep, and the Divine: Notes on Thick Therapeutics in Peri-Urban Senegal." *Culture, Medicine, and Psychiatry* 43, no. 4: 663–85.

Mahone, Sloan, and Megan Vaughan, eds. 2007. *Psychiatry and Empire*. New York: Palgrave Macmillan.

McCulloch, John. 1995. *Colonial Psychiatry and the African Mind*. Cambridge: Cambridge University Press.

Ndiaye, Amadou M. 1979. "Des 'fléaux sociaux' aux 'encombrements humains': Essai d'approche de l'évolution de la sensibilité aux questions sociales à travers la presse quotidienne sénégalaise de 1960 à 1975." PhD diss., University of Dakar.

Nugent, Paul. 2004. *Africa since Independence: A Comparative History*. New York: Palgrave Macmillan.

O'Brien, Donal B. C., Mamadou Diouf, and Momar-Coumba Diop, eds. 2002. *La construction de l'État au Sénégal*. Paris: Karthala.

Olivier de Sardan, Jean-Pierre. 1994. "Possession, affliction et folie: Les ruses de la thérapisation." *L'Homme* 34, no. 131: 7–27.

Ouango, Jean-Gabriel, Kapouné Karfo, Moussa Kere, Marcelline Ouedraogo, Gisèle Kaboré, and Arouna Ouédraogo. 1998. "Concept traditionnel de la folie et difficultés thérapeutiques psychiatriques chez les Moosé du Kadiogo." *Santé mentale au Québec* 23, no. 2: 197–210.

Ozouf, Patrick, René Collignon, and Omar Sylla. 1977. "Thiaroye ou les avatars d'une institution." *Psychopathologie Africaine* 13, no. 1: 81–111.

Parle, Julie. 2014. "Family Commitments, Economies of Emotions, and Negotiating Mental Illness in Late-Nineteenth to Mid-Twentieth-Century Natal, South Africa." *South African Historical Journal* 66, no. 1: 1–21.

Petit, Véronique. 2018. "Retours contraints de migrants internationaux au Sénégal: Dilemmes familiaux face à la maladie mentale." *Revue européenne des migrations internationales* 34, no. 2–3: 131–58.

Petit, Véronique. 2020. "'Tu peux être en vie et déjà mort': Le quotidien ordinaire d'une personne atteinte de troubles mentaux au Sénégal." *Politique Africaine* 157, no. 1: 39–69.

Povinelli, Elizabeth A. 2013. *Economies of Abandonment: Social Belonging and Endurance in Late Liberalism*. Durham, NC: Duke University Press.

Quarshie, Nana Osei. 2011. "Confinement in the Lunatic Asylums of the Gold Coast from 1887 to 1906." *Psychopathologie Africaine* 36, no. 2: 191–226.

Quinn, Neil. 2007. "Beliefs and Community Responses to Mental Illness in Ghana: The Experiences of Family Carers." *International Journal of Social Psychiatry* 53, no. 2: 175–88.

Read, Ursula M. 2012. "Between Chains and Vagrancy: Living with Mental Illness in Kintampo, Ghana." PhD diss., University College London.

Read, Ursula M., and Solomon Nyame. 2019. "'It Is Left to Me and My God': Precarity, Responsibility, and Social Change in Family Care for People with Mental Illness in Ghana." *Africa Today* 65, no. 3: 3–27.

Revel, Jacques. 1996. *Jeux d'échelles: La micro-analyse à l'expérience*. Paris: Gallimard.

Rodet, Marie, and Romain Tiquet. 2018. "Reforming State Violence in French West Africa: Relegation in the Epoch of Decolonization." In *Africans in Exile: Mobility, Law, and Identity*, edited by Benjamin N. Lawrance and Nathan R. Carpenter, 118–44. Bloomington: Indiana University Press.

Sadowsky, Jonathan. 1999. *Imperial Bedlam: Institutions of Madness in Colonial Southwest Nigeria*. Berkeley: University of California Press.

Sifou, Fatiha. 2004. "La protestation zlgérienne contre la domination française: Plaintes et pétitions (1830–1914)." PhD diss., University of Aix-Marseille.

Sow, Alpha Ibrahim. 1978. *Les structures anthropologiques de la folie en Afrique noire*. Paris: Payot.

Storper-Perez, Danielle. 1975. *La folie colonisée*. Paris: Maspero.

Sylla, Aïda, Ndèye D. N. Ndongo, Lamine Fall, and Momar Guèye. 2011. "Difficultés de réinsertion familiale de malades mentaux ayant élu: Domicile à l'Hôpital Psychiatrique de Thiaroye." *Psychopathologie Africaine* 26, no. 3: 317–34.

Thiam, Mamadou Habib, and Moro Marie Rose Moro. 2014. "Présentation." *L'Autre* 15, no. 2: 137–40.

Tiquet, Romain. 2018. "Service civique et développement au Sénégal: Une utopie au cœur des relations entre armée et pouvoir politique (1960–1968)." *Afrique Contemporaine* 260:45–59.

Tiquet, Romain. 2019. "Le renouveau de la 'mission civilisatrice'? Développement et mobilisation de la main-d'œuvre au Sénégal (années 1960)." *Relations Internationales* 177:73–84.

Vaughan, Megan. 1983. "Idioms of Madness: Zomba Lunatic Asylum, Nyasaland, in the Colonial Period." *Journal of Southern African Studies* 9, no. 2: 218–38.

White, Luise. 2015. "Suitcases, Roads, and Archives: Writing the History of Africa after 1960." *History in Africa* 42:265–67.

Whyte, Susan R. 2012. "Chronicity and Control: Framing 'Noncommunicable Diseases' in Africa." *Anthropology and Medicine* 19, no. 1: 63–74.

Zempleni, Andràs. 1968. "L'interprétation et la thérapie traditionnelle du désordre mental chez les Wolof et les Lebou (Sénégal)." PhD diss., University of Paris.

Nancy Rose Hunt 10

Lorry Dreams and Slave Ship Disintegrations

Motion, Madness, and Incongruent Planes in History

Two words incite this investigation into disturbance among Africans from two historical planes, to use Simmel's (1980: 128; Hunt 2018) word. Each suggests incongruent kinds of motion, one from 1950s West Africa and another from the late eighteenth-century Atlantic. This chapter aims not at systematic comparison, nor does it unfold sequentially. Rather, it is an experiment in historical writing working through a structure of discontinuity (some would say anachrony; Hunt 2018). It also operates through particular historical materials and counterpoint. The incongruences disclose matters of psychopathology in relation to speed, racist formations, and technologies of motion.

The first word is *vernacular*, a lexeme that displaces the purified, reified, and continual senses to the *traditional* (Ranger 1983) and signals the residual. Vernacular hails from language, and has been on an uptick since, say, 2005 (Larson 2009; Hunt 2016; Mukharji 2016; Orsini 2020). The word also sidesteps the *popular*, a useful word that flourished in relation to African genres and cultural production (Fabian 1996; Barber 2007) yet speaks less to past residuals alive in a present.

Vernacular goes with registers and amalgams of practice, yet with residual traces, even if these are sometimes denigrated or romanticized. Lurking in racialized milieus, vernacular bits may be quarried from traces, spaces, or encounters as residual elements that persist. Sometimes mixed with catastrophes big or small, the vernacular also may yield nightmares, deliria, or dissociation.

Madness is the second word. This capacious, often metaphorical term opens the eccentric, the imbalanced, the pathological, and the psychopolitical.[1] Ernesto de Martino (2012) spoke of *crises of presence* to reckon with madness. His expression, avidly used by anthropologists (Beneduce 2017), contains promise within and beyond trance. De Martino's ethnographic investigations in 1940s southern Italy align well with Africa's *zar* (Leiris 1938; Boddy 1989),[2] among other forms of spirit possession (Lambek 1981). The phenomenological emphasis of de Martino insists on the historicity of subjects and their concrete worlds (Charuty 2018) and aligns well with this chapter's investigation of two juxtaposed milieus.

Something similar unfolds here. I draw on Canguilhem's milieu (Canguilhem 2012; Hunt 2016) for concrete spaces that may turn beneficial or toxic. In late colonial Gold Coast, the everyday appears as plentiful, mobile, and animated, and sometimes as anguish or sorrow. Middle Passage ships—as a formation and milieu—spawned terrible crises of presence. With this juxtaposition, I aim at reformatting histories of madness in Africa.

Psychiatric histories have long been dominated by archives easily found: those generated by asylums. The risk of staleness comes from being wedged toward psychiatrists and modernity. Africa's early psychiatric histories circled around asylums (Vaughan 1983; Marks 1999; Sadowsky 1999; Jackson 2018), often in innovative ways. Other traces—like Zulu nightmares (Callaway 1885) or Obeah disruptions (Senior 2018)— yield racialized forms of "double consciousness" (Du Bois 1903). From early modern madness to modern lunacies (Midelfort 1999; de Martino 2012), it is possible to recover the ordinary, unofficial, and street-based forms of discord or authorial complexities. Such veins, strata, and folds bring near Ian Hacking's (1998) "ecological niches." Archival mining may press for witnessing, mediations, vernacular bits, or "ego-documents" (von Greyerz 2010; Natermann 2018).[3]

Foucault's (1978, 148) "threshold" to modernity came to embrace madness, prisons, and asylums. The word *modernity*, freed from chronology, may inspire histories of "contacts between different parts of the world" (van der Veer 1998, 290) or "connected histories" with imperial "entanglements" (Steinmetz 2013; Perneau and Wodzicki 2017; Capan 2020). A creative, "entangled" historical ethnography—of Senegal's famous psychiatric clinic, Fann—complicates the presumed (Kilroy-Marac 2019). Traces, when pressed, yield disparities and ironies (Hunt 2016; Lovell and Diagne 2019). Language and densities interrogate subjects and times. Regardless, human disturbances and trembling open perplexities about causes, interiorities, and presence. Histories decentering the powerful also remain important. I broach modernity less as epoch than disposition. "Cases" (Forrester 2017) (with the microscopic) are mined for clashes, perceptions, and crises of presence. This chapter offers two *seams* to madness, widely separated by time and tone. One interposes a late colonial *vernacular*, mediated by a colonial anthropologist: "new" shrines with much residual referencing and emergent mammy wagons[4] of the British Gold Coast. This postwar milieu exudes a swift, animated pulse beside the intimate. The tenor of lorry-infused dreaming was not languorous, unlike those slow ships of dread. Middle Passage suicides tell of consciousness and refusal. This eighteenth-century crucible combines African and Atlantic forms of madness with insurgencies and cruelties. Margaret Field's readings add in West African convivialities, grief, and decolonizing motion (Washbrook 1998; Thomas 2011; Hunt 2016).

Bits mined from cases are departures, parsed here in relation to "necropolitics" (Mbembe 2019) but also velocities (Virilio 1986; Hunt 1999). Canguilhem's concept of milieu is powerful for thinking about spaces of violence, suffering, and disintegration. Those managing slave ships stand here beside Field's colonial ethnography. Both knew scribes and expert witnesses. Their observations bare lived worlds, African subjects, psychopathologies, and, as Frantz Fanon found, alienation and practices of freedom (Fanon 2021). A singular iconic madman as the "voice of history" is absent, but "signs and categories" extend clues about "historical consciousness" (Comaroff and Comaroff 1987).

These disparate milieus enable sizing up matters of space, crisis, presence, and diagnostics. In late colonial Gold Coast, the everyday surged forth as plentiful, mobile, animated, yet not without grieving and haunted dreams. Madness burst forth from Atlantic ships, acute and devised spaces of compulsion and death. Lest the impulse to mull over two discordant milieus seems baffling, the rewards deserve underscoring. This is not an exercise in seriality. These disordered swaths speak across centuries, with a register about modernity, motion, and crises of presence. Themes from this volume's introduction resurface in this concluding chapter. A central message is that milieus, like transport conveyances, matter to mental health. The textures went with penchants to document, attest, and witness.

Within this incisive pair, mobility (Hunt 1999) and madness surface alongside technologies: 1950s lorries and the slave ships. Psychopolitical crises and blockage surface too, just as these conveyances ignited imaginaries and experiences of cruelty, anguish, and reverie. That the two slices or planes pertain to West Africa did not motivate conjoining them in this inquiry. Yet the juxtaposition enables grappling with eruptions and interpretations. The modes of locomotion—coerced, carceral, voluntary, or dreamlike—yield derangement and diagnoses. Above all, allied resonances—involving tonalities, traffic, and passages—suggest a significant distance between causation and experiences.

I turn first to the twentieth-century milieu. The Middle Passage follows. Together, this formal experiment forces a *temporal distortion* (Todorov 1984, 60, 100; see also Guerlac 1980) and draws attention to a discordant narrative ordering despite a sequence in historical time. Why do such a thing? Why invert two large swaths of history? These are important questions. In sum, such an experiment disrupts our narrative expectations in history, and it also enables rethinking two planes of time, whose import grows through being thought about not as sequence but as a diagnostic tandem.

Milieu 1: New Shrines and Lorry Dreams

Margaret Field (1937) first went to the Gold Coast in the 1930s as a colonial anthropologist and studied Ga religion and medicinal practices. She returned to Britain during the war years, adding a medical degree and some psychiatric training to her credentials. She returned to the Gold Coast in the 1950s to study mental illness in Akan villages and towns. Already in the 1930s, she noticed a proliferation within this cocoa-growing country of a new kind of commercial shrine where many went to resolve their problems. In the 1950s, Field parked herself for months near one such new shrine, and from this perch documented over a thousand cases. Of these, she published some 150, telling of symptoms and lives lived that were vital to her "ethno-psychiatric study" (Field 1960a; Littlewood 2017).

Field collected a rich record of stories and symptoms about people exiting from these commercial and sacred spaces. She attended to emic vocabularies and practices: matters of shrine organization, deities, and the interlinked importance of fame and lorries. Field also pursued individuals' uneasy, nocturnal dreams. In her field notes, written per "patient," she included social observations, kinship analysis, and illness biographies. Her readings were emic but relentlessly translated the somatic and emotional into psychiatric categories of her day. Culturally sensitive for her era, Field mixed psychiatric and anthropological knowledge. As experienced as she was in southern Gold Coast worlds, she made observations in keeping with the earnest, fraught, and often patronizing British colonial social anthropology of her day (Asad 1973).

She came to know twenty-four new shrines within twenty-one miles of her village and field base. The format of her life stories suggests a transcultural psychiatric determination, stilted but unusual for her time. Her interpretations veered into witchcraft "folklore" and colonial projections about "young literates" at risk of schizophrenia or mental breakdown. She was no Wulf Sachs, nor a J. C. Carothers: she stayed far from asylums and did not make the kind of paternalist or racist judgments found among many of Africa's postwar psychiatrists (McCulloch 1995). Still, she rarely quoted the voices of informants. Field's penchant for listening came alive from her field site near a new shrine and also through seeking dreams. She let Gold Coast's lorries speak through autobiographical accounts of ailments and aspirations. Her interdisciplinary knowledge was generative, joining diagnostic skill with a mélange of elements, some modern, some surely autobiographical, with much respect for the residual and the vernacular. Her inclination to listen enabled the "dialogic and processual" with an "interpenetration" of expert perspectives and domains (Steinmetz 2017, 514).

Psychiatric Ethnographer with Cases

Ama was about fifty-five years old when she began dreaming about someone dying, with an image of herself crying at the funeral. When she went to the shrine, four women knelt beside her. The friends had come to know each other through many shared lorry journeys together. Lorry time produced veins of sociality. Yaa, also about fifty-five years old, had a son nicknamed "lorry-driver's mat." Despite bribing some police, this young man had not passed his driving test. He blamed Ama for his bad luck. The accusation had his mother saying that the Tigari deity had "caught" her in a sorcery embrace (Field 1960b, 159).

Another Ama, some fifty years old, confessed at the shrine. She and her son had been in a lorry accident, landing them in hospital for a week. While there, Ama dreamed of traveling to her mother's town and getting frightened. She wanted to shout but could not. The next day, she found burns all over her scalp and belly. Restless, feeling useless, she could not work. Later, she felt herself a witch who caused a lorry accident. She confessed at the shrine. A night later, she dreamed she was in a shabby, unpainted lorry "running away with her" until frightened, "she . . . jumped out." Ama got worse. Mute, full of remorse, sometimes not eating, she did her washing until her bar of soap was gone (Field 1960b, 151–52).

Saving oneself by jumping out of a runaway lorry was a familiar dream, often a sign of auspiciousness: "they feel they have taken active steps to get out of their troubles" (Field 1960b). Akosua had disturbing dreams of an obosom deity that "caught" her (defining her as a witch), of cows chasing her, or walking into a stream after catfish, or a stream sweeping her away. Akosua's first husband was an illiterate Christian driver who lost his two big trucks from drinking too much. Afterward, he stopped aspiring to own one, abandoning his dreams of fame. He died when his children were young. When Field met his widow, Akosua was about fifty years old with a son: a lorry driver who drank too much and accused her of witchcraft. Three times, the son received police fines for driving his lorry into a ditch. Another son was a driver who doubled as a dispenser-in-training at a mission hospital. Another son was a motor mechanic. Akosua's troubles began twenty years before with her first husband when she began to have illness dreams about being hounded. These alternated with dreams where cows chased her, and others where policemen harassed her. She read these "danger dreams" as if a deity caught her. When she found a new lorry driver husband, he was constantly on the move between the colony's ports and towns, and his mobilities and absences filtered into Akosua's worries.

Field painted a picture of conscientious Akan mothers who raised many children and paid their school fees from monies earned trading, gardening, and farming. As they aged, these postmenopausal women felt their husbands passed them by for youthful women. In Field's words, many were depressed and would enter a shrine with guilt feelings and confess their wrongdoing. In the process, she showed how lorry culture intruded into the self-understandings, sorrows, and dreams of these women.

Akan and Ga messages blaring from the fronts and rears of mammy wagons have long charmed expatriates in Ghana. Field assembled a long list of lorry slogans about fortune and misfortune, an important section in her book. Her cases suggest patterns to symptom and resort, with aging women turning to deity shrines for relief from self-reproach, stress, and sadness. Field categorized many cases under "depression," translating residual elements into a fairly recent psychiatric category. Her engagements stemmed from psychiatry and anthropology: two forms of knowledge anchored in her dialogical interactions in a colonial field that she had been studying since the 1930s.

The value of Field's ethnography within anthropology and early transcultural psychiatry lies in her textured descriptions despite a sometimes condescending or dissonant edge, like when she joined psychiatrists of her time in glossing literate, urban Africans as deracinated and unstable (Field 1960b). As an acolyte of C. G. Seligman, the key British anthropologist of colonial dreaming, she had the good sense to document these. She also cautioned that the insensitivities of colonial administrators could ignite nationalist uprisings among Gold Coast's postwar generation. While biographical elements on Field are still emerging (McCulloch 1995; Linstrum 2016; Littlewood 2017), new archives might still be found and etched in.[5]

Field's findings on melancholia and sorcery-based self-accusations among rural Akan women were significant at the time. She shared her findings in a major African mental health conference in 1959 Bukavu (Field 1960b). Declaring depression a serious problem among women—but not male lorry drivers—her findings went against psychiatric truisms of the time, which held this diagnosis to be rare in Africa (Vaughan 2010; Sadowsky 2021). Field's facts and impressions live on, even if their value for histories of this region, their vehicles, and aspirations have eluded some (Hart 2016). Though her writing leaned toward the stoic and the spare, the details on lorries and dreams suggest her imaginative sense of irony.

Velocity, Dreams, Translation

Field's canny eye yields specificities. Lorry drivers were a hurried, avid clientele of those shrines as were dejected wives and widows. The drivers would depart so quickly that Field could meet few of them. The shrines remind that any pattern of resort, which is a healing form alluding to a vernacular past, may mushroom quickly in response to new needs and energies. These places surely sustained older Akan ways of treating madness. Yet, as Field explored, the Gold Coast cash crop economy in cocoa with speedy mammy wagons made shrines apt for quick fixes and relief. The vehicles swept in as new media, promising fortune yet producing road accidents and other calamities.

There was a simultaneity to these shrines bursting forth in the 1950s, just when the observant Field was studying fixations and pulses to southern Gold Coast lives. Her key book (1960a) highlights shrines and lorries, hunger for fame, and the tendency to self-blame. Many idioms revolved around passenger trucks, whose ownership and presence lifted egos and economies, and shaped experiences and friendships. This modernizing milieu dominates her ethnography with colorful stories and slogans about luck and hardship. Lorries were infecting lives, selves, and spirits. At the same time, nightmares, dreams, and longing vied with these experiences of modernity, speed, traffic, and socialities.

As decolonization approached, Field was suggesting how these vehicles moved in parallel with depression and mental troubles. That lorries went with feeling caught, trapped, or mixed up with human harm—witchcraft— is significant. The vehicles issued in new intensities of travel, fashion, shrines, and commercial farming, within worlds teeming with phobias and grandiosity.

Ethnography suggests ways to attend to *impure* vernacular and colonial historicities. Field exposes Akan idioms through painted signs, deities, and style. Lorries were a key "vector" within this "ecological niche," to return to Hacking's language, though they were also metaphors for an ebullient modernity. As Field detailed dozens of cases, she mined these ego-documents with dreams to ask questions about diagnosis within an analysis structured by psychiatric categories (from schizophrenia to paranoia and depression), interlaced with sorcery idioms.

Her project in cultural translation moved from patient words and appearances to clinical terms. Field's items, some residual, some emergent— lorries, deities, cows, wild animals, fairies, botanicals—speak to the subtlety of her work. Not all were material objects or technologies, though imagined, religious elements were many. Still, Field diagnosed how the lorry became a critical meta-object. This technology, central to marriages, reproduction, and domestic economies, was omnipresent in gladness, sleeping, sorrow, and material and psychic worlds.[6] Also present were hierarchies of chance and visibility, reputation and ignominy, power and diminution. The "catching" idiom for witchcraft, like those "caught," knew forms of accusation and affliction tethering the modern to pasts. Yet the paramount technology seems to have been partially romanticized lorry trucks. Their drivers, passengers, and dreams evoked futures. Lorries engrossed some, excluded others, and their fortune-to-calamity spectrum mirrored psychiatric troubles in late colonial Gold Coast.

An Interlude: Counterpoint, Not Comparison

This chapter's seemingly strange juxtaposition engages movement, madness, and racialized contexts. Paul Virilio (Dercon 2016, 175; cf. Virilio 1986) once said: "When we think of speed, we say it's the means of getting from here to there fast. . . . But I say no to this. Speed is a milieu, and a milieu in which we participate only indirectly." The southern Gold Coast's new shrines and lorries provide entry to one 1950s milieu, with speed generating dreams of fame and futures as well as mental suffering. Madness was not part of the professional vocabulary of a colonial expert like Margaret Field, but the lorries do suggest her detecting a touch of social madness.

This chapter shifts with the next section to late eighteenth-century slave ships and their slowness. These grim technologies generated feelings of loss and anguish as well as suicidal ideations and death. There were no ethnographers aboard those ships, though Guinea captains and Guinea surgeons testified before a British investigative body in the 1790s. Their words— however condensed, standardized, and distorting—yield many insights, including about slave acts of refusal and despair.

Working by counterpoint in historical analysis and writing aids philosophical and historiographical reflection. So it is in this chapter, which juxtaposes incongruent situations or unexpected events, spaces, or forms, sometimes schematically so. It is quite different than pursuing a systematic comparison within a common decade or era. Historians rarely mix epochs, but there is value in doing so. In this case, working through a seemingly anomalous and jarring counterpoint helps identify reverberations around motion, tenor, and milieu. The value of the sensory as knowledge about madness is signaled.

This chapter also brings side-by-side disparate sources, regions, and eras. Unlike milieus, vectors, cases, tonalities, and categories can be parsed.

The next seam to this chapter moves backward some 150 years to the West African coast with ships plying Atlantic waters. A slave ship was an overpacked crucible, a place of punishment, in some senses, not unlike psychiatric asylums (Goffman 1961; Foucault 2006). These cruel sites of racialized modernity (Gilroy 1993; Rediker 2007) entailed a full spectrum of the sensory (Mrázek 2020) and generated many shades of madness. A slave ship produced the emaciated of "camps," spaces of "bare life" (Agamben 2000),[7] and it subjected captives to noxious smells, violent terrors, and death (Mbembe 2019).

The idea here is not to compare empirical detail but to establish an indirectness in knowing, through an arresting counterpoint, a form of archival historicity that opens new ways of thinking history. In laying out contexts, atmospheres, or moods in relation to, in this case, motion and disturbances, all emerging from starkly unlike worlds, my approach encourages a juxtaposed form of alert participation in two milieus. The partaking is less sure than sensed and indirect. Many facts are laid bare, in keeping with Virilio's words (Dercon 2016, 175; cf. Virilio 1986) about milieu, motion, and haste, as matters "in which we participate only indirectly."

In musing with Hartog (2015), the practice is not about presentism, except some readers might make this case material intelligible through the contemporary lens of, say, Black Lives Matter. Some resonances are obvious there. The tactic here is more about archive-based experiences of time. The order of time is even irreverent, while it is necessarily dual. Any conventional ordering of time is inverted: readers will sense that narrative time is loosened, undone.

The result in this meditation on race and madness is mediated by speed, motion, and cruelty. The stance gives form to two sets of experiences of time, and those familiar modes: the present, past, and future. We are far from any old regime of historicity here, one still sustained in many circles as a narrative history of big events. The regime of historicity proposed here relies for its intelligibility on slices of time, and their temporal inversion into counterpoint: as anachrony. Neither memory nor heritage matter, but a taste (Farge 1989) for time, the archival and the microscopic do, as well as that unruly disordering of time that tells much.

Milieu 2: On Slave Ships

How to bring analytically *near*—to use that Benjaminian word (Hunt 2016; Rouleau 2017)—incidents and traces of madness? This section turns to disturbances and suicide through a close reading of captains' and medics' witnessing about these vessels. The enslaved became patients, with those at risk of death to be kept alive at all costs.

What should we do with such sources containing no patient "voices"? Ferreting out the silenced within a source is old within the historical craft, though the method when applied to texts spoken or authored by European strangers has risks (Hunt 2016). By reading among lines and sounds, how ailing slaves impressed themselves on European witnesses—into their words and memories—may be discerned. Conceptualizing such a shift reminds of that old, knotty discussion about patient voices being absent from medical histories (Porter 1985). This view needs to be triangulated with that of historians of Africa who have long worked with compensatory, anti-reifying moves, with and against the voices of memory work (Hunt 1999; White, Miescher, and Cohen 2001).

The vernacular need not be another way of locating voices. It may be combined with early modernist and anthropological sensibilities, listening from beneath and beside for the residual in a present, sensing hues, especially when words are not easily had (Ginzburg 1980; McCaskie 2000). The testimony here emerged from processes of assembly and abridgment in the 1790s as part of an official British process investigating the slave trade. The witnesses knew an array of positions on the ships. John Knox was a commander for seven to eight years and for an equal duration a surgeon. Thomas Trotter, a royal navy surgeon, engaged in work on the iconic slave ship, the *Brookes*. Alexander Falconbridge participated in four voyages to Africa, with three to the West Indies in the 1780s. James Towne was a carpenter. All worked for money, and surgeons earned more for each enslaved person who survived (Watson 1969; Sheridan 1981).

The almost seven hundred pages of abridged testimony by dozens of witnesses offers an array of uncodified, madness-linked words: mad, turbulent, insane, insanity, dejection, sulkiness, and melancholia. The testimony suggests a trajectory from departure to arrival. Implicit are African beginnings, waiting to fill a ship and depart; then literal—male—ups and downs within the ship, from sleeping and holding areas to decks above;

eating time, up on deck; so-called jumping or dancing with whipping; and on arrival in the West Indies, a time of chaotic sales and also terror about kin separations for the enslaved.

Texture is rare in this testimony. I privilege the sensory and those cases suggesting an event, thus incidents, confrontations, or minuscule aspects suggesting refusals by the enslaved. Enunciated by those managing a ship, the archive tells of moments where care was not primary. I argue that this refractory source, with no ethnographic register, is invaluable. Yet I show this by combing for grains about remembered, if nameless, enslaved figures. It is in extracting microscopic episodes that a mixture of violence, desperation, anger, and the suicidal comes searingly into view.

"Mad" Slaves

On his first voyage, Falconbridge (*Abridgment of the Evidence* [hereafter AE] 1792, 232) "saw at Bonny on board the Emilia, a woman chained on deck who the chief mate said was mad." Later, during "a lucid interval," they sold her off in Jamaica. Other enslaved persons moved in and out of states of madness and lucidity, amid extreme violence. Clement Noble, with nine voyages to Africa as mate and master, recalled a man "on board his ship attempting to destroy himself, and believes the man was perfectly mad." He did not "appear so at first." Yet this enslaved person "stormed and made a great noise, worked with his hands, etc. and shewed every sign of being mad." Noble (AE 1792, 52) was not sure if he "generally refused sustenance," though recalled speaking with him "at times when he seemed to be rather better than at others." This slave "gave no reason at all for his violent conduct," though they "could seldom get him to speak." He also remembered an "insane and very troublesome" woman who jumped overboard. He ordered her "confined to prevent her from doing it again, but punished her no other way." Noble (AE 1792, 48) claimed to "not recollect whether she died or not."

Such strands suggest faulty memories, since madness went with noise, violence, and refusing to eat. Historians have treated such as "evidence" (Sheridan 1985), collected by the British Privy Council, more than as motivated testimony. The sources are unlike the testimonies and memoirs of the enslaved or once enslaved produced within abolitionist circles. Political energies led to the Council's investigative process, with pro- and antislavery attitudes and ambiguities regarding paternalism and cruelties. Curious are the flatness and repetition. How the collection and abridgements (used here and by others)[8] were orchestrated, assembled, and truncated is opaque, with questions and questioners effaced.

I expected vivid stories, with European self-images and suggestions, and to work with them along the lines of Alex Bontemps, who drew out psychological complexities from the refractory sources generated by planters of the American South: ads for fugitive slaves. I found some person-specific storylines with "divided selves" (Bontemps 2001), "disintegrated selves" (Vaughan 1993, 48), and forms of assertion among the enslaved. The Guinea testimonies go beyond "agency" (Johnson 2003). Rather, the witnessing enables mining white-delivered narratives about selves on the edge.

Fits, Dejection, and Jumping Overboard

Isaac Wilson (AE 1792, 220), a majesty's navy surgeon, knew some slaves to "fall overboard by accident" but generally they were picked up from the waters. He remembered one who fell free of his chains "in a fit," before drowning. Trotter (AE 1792, 38) recalled an enslaved man jumping overboard who drowned, another "taken up," and a woman "chained to the mainmast, after being taken up." On the Alexander, one enslaved man forced his way through "netting when brought on board," who was "devoured by the sharks" (Falconbridge, AE 1792, 232).

The odds varied, but many drowned due to accidents, fits of madness, or seeking death. If some were individual acts, some became collective events. Falconbridge (AE 1792, 234) witnessed a "scramble on board" where forty or fifty "leaped into the sea," though most were "taken up again." During the same voyage, "near 20 jumped overboard." Some disappeared discreetly, as Falconbridge (AE 1792, 232) recalled, when "missing a sick man in the Alexander," he concluded "must have got overboard." Ships were outfitted to prevent jumping off. Many slaves still did, or tried to do so, leading to lacerations, death, and punitive forms of prevention.

Dejection was a diagnostic word for suicidal willfulness, suggesting derangement and misery. "A woman on board the Alexander was dejected, taken ill of a dysentery, and refused both food and medicine. Being asked by the interpreter what she wanted, she replied nothing but to die" (Falconbridge, AE 1792, 229). Falconbridge recalled "a fine young woman brought on board, cried continually, refused her food, and wasted much in

3 or 4 days." When "sent on shore to Bonny" to recover, she "soon became cheerful, but hearing she was to be sent again onboard" she "hung herself" (Falconbridge, AE 1792, 232).

Suicide involved cleverness, forethought, force, and skill. Wilson (AE 1792, 221) told of another woman who "hanged herself by tying rope-yarn to a batten, near her usual sleeping place, and nipping off the platform. The next morning, she was found warm." Another woman "found means to get rope yarn the night preceding, which she tied to the head of the armourer's vice, then in the woman's room, she fastened it round her neck, and in the morning was found dead, whence it appeared, she must have used great exertions to accomplish her end." A seasick Ebo woman, "seeming to pine and waste," was sent ashore. James Frazer (AE 1792, 22), with twenty years as mate and commander, learned she hanged herself. Food, diet, and ingestion stoked conflict and mingled with the suicidal. Wilson (AE 1792, 220) testified that it was "common for slaves to refuse sustenance." It was also a common practice to "induce" eating. One surgeon knew "many instances of their refusing to take medicines" because they wished to die (Falconbridge, AE 1792, 229).

Some incidents were polished through official witnessing. Frazer (AE 1792, 21) elaborated a memory of being sick in his cabin one day when "the chief mate and surgeon once and again came to inform him that there was a man upon the main deck that would neither eat, drink, or speak." He spoke about the importance of speech, of getting this enslaved man to express himself and securing the help of other slaves in making him speak. As one remained "obstinate," the urgency became food. Diagnosis was thorny: "not knowing whether it was sulkiness or insanity." Frazer ordered the chief mate and surgeon to present the enslaved man "with a piece of fire in one hand and a piece of yam in the other." Such an enforcement of reason suggested an absence of cruelty. He claimed "that the man took the yam and ate it, and threw the fire overboard." Later, Frazer's colleagues showed off the rescued man with a rare sartorial reference to his "frock and trousers," received from ship sailors for "washing and mending their clothes." This enslaved person was somehow special, and Frazer's story ended with the high sum he yielded as a domesticated slave when sold off in Grenada.

Such idealized evidence is rare. Usually those who refused to eat met violence, as can be seen in another brief story. Wilson (AE 1792, 221–22) recalled that, after trying to make one enslaved man "understand that he should have anything he wished for, but he still refused to eat," they used a "cat"—whip—"with as little success." With the slave keeping his teeth closed, "it was impossible to get anything down." They tried to force open his mouth. After several days, "he was brought up as dead, to be thrown overboard," yet then recovered. Then, two days later, the process repeated. They helped him move toward "the fireplace, when in a feeble voice, in his own tongue, he asked for water." Yet soon the enslaved man shut his teeth again, "as fast as ever and resolved to die." Refusing food alternated with apparent moments of recovery, but the slave's determination to die would win out in the end.

Noble (AE 1792, 52) remembered the thinness of a young slave not long on board. He refused all food, "mild means were used to divert him," yet "weakness and fainting" ensued. Noble had seen some die a few minutes after being brought up from the lower deck of "corrupted air and heat." He had seen some go "down apparently quite well at night," yet were "found dead in the morning." Wishing to escape and refusing food went with the revolting, pestilential, foul air that killed.

Trotter (AE 1792, 38) recalled a woman "repeatedly flogged," who had "victuals forced into her mouth" yet nothing "could make her swallow." She lived her last days "in a state of torpid insensibility." Many were determined to outdo those in charge, and some outwitted "even in the act of chastisement." Noble (AE 1792, 52) saw many refusing food who would "look up at him with a smile, and in their own language say 'presently we shall be no more.'" If the grins on emaciated bodies haunted captains, mates, and surgeons, they also suggest some pleasure in achieving a disappearance into death.

The testimony speaks to dissent and the suicidal, while money motivated efforts to save enslaved lives. The milieu was miasmatic, polluted, repulsive to the core, making the prevention of death a medical and monetary challenge. All was compounded by unstable mental conditions—forms of madness— among those striving to escape from these slow-moving containers.

Tonality and Space

How did witnesses characterize mental states? Trotter (AE 1792, 40) spoke to "the contaminated atmosphere" that depressed "passions" among those "torn from all that is to be valued in life." Death, mourning, few diversions, and sadism were everyday occurrences on these ships, with sometimes an ugly "vivacity" (to invert the festive usage for early modern madness of Foucault 1961, 197; Megill 1979, 478). Suicide was a constant risk. Conditions, technologies, and practices speak to how the ships generated crises of presence. Some saw escape through death or went to lengths in securing a suicide. Many wasted away by refusing food. Some stormed with fury and vengeance, dying in the process.

Some Guinea witnesses seemed keen to show off their humanitarian sides, admitting tearful reunions among enslaved kin. Some slaves were terrified when separated from "husbands, wives, mothers, children" (Noble, AE 1792, 51). Falconbridge (AE 1792, 234) heard of a white purchaser who refused to buy a man's wife, only to learn the next day that "the man had hanged himself." Once, at Cape Coast Castle when choosing enslaved persons for his ship, Falconbridge objected to a "meagre" man. Later, he "observed him to weep" and "conceal" his tears because "he was to be parted from his brother." In the end, this surgeon who veered toward abolitionism (AE 1792, 238) took the thin brother along. Isaac Wilson (AE 1792, 222), a majesty's navy surgeon, related an instance of two siblings unexpectedly meeting up on board. Their joyful embrace "induced him to believe" that African slaves "were as affectionate as most other people." Falconbridge (AE 1792, 232) recalled the enslaved being "in great distress and making grievous outcries" during one "sale by scramble," when a voyage ended in the West Indies. The clamor stemmed from departing the now familiar ship space, when slaves would sound with "a general cry and a noise throughout the whole ship."

Madness also appeared through stories of supervising the deathlike lower deck. Trotter (AE 1792, 40) recalled being "thwarted" in tending the sick, "who in violent bursts of anger" refused his medicines in this congested space. It was pathological, and surgeons knew the risks. Wilson (AE 1792, 220) "took off his shoes before going down, and was very cautious how he walked." Joy was contrived in such a space of whipping, punishments, and noxious air. A tone of ferocious anger would often swell up. Still, childbearing could punctuate these ship scenes. Falconbridge (AE 1792, 238) noted that "out of 4 or 5 deliveries on shipboard two had twins."

Diagnostic Words

Slaves were "apt to quarrel" and seemed "implacable" (Frazer, AE 1792, 12). Henry Ellison (AE 1792, 146) recalled some enslaved women who disturbed a captain dining. Suddenly, a chief officer "came out, and with a wire cat began to flog away," so violently that six women jumped overboard and five drowned. The captain tortured another, submerging her in water "up and down a dozen times." She died the next day.

Turbulent was part of the lexicon for madness on these ships. It went with rage and revenge. Ellison recounted a slave who "disobliged the second mate." He "gave her a cut or two" with a cat-o'-nine-tails until she "flew at him with great rage." He pushed her away, "giving her three or four final strokes." Soon the woman was no more. Ellison (AE 1792, 147) thought that being deprived of "revenge" set her off. Abruptly, she "dropped down dead." Within a half an hour, he narrated, her corpse was overboard, likely "torn to pieces by sharks."

Turbulence alternated with cruelties. Falconbridge (AE 1792, 231) spoke about shackling the enslaved together, a measure provoking rows. Such human pairs "find it difficult to get over other slaves." One "companion" would refuse to move, causing "great disturbance." The toxic air and over-crowding made fights worse, and death was ever lurking in this subterranean zone. Falconbridge (AE 1792, 231) witnessed shackled slave companions, often with "a dead and living slave found in the morning shackled together."

The Middle Passage entailed ruptures in practice and speech: *melancholia* came into play beside self-destruction. Frazer (AE 1792, 25) recalled a "man who attempted to cut his own throat," who had "all the appearance of a sullen melancholy, but was by no means insane," even if "a degree of delirium might come on before death." The transformation was striking since "when he came on board," he seemed to be "in his perfect senses." Melancholia endured as a category on these ships and within the practices of Guinea surgeons. In the eighteenth century, psychiatric knowledge was not strongly codified. Still, in these pestilential, miasmatic ships, diagnostic distinctions were many. When Falconbridge (AE 1792, 231) listed causes of shipboard deaths, he began with "a diseased mind." Other reasons followed: "sudden transitions from heat to cold, a putrid atmosphere, wallowing in their own excrement, and being shackled together." In placing mental pathology first, yet with being shackled and kept below deck as important, he noted that "men die in twice the number of women" with the latter not shackled or housed below. No one suggested suicide was pathological. The pestilential explained the wish to escape, yet witnesses fashioned a religious dimension for the wish to return home and to ancestors.

Wilson (AE 1792, 219) could not "recollect ever to have cured any" from melancholia. Surgeons used the word to evoke dejected moods in keeping with the term's polysemy, as Robert Burton ([1624] 1972) long ago insisted in his *Anatomy of Melancholy*. Melancholy on ships had types (Mallipeddi 2014). The label went with forced separation, loss, and longing for death. Trotter (AE 1792, 37) linked sullen melancholy to being "torn from their connections and their country." Wilson (AE 1792, 225) spoke of "grief." The carpenter James Towne (AE 1792, 11) thought the sickness seemed due less to "their crowded state" than "being carried away from their country and friends." The diagnostic register included the word *sulky*. Surgeons and captains distinguished sullen from fixed melancholy, and the mad from the insane. Fixed melancholy entailed "lowness of spirits and despondency" and "refusing nourishment," so "the stomach gets weak, fluxes ensue, and, from a debilitated state, soon carry them off."

Sound, Choking, and an Antivernacular

Melancholia sounded. Frazer (AE 1792, 25) spoke of ship vibrations and "signs of extreme distress and despair" when the enslaved first came on board: "a feeling of their situation, and regret at being torn from friends and connections." Slaves could be "heard in the night, making a howling melancholy noise, expressive of extreme anguish." A woman interpreter inquired into their wailful lamentations since some "dreamed they were in their own country" and when awaking would find themselves in the ship's hold.

Song was everyday with "some tune or other in their own way" or "mournful tunes in the night" (Ellison, AE 1792, 147). They "sing, but not for their amusement," said Ecroide Claxton (AE 1792, 20). When a captain "ordered them to sing," some "sang songs of sorrow" about "sickness, fear of being beaten, their hunger, and the memory of their country." Sometimes sounds or their effacement dominated departures: "They sailed after dark in the night, when the Naves were secured below, to prevent their shewing signs of discontent at leaving the coast." Trotter (AE 1792, 37) added that all ships left at night.

Sound and song suggest the sensory. The testimony suggests a grieving soundscape, present for all. Europeans found the timbres and reverberations stirring, wrenching. They could neither control slave disappearances nor the ways they joined in making a ship sound. The soundings and wailing became like a vernacular, yearning for a past known, born of these harrowing vessels and carried far—perhaps even into the emergence of the blues in America (Baraka 1963).

Dance belongs to gesture. Claxton named a fictive dimension: "dance, as they call it" (AE 1792, 18). Noble (AE 1792, 52) described the practice well: "a drum is beat, and they jump or dance to it, as well as their situation will admit," since "the stout men are all in irons, and a right leg and a left, and their hands the same: a chain fastens the greatest part of them to the deck, a few days before leaving the coast, and a few days after." Dancing kept the enslaved moving and perhaps in better health, though the testimony suggests it was rarely pleasant, and mixed with frenetic punishment. A drum was nearby, but so were punitive cat-o'-nine-tails. Falconbridge (AE 1792, 232) claimed that "dancing by slave-dealers has been often desired in every ship."

Some recalled glimpsing from afar Africa's slaving coasts, like Weuves (AE 1792, 37) who saw possible victims "dressed and dancing cheerfully." Drumming and dance go to the core of African healing (Hunt 2013), as John Janzen (1982, 118) long ago suggested with *Lemba*, a mobile, seventeenth-century "cult of affliction" from the lower Congo region. Lemba's mercantile organizers were members of an elite who became wealthy from the export trade. Women sensing barrenness sought Lemba for reproductive and mental problems. A common refrain went: "That which was a 'stitch' of pain, Has become the path to the priesthood. . . . What Lemba gives, Lemba takes away. What the sun gives, the sun takes away." The lyrics spoke to harassing spirits, nightmares, and pain. People were trying to "imaginatively . . . cope with a force that transformed" everything: capitalism and the Atlantic trade. Lemba grew as fifteen thousand slaves were shipped out annually in the eighteenth century. About calming or *lembikisa*, Lemba illness involved heads, hearts, abdomens, spirit possession, and a "stitch, or breathing with difficulty." Many of those afflicted—chiefs, judges, traders, healers—were busy in trade and vulnerable to envy and witchcraft. An obsession with fame deepened Lemba's illness, which surfaced where many were on the move along trade routes. Lemba could temper fame and also bring wealthy traders down to size.

Guinea surgeons were probably unaware of the expression for being caught, breathing with difficulty, and choking on the verge of death. Yet parallel idioms—choking and feeling caught—entered the lower and upper decks. Dancing became general across ships, as Noble (AE 1792, 52) observed. It was not elaborated as warmth or sociality in the testimonies. It remained vague, a guilty realm, construed as helpful for slave health, but turned grim and punitive. The violence of dance became a fixation. Trotter

(AE 1792, 40) found it "necessary for their health." George Millar (AE 1792, 157) clarified a difference: dancing in irons was impossible, yet to "jump up and down" remained feasible. Trotter (AE 1792, 39) described the enslaved "in irons" as those "ordered to stand up, and make what motions they could," yet those "out of irons" could "dance round the deck." Falconbridge (AE 1792, 232) recalled dancing as a coerced, morning, upper deck activity. He would examine the "irons of male slaves . . . as they come up in the morning" and were "made to jump."

Dancing could go fictive or be romanticized, as in the kindness, movement, and brandy found in a famous Guinea surgeon's *vade mecum* (Aubrey 1729). Noble (AE 1792, 52) had many slaves "very fond of dancing, except a few sulky ones." Persuasion and force, he implied, were routine: "the means used to compel them to dance." Most admitted dancing as "compelled by the cat" (John Ashley Hall, AE 1792, 208). Keeping the enslaved crowded below deck made "them faint through heat, the steam coming through the gratings like a furnace." Dancing "by the cat" (Wilson, AE 1792, 220) may have enabled better breathing. The tension between softness and violence was ubiquitous.

So banal and twisted did forced dancing become that it almost suggests an *antivernacular*—one destructive of enduring African practices. Distortion and hate appear in this violent realm of force and conflict. Whipping ran contrary to the convivialities of African rituals and festivities, drumming and dancing. Shipmasters justified whipping: "Never had any slaves die on board in consequence of correction," said Clement Noble (AE 1792, 48). Virtually absent are mediating African figures who labored on these ships, yet the wrath and guilt of European personnel are clear. If dancing began as a way of shaking off melancholia (Mallipeddi 2014), it marked captain and surgeon testimony as a time of compulsion and revenge.

In this archive of witnessing, the names of the enslaved are absent: their voices, words, and speech rare. The gestural and the seen, like displeasure and refusals, marked the remembrances of ship operators and medics. Traces of volition and breakdown are etched into memories, showing the methodological importance of *disembedding* figures, clashes, and emotions. Vocabularies for agitated and grieving states of mind varied. Yet shades of madness continually creeped in. The paradoxes of quasi-dancing and lashing suggest how convoluted and harmful this coerced vernacular became. These efforts from above to recreate something familiar, yet as a contrived, twisted ambit, suggest a mimetic aspiration toward life, survival, and wealth. But the mimesis was untenable: forms of suicide and madness came dashing back in.

Discussion

This chapter effaced that conventional motif of psychiatric histories: asylums. By insisting on slave ships as terrible enclosures (Goffman 1961), the psychopathologies of these awkward, violent containers, their sounds and organization, have been exposed. Akan new shrines of the 1950s canceled out asylums, too. Field's rural cases moved beyond the homicidal of psychiatry's late colonial "hospital picture" (Field 1960b).

Although startling, by juxtaposing 1950s lorries and commercial shrines with 1790s Guinea ships, the central counterpoint of this chapter yields much. Gold Coast mammy wagons joined shrines in prying open elements of a modern, emergent vernacular. The anthropologist listened and sometimes imposed while observing worlds motivated by fame and deities. Within the Guinea testimony, shrines, religiosity, and deities are absent, even if witchcraft surfaces. Residual healing moved with the furtive materialities of slave life as they recreated Obeah, Lemba, conjuration, and other terror-based therapies in the Americas (Janzen 1982; Fett 2002; Palmié 2002; Senior 2018).

Virilio's (1986) words about *speed-as-milieu* are precious. Field encountered depressed women enmeshed in dreams, fast lorries, and vulnerabilities. A slave ship was a slow-moving milieu that generated suicide and dejected states of mind. Songs of lament vied with distorted dances on these vessels. Surgeons said little about amulets, clothing, or bodily decorations. Yet they learned about aversions and sinking moods. The will to escape was pervasive: many captives hastened to die. A key antivernacular lay in the contrived, perverse refashioning of African dancing—away from pleasure and healing—into twisted, coerced jumping. Psychiatric lexicons surfaced, from Field's modern psychiatric categories to Guinea witnesses sizing up the morose. Madness on ships stemmed from carceral, cruel conditions, even if insurgency or death could seem resplendent for some slaves.

This chapter disordered time with two planes to history, with a pair of incongruent milieus calling out for hermeneutic technique. With sounds, objects, and dreams, the sensory may surface from the archival and mark milieus. The acoustic and affective have been remaking interpretations over a wide scale in historiography (Stewart 2007; Hunt 2013, 2016; Mrázek 2020). Dirge-like sounds suggest mourning. A ship's "acoustic register" (Hunt 2008) troubled memories. Field listened yet rarely quoted vernacular speech. Her ethnographic objects—lorries and cloth—entangled fame and dreams. On slave ships, material objects speak to subjugation, while the enslaved in dreaming went with longing to exit from the nightmarish vessels.

Histories of madness may generate knowledge from minutiae, yet as this experiment has shown, historians of medicine or psychiatry do not necessarily require patient "voices." Cases and the microscopic yield plenty. Nor need the vernacular be a driving fixation, yet when residual elements are there they can tell us much. Likewise, silences and absences are telling. Without obvious ego-documents, even mediated ones, a telling patchwork still emerges.

This chapter suggests the value of what we might call *faint archives*. Microscopic bits allow sensing collective or individuated psychic states, dreams, or nightmares. Slight, indirect evidence, where some speak for those at a fringe or lower stratum, tells of faintness. Two cases—melancholic Akan women of the 1950s, and disintegrating slaves of the 1790s—are profoundly unlike, with different cadences, severities, and psychopathologies. The contrast speaks to diagnostic codes and ways of knowing selves and states. Margaret Field did not use the word *melancholia* but that late twentieth-century word, *depression*, when few psychiatrists in Africa did (Vaughan 1991, 2010; Sadowsky 2021). Though having long studied Akan religion, her postwar psychiatric lexicon embraced categories like schizophrenia. Field, who trained in the anthropology of dreams, elicited many. Yet the sole explicit dream in ship testimony evoked a return to Africa, a daydream turned nightmarish repeatedly. Postmenopausal women dreamed of lorries and suffered in worlds of marital neglect and motorized speed. Slaves, long held on rough seas, would be moved into an upper deck then down to a pestilential level. Self-death and "dissociative drift" (Burraway 2018, 479, 475; de Martino 2012) resonate with Akan witch identifications. Some dissociated amid fearful lorry nightmares. That many hanged or starved themselves on slave ships opens wide a weighty suicidal box of global modernity.

This chapter, the volume's last, has returned us to matters of the book's introduction: madness and vernacular elements, racist machinations, and psychopolitics in spaces of social harm and moneymaking perversities. The two milieus hail from West African zones. Yet the impulse here never came from equivalence but in making two milieus speak through counterpoint.

The result renews mobility and movement technologies (Hunt 1999) as a crucial domain for African histories of psychiatry. Motion and immobility converged around transport conveyances and also in states of mind. Passenger lorries of the 1950s, like late eighteenth-century slave vessels, ignited imaginaries and experiences.

This experiment in historical writing structured a strange set of images, events, and contexts whose discontinuities may have unsettled narrative expectations. Narrative, rendering madness in two zones of time, has been more important here than chronology. A certain autonomy in historical form derived its power from challenging expectations, and seeking intelligibility on different planes. The chapter worked through an inverted series of events and textures with suffering, paranoia, and deliria. This inquiry into madness tracked modes, tones, and categories. Diverse facets—the carceral, the oneiric, and the technological—released fancy, derangement, and suicide. As selves trembled and disintegrated, stark disparities, by epoch and by racialized intentions, enabled coming to know these utterly asymmetrical milieus.

Acknowledgments

My thanks to Hubertus Büschel, and also to my dear friend Tom McCaskie, for the astute readings.

Notes

1   The multiple connotations of madness—religious, social, and political among them—have shifted through time and place. Among a spectrum of interpretations, see Foucault (2006, 2011) and Fanon (2021), as well as Wing (1978), Vaughan (1993), Staub (2011), and Hunt (introduction to this volume). Hokkanen (2018) argues that *madness* is not the best term for African colonial historical episodes with extreme emotions. I rather embrace the term's polysemic potential here.

2   A fluid set of religious, healing, and performative practices found in parts of North Africa, the Middle East, and the Horn of Africa (Djibouti, Eritrea, Ethiopia, and Somalia). *Zar* embraces dance, trance, and usually forms of fe-

male mental illness involving spirit possession via a spirit category. The term derives from the Arabic language. Psychologists see *zar* as a "culture-bound syndrome" involving dissociative, somatic, and affective symptoms: shouting, laughing, apathy, or refusing to perform daily tasks (APA Dictionary of Psychology, https://dictionary.apa.org/zar, 27 August 2023). Anthropologists focus on how people experience this healing complex with spirits, rituals, an initiatory path, communities, song, and music. When jinn (spirits) possess humans, afflicting them with trouble, a *zar* initiation is often sought out (El Hadidi 2016).

3   The category, ego-document, has thus far been little used by historians of Africa. Yet, consider the fine analysis of whiteness, ego-documents, and imperial lives in Congo Free State and German East Africa (even if it suggests naively that "nothing can be done about the regrettable lack of indigenous voices") (Natermann 2018, 229; Hunt 2016).

4   A passenger and transport vehicle with lorry chassis and a wooden frame built and decorated on top, known in Ghana as a *tro-tro* from an old Ga meaning three pence (a currency unit during British colonial rule). For some time, such a three pence piece was the going rate for a single ride.

5   Field wrote a novel, published under a pseudonym; it combined madness and decolonization, suggesting politics edged with fear (Linstrum 2016). Her turn to modernization as a psychological theory has been critiqued (Büschel 2015). Her field notes and other papers seem to have vanished, though she may have sent her papers to Professor Ivor Wilks in Evanston, Illinois, late in her life (Tom Mc-Caskie, personal communication, May 20, 2021). Still, her papers—I contacted Northwestern, SOAS, and the Rhodes House—have not yet resurfaced.

6   Lorries were not unlike bicycles in interwar Congo: pivotal to moral imaginations, rank, and dreams (Hunt 1999).

7   Scholarship on slave ships and the Middle Passage is vast, as is work on travels in and reworkings of African healing practices. Scholars have explored social, therapeutic, religious, affective, economic, and psychiatric dimensions: Janzen (1982), Fett (2002), Rediker (2007), Smallwood (2007), Snyder (2015), Mustakeem (2016), Kananoja (2018), and Senior (2018). My fixation here draws from one source: testimonies found in the *Abridgment* papers (AE 1792). Some scholars have touched on this source extensively (Watson 1969; Sheridan 1981; Stevenson 2018), while others have used them hardly or not at all.

8   Like Sheridan (1981) and Watson (1969). In an excellent parallel analysis, Mallipeddi (2014) draws on the British Parliamentary House of Commons Sessional Papers; see also Lovejoy and Oliveira (2013).

Sources

Abridgment of the Evidence Delivered before a Select Committee of the House of Commons, in the Years 1790 and 1791, on the part of the petitioners for the abolition of the slave-trade (hereafter AE). 1792. London: James Phillips. Complementary digital versions used: https://babel.hathitrust.org/cgi/pt?id=dul1.ark:/13960 /t5w679c6h&view=1up&format=plaintext&seq=5 and https://archive.org/details /abridgementofmin34grea/mode/1up?ref=ol&view=theater.

Agamben, Giorgio. 2000. "Qu'est-ce qu'un camp?" In *Means without End*. Minneapolis: University of Minnesota Press.

APA Dictionary of Psychology. 2023. https://dictionary.apa.org.

Asad, Talal, ed. 1973. *Anthropology & the Colonial Encounter*. New York: Humanities Press.

Aubrey, Thomas. 1729. *The Sea-Surgeon or the Guinea Man's Vade Mecum: In which is laid down, the method of curing such diseases as usually happen abroad, especially on the coast of Guinea; with the best way of treating negroes, both in health and in sickness, written for the use of young sea surgeons*. London: John Clarke.

Baraka, Amiri. 1963. *Blues People: Negro Music in White America*. New York: William Morrow.

Barber, Karin. 2007. *The Anthropology of Texts, Persons and Publics: Oral and Written Culture in Africa and Beyond*. Cambridge: Cambridge University Press.

Beneduce, Roberto. 2017. "History as Palimpsest: Notes on Subalternity, Alienation, and Domination in Gramsci, de Martino, and Fanon." *International Gramsci Journal* 2, no. 3: 134–73.

Boddy, Janice. 1989. *Wombs and Alien Spirits: Women, Men, and the Zar Cult in Northern Sudan*. Madison: University of Wisconsin Press.

Bontemps, Alex. 2001. *The Punished Self: Surviving Slavery in the Colonial South*. Ithaca, NY: Cornell University Press.

Burraway, Joshua. 2018. "Remembering to Forget: Blacking Out in Itchy Park." *Current Anthropology* 59, no. 5: 469–87.

Burton, Robert. (1624) 1972. *The Anatomy of Melancholy*. London: Dent.

Büschel, Hubertus. 2015. "Die Moderne macht sie geisteskrank! Primitivismus-Zuschreibung, Modernisierungserfahrung, Entwicklungsarbeit und Globale Psychiatrie im 20. Jahrhundert." *Geschichte und Gesellschaft* 41, no. 4: 685–717.

Callaway, Henry. 1885. *The Religious System of the Amazulu: Izinyanga zokubula; or, Divination, as Existing among the Amazulu, in Their Own Words*. Springvale, Natal: J. A. Blair.

Canguilhem, Georges. 2012. *Writings on Medicine*. New York: Fordham University Press.

Capan, Zeynep Gulsah. 2020. "Beyond Visible Entanglements: Connected Histories of the International." *International Studies Review* 22, no. 2: 289–306.

Charuty, Giordana. 2018. "Être ensemble dans la même histoire: L'œuvre-vie d'Ernesto de Martino." In *Bérose: Encyclopédie internationale des histoires de l'anthropologie*. Paris: IIAC-LAHIC, CNRS.

Comaroff, Jean, and John L. Comaroff. 1987. "The Madman and the Migrant: Work and Labor in the Historical Consciousness of a South African People." *American Ethnologist* 14, no. 2: 191–209.

De Martino, Ernesto. 2012. "Crisis of Presence and Religious Reintegration." *HAU, Journal of Ethnographic Theory* 2, no. 2: 431–50.

Dercon, Chris. 2016. "Speed-Space: Paul Virilio Interview." In *Impulse Archaeology*, edited by Eldon Garnet, 175–79. Toronto: University of Toronto Press.

Du Bois, William Edward Burghardt. 1903. *The Souls of Black Folk: Essays and Sketches*. Chicago: A. C. McClurg.

El Hadidi, Hager. 2016. "Introduction." In *Zar: Spirit Possession, Music, and Healing Rituals in Egypt*. Cairo: American University in Cairo Press.

Fabian, Johannes. 1996. *Remembering the Present: Painting and Popular History in Zaire*. Berkeley: University of California Press.

Fanon, Frantz. 2021. *The Political Writings from Alienation and Freedom*. Edited by Jean Khalfa and Robert J. C. Young. Translated by Steven Corcoran. London: Bloomsbury Academic.

Farge, Arlette. 1989. *Le goût de l'archive*. Paris: Editions du Seuil.

Fett, Sharla M. 2002. *Working Cures: Healing, Health, and Power on Southern Slave Plantations*. Chapel Hill: University of North Carolina Press.

Field, Margaret Joyce. 1937. *Religion and Medicine of the Ga People*. Oxford: Oxford University Press.

Field, Margaret Joyce. 1960a. *Search for Security: An Ethno-Psychiatric Study of Rural Ghana*. Evanston, IL: Northwestern University Press.

Field, Margaret Joyce. 1960b. "Mental Illness in Rural Ghana." In *Désordres mentaux et santé mentale en Afrique au sud du Sahara*. WHO Meeting of Specialists on Mental Health, Bukavu, Congo, 1958. London: CCTA.

Forrester, John. 2017. *Thinking in Cases*. Cambridge, UK: Polity.

Foucault, Michel. 1961. "La folie n'existe pas que dans une société." In *Dits et écrits I: 1954–1975*, 195–97. Paris: Editions Gallimard.

Foucault, Michel. 1978. *The History of Sexuality*. New York: Pantheon.

Foucault, Michel. 2006. *History of Madness*. Translated by Jean Khalfa. London: Routledge.

Foucault, Michel. 2011. *Madness: The Invention of an Idea*. New York: Harper Perennial.

Gilroy, Paul. 1993. *The Black Atlantic: Modernity and Double Consciousness*. Cambridge, MA: Harvard University Press.

Ginzburg, Carlo. 1980. *The Cheese and the Worms: The Cosmos of a Sixteenth-Century Miller*. Baltimore, MD: Johns Hopkins University Press.

Goffman, Erving. 1961. *Asylums: Essays on the Social Situation of Mental Patients and Other Inmates*. Chicago: Aldine.

Guerlac, S. 1980. Review of *Narrative Discourse, an Essay in Method*, by G. Genette and J. E. Lewin. *Modern Language Notes* 95, no. 5: 1414–21.

Hacking, Ian. 1998. *Mad Travelers: Reflections on the Reality of Transient Mental Illnesses*. Charlottesville: University Press of Virginia.

Hart, Jennifer A. 2016. *Ghana on the Go: African Mobility in the Age of Motor Transportation*. Bloomington: Indiana University Press.

Hartog, François. 2015. *Regimes of Historicity: Presentism and Experiences of Time*. New York: Columbia University Press.

Hokkanen, Markku. 2018. "Madness, Emotions and Loss of Control in a Colonial Frontier: Methodological Challenges of Crises of Mind." In *Encountering Crises of the Mind*, 277–95. Leiden: Brill.

Hunt, Nancy Rose. 1999. *A Colonial Lexicon: Of Birth Ritual, Medicalization, and Mobility in the Congo*. Durham, NC: Duke University Press.

Hunt, Nancy Rose. 2008. "An Acoustic Register, Tenacious Images, and Congolese Scenes of Rape and Repetition." *Cultural Anthropology* 23, no. 2: 220–53.

Hunt, Nancy Rose. 2013. "Health and Healing." In *The Oxford Handbook of Modern African History*, edited by John Parker and Richard Reid, 378–95. Oxford: Oxford University Press.

Hunt, Nancy Rose. 2016. *A Nervous State: Violence, Remedies, and Reverie in Colonial Congo*. Durham, NC: Duke University Press.

Hunt, Nancy Rose. 2018. "History as Form, with Simmel in Tow." *History and Theory* 57, no. 4: 126–44.

Jackson, Lynette. 2018. *Surfacing Up: Psychiatry and Social Order in Colonial Zimbabwe, 1908–1968*. Ithaca, NY: Cornell University Press.

Janzen, John M. 1982. *Lemba 1650–1930: A Drum of Affliction in Africa and the New World*. New York: Garland.

Johnson, Walter. 2003. "On Agency." *Journal of Social History* 37:113–24.

Kananoja, Kalle. 2018. "Melancholia, Race, and Slavery in the Early Modern Southern Atlantic World." In *Crises of Mind: Cultural and Institutional Approaches to Insanity*, edited by Jari Eilola, Markku Hokkanen, and Tuomas Laine-Frigren, 88–112. Leiden: Brill.

Kilroy-Marac, Katie. 2019. *An Impossible Inheritance: Postcolonial Psychiatry and the Work of Memory in a West African Clinic*. Berkeley: University of California Press.

Lambek, Michael. 1981. *Human Spirits: A Cultural Account of Trance in Mayotte*. Cambridge: Cambridge University Press.

Larson, Pier M. 2009. *Ocean of Letters: Language and Creolization in an Indian Ocean Diaspora*. Cambridge: Cambridge University Press.

Leiris, Michel. 1938. "La croyance aux génies zar en Éthiopie du nord." *Journal de psychologie normale et pathologiques* 35:108–25.

Linstrum, Erik. 2016. *Ruling Minds: Psychology in the British Empire*. Cambridge, MA: Harvard University Press.

Littlewood, Roland. 2017. "Search for Security: An Ethno-Psychiatric Study of Rural Ghana, by Margaret Joyce Field: London, Faber and Faber, 1960." *Anthropology and Medicine* 24, no. 2: 236–38.

Lovejoy, Paul E., and Vanessa S. Oliveira. 2013. "An Index to the Slavery and Slave Trade Enquiry: The British Parliamentary House of Commons Sessional Papers, 1788–1792." *History in Africa*, 40, no. 1: 193–255.

Lovell, Anne M., and Papa Mamadou Diagne. 2019. "Falling, Dying Sheep, and the Divine: Notes on Thick Therapeutics in Peri-Urban Senegal." *Culture, Medicine and Psychiatry* 43, no. 4: 663–85.

Mallipeddi, Ramesh. 2014. "'A Fixed Melancholy': Migration, Memory, and the Middle Passage." *The Eighteenth Century* 55, no. 2–3: 235–53.

Marks, Shula, ed. 1987. *Not Either an Experimental Doll: The Separate Worlds of Three South African Women*. Bloomington: Indiana University Press.

Marks, Shula. 1999. "'Every Facility That Modern Science and Enlightened Humanity Have Devised': Race and Progress in a Colonial Hospital, Valkenberg Mental Asylum, Cape Colony, 1894–1910." In *Insanity, Institutions and Society, 1800–1914: A Social History of Madness in Comparative Perspective*, edited by Joseph Melling and Bill Forsythe, 268–92. London: Routledge.

Mbembe, Achille. 2019. *Necropolitics*. Durham, NC: Duke University Press.

McCaskie, T. C. 2000. *Asante Identities: History and Modernity in an African Village, 1850–1950*. London: Edinburgh University Press.

McCulloch, Jock. 1995. *Colonial Psychiatry and "the African Mind."* Cambridge: Cambridge University Press.

Megill, Allan. 1979. "Foucault, Structuralism, and the Ends of History." *Journal of Modern History* 51, no. 3: 451–503.

Midelfort, H. C. Erik. 1999. *A History of Madness in Sixteenth-Century Germany*. Stanford, CA: Stanford University Press.

Mrázek, Rudolf. 2020. *The Complete Lives of Camp People: Colonialism, Fascism, Concentrated Modernity*. Durham, NC: Duke University Press.

Mukharji, Projit Bihari. 2016. *Doctoring Tradition: Ayurveda, Small Technologies and Braided Sciences*. Chicago: University of Chicago Press.

Mustakeem, Sowande M. 2016. *Slavery at Sea: Terror, Sex, and Sickness in the Middle Passage*. Champaign: University of Illinois Press.

Natermann, Diana Miryong. 2018. *Pursuing Whiteness in the Colonies: Private Memories from the Congo Free State and German East Africa (1884–1914)*. Historische Belgienforschung 3. Münster, Germany: Waxmann.

Orsini, Francesca. 2020. "Vernacular: Flawed but Necessary?" *South Asian Review* 41, no. 2: 204–6.

Palmié, Stephan. 2002. *Wizards and Scientists: Explorations in Afro-Cuban Modernity and Tradition*. Durham, NC: Duke University Press.

Perneau, Margrit, and Luc Wodzicki. 2017. "Entanglements, Political Communication, and Shared Temporal Layers." *Cromohs (Cyber Review of Modern Historiography)* 21, no. 1: 1–17.

Porter, Roy. 1985. "The Patient's View: Doing Medical History from Below." *Theory and Society* 14, no. 2: 175–98.

Ranger, Terence. 1983. "The Invention of Tradition in Colonial Africa." In *The Invention of Tradition*, edited by Eric Hobsbawm and Terence Ranger, 211–62. Cambridge: Cambridge University Press.

Rediker, Marcus. 2007. *The Slave Ship: A Human History*. New York: Viking.

Rouleau, Martine. 2017. "The Trace Is the Appearance of Nearness." *UCL Culture Blog*, May 30. https://blogs.ucl.ac.uk/museums/2017/05/30/the-trace-is-the-appearance-of-nearness/.

Sadowsky, Jonathan. 1999. *Imperial Bedlam: Institutions of Madness in Colonial Southwest Nigeria*. Berkeley: University of California Press.

Sadowsky, Jonathan. 2021. *The Empire of Depression: A New History*. Cambridge, UK: Polity.

Senior, Emily. 2018. *The Caribbean and the Medical Imagination, 1764–1834: Slavery, Disease and Colonial Modernity*. Cambridge: Cambridge University Press.

Sheridan, Richard B. 1981. "The Guinea Surgeons on the Middle Passage: The Provision of Medical Services in the British Slave Trade." *International Journal of African Historical Studies* 14, no. 4: 601–25.

Sheridan, Richard B. 1985. *Doctors and Slaves: A Medical and Demographic History of Slavery in the British West Indies, 1680–1834*. Cambridge: Cambridge University Press.

Simmel, Georg. 1980. *Essays on Interpretation in Social Science*. Translated by Guy Oakes. Totowa NJ: Rowman and Littlefield.

Smallwood, Stephanie E. 2007. *Saltwater Slavery: A Middle Passage from Africa to American Diaspora*. Cambridge, MA: Harvard University Press.

Snyder, Terri L. 2015. *The Power to Die: Slavery and Suicide in British North America*. Chicago: University of Chicago Press.

Staub, Michael E. 2011. *Madness Is Civilization When the Diagnosis Was Social, 1948–1980*. Chicago: University of Chicago Press.

Steinmetz, George, ed. 2013. *Sociology and Empire: The Imperial Entanglements of a Discipline*. Durham, NC: Duke University Press.

Steinmetz, George. 2017. "Field Theory and Interdisciplinarity: History and Sociology in Germany and France during the Twentieth Century." *Comparative Studies in Society and History* 59, no. 2: 477–514.

Stevenson, Robert L., Jr. 2018. "Jumping Overboard: Examining Suicide, Resistance, and West African Cosmologies during the Middle Passage." PhD diss., Michigan State University.

Stewart, Kathleen. 2007. *Ordinary Affects*. Durham, NC: Duke University Press.

Subrahmanyam, Sanjay. 1997. "Connected Histories: Notes towards a Reconfiguration of Early Modern Eurasia." *Modern Asian Studies* 31, no. 3: 735–62.

Thomas, Lynn M. 2011. "Modernity's Failings, Political Claims, and Intermediate Concepts." *American Historical Review* 116, no. 3: 727–40.

Todorov, Tzvetan. 1984. *The Conquest of America: The Question of the Other*. New York: Harper and Row.

Van der Veer, Peter. 1998. "The Global History of 'Modernity.'" *Journal of the Economic and Social History of the Orient* 41, no. 3: 285–94.

Vaughan, Megan. 1983. "Idioms of Madness: Zomba Lunatic Asylum, Nyasaland, in the Colonial Period." *Journal of Southern African Studies* 9, no. 2: 218–38.

Vaughan, Megan. 1991. *Curing Their Ills: Colonial Power and African Illness*. Cambridge, UK: Polity.

Vaughan, Megan. 1993. "Madness and Colonialism, Colonialism as Madness." *Paideuma* 39:45–55.

Vaughan, Megan. 2010. "Suicide in Late Colonial Africa: The Evidence of Inquests from Nyasaland." *American Historical Review* 115, no. 2: 385–404.

Virilio, Paul. 1986. *Speed and Politics: An Essay on Dromology*. New York: Columbia University Press.

Von Greyerz, Kaspar. 2010. "Ego-Documents: The Last Word?" *German History* 28, no. 3: 273–82.

Washbrook, David. 1998. "The Global History of 'Modernity': A Response to a Reply." *Journal of the Economic and Social History of the Orient* 41, no. 3: 295–311.

Watson, W. N. Boog. 1969. "The Guinea Trade and Some of Its Surgeons (with Special Reference to the Royal College of Surgeons of Edinburgh)." *Journal of the Royal College of Surgeons of Edinburgh* 14:203–14.

White, Luise, Stephan Miescher, and David William Cohen. 2001. *African Words, African Voices: Critical Practices in Oral History*. Bloomington: Indiana University Press.

Wing, John Kenneth. 1978. *Reasoning about Madness*. Oxford: Oxford University Press.

Hubertus Büschel

CODA

On the Importance of Suffering

Mr. Ogundeji—his full name is unknown—became an artist in a Nigerian colonial asylum for the insane. He painted with fine brushstrokes and shiny watercolors. He portrayed birds and young animals with cloudy or colorful shadows, and also children, women, and even himself as a small, yet voluminous and friendly man, though without a face. In the early 1940s, Ogundeji suffered from dark dreams about a large red bird that was trying to kill him. Another dream tortured him often: it was about him murdering his own child (Beier 1982, 84–85).

Ogundeji came from Otta, a Yoruba town. The king of Otta and his Native Council came to the conclusion that Ogundeji was the victim of an "evil witch." They advised him to consult a "witchdoctor" specialist of healing, ritual, and perhaps cursing, or simply to ignore his scary dreams. This situation changed in 1942 when the British colonial government in Nigeria abolished the judicial powers of this Native Council. At the same time, an English judge and a

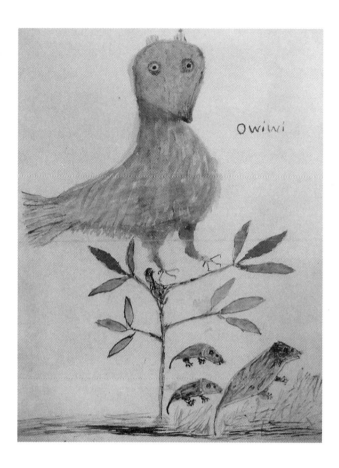

Owiwi

C.1   A mental health patient, Ogundeji from Otta, painted
       this owl with mice at the Lantoro Mental Asylum, Abeo-
       kuta, Nigeria, December 1950. (Ulli Beier Collection,
       Iwalewa House, Bayreuth: see Beier 1982, 13.)

government doctor intervened and decided that Ogundeji was insane. They
interned him, forcefully, in the Lantoro Mental Asylum in Abeokuta, where
the man stayed for the next ten years (Beier 1982, 84).

In 1950, Ogundeji met the German anthropologist and art historian
Ulli Beier. This quite bohemian thinker and writer worked as an assistant
lecturer at the University of Ibadan, close to Abeokuta. Out of coincidence
and also out of curiosity, Beier visited Lantoro Mental Asylum, as he later
wrote: "The doctor conducted me through the mental home. A large hot,
dusty courtyard, surrounded by a high fence. A large shade tree stood in

the center, otherwise everything was exposed to the glaring sun. The barracks were built of raw cement blocks. Everything was monotonously grey, a desolate sight. A few patients sat tired and bored under the tree. Some stood up, laughed and shook my hand. Others appeared not so nice to us and stared sadly into the sand" (Beier 1982, 82).

Beier also visited an occupational therapy class at the asylum, where he saw that the only activity of the patients seemed to be weaving mats from coconut fiber. He received permission from the doctors to give these inmate-like patients colored pens and paper for a "mural class" every Thursday. Most patients—they were all men—had never painted before. Among the Yoruba, painting tended to be a female ritual craft preserved for decorating holy shrines. Despite any reservations they may have had, these men got busy in these painting classes. Ogundeji had a friend named Titus, who had killed a woman and then been transferred out of lifelong imprisonment to the mental asylum. Titus painted palm trees, horses, riders, and Yoruba kings, all in bright colors with thick charcoal strokes and many enigmatic shapes. There was also Godwin, who suffered from threatening and suddenly occurring hallucinations. Godwin painted his inner world from where he lived, mixing trees with grapevines, olive trees, palm trees, and human beings whose leopard-like bodies could amuse. He placed all these figures among flowers, flower beds, even fields of flowers that floated as if above the ground.

Also present were Demuja, Gbadamosi, Abu, Raij, Nze, Joseph, Oseke, John, and Peter, among many others—all men who had never before held a colored pencil or a piece of drawing paper in their hands and who now portrayed worlds of color, form, and wonder within Ulli Beier's painting classes. When each left Lantoro, either to return to their villages as "cured" or to be transferred to another mental asylum or prison, they left their works of art behind (Beier 1982, 85).

It is impossible to know whether these men were ashamed before their families, since they were carrying out a female activity in an asylum, or if they wanted to hide their art along with their "inner worlds" from the doctors, wardens, or prison guards. Nor do we know whether Beier induced them to leave their artworks or to donate it to him. In any case, these works of art reached—in large numbers—the Iwalewa House in Bayreuth, Germany, where parts of Ulli Beier's papers have been kept since his death. That some of these paintings are currently being returned to museums in Nigeria is interesting. Yet, until today, research on these "mad" artists of Lantoro and their art has been lacking.

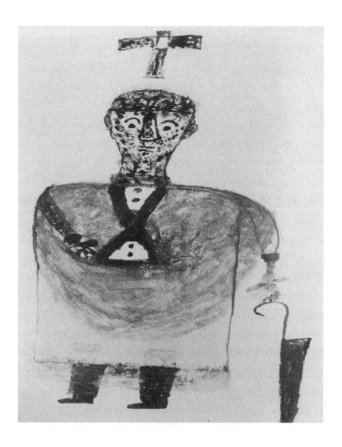

C.2 Ogundeji's asylum friend, Titus, painted this image at the Lantoro Mental Asylum, Abeokuta, Nigeria, December 1950. (Ulli Beier Collection, Iwalewa House, Bayreuth: see Beier 1982, 30.)

These Lantoro artworks, like their creators, are examples of some of the many blind spots in the history of mental illness, psychology, psychiatry, and what may be glossed as madness in Africa and other regions of the Global South. In Europe, such artwork, created in psychiatric institutions by patients, has been excellently conserved and also researched in relation to their social, cultural, symbolic, oneiric, and historical dimensions (Von Beyme and Hohnholz 2018). Yet scholars have so far rarely devoted time to researching African and other forms of non-European *art brut*. In Germany and within German-speaking psychiatric institutions, the psychiatrist Hans

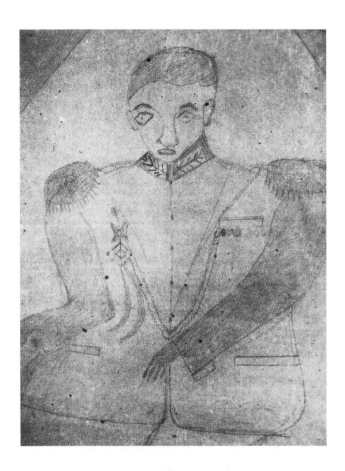

C.3   A self-portrait by Abu, a patient in the Lantoro Mental
Asylum, Abeokuta, Nigeria, imagining himself in this
painting as a general, November 1950. (Ulli Beier Collection, Iwalewa House, Bayreuth; see Beier 1982, 49.)

Prinzhorn of the Heidelberg University Hospital is known for creating a now
world-famous collection of such artwork between 1919 and 1921. By the time
he left Heidelberg, Prinzhorn had amassed over five thousand paintings,
sculptures, and objects created by mentally ill persons from all over Germany, Switzerland, and Austria. In 1922, he published the first—and later
very intensively appreciated—study on the *Bildnerei der Geisteskranken*
(Prinzhorn 1922). Despite a growing sophistication in interpreting clinical
photographs of internees from South African asylums (Du Plessis 2022),

little comparable research on art, visuality, and asylums for Africa exists (though for recent projects, see Fortier 2011). We know little about how often Africa's asylum patients drew or painted, and whether under involuntary or voluntary conditions within the continent's colonial and postcolonial asylums, even if we can sense that professional practices of art therapy in Africa issued in a new era (Fortier 2011).

Still Too Few: Patient Experiences

This relative void in research and care is all the more remarkable in relation to what can be stated for those persons who came to be placed and diagnosed within a psychiatric category of some kind and then often interned in an asylum. Although historians can sometimes sense deliria or read patient traces from their texts, as we see clearly in this volume (chapters 1, 3, and 5), they too often seem silenced, unseen, or as if unable to speak out or make themselves heard.

Yet sometimes, at least at Lantoro, the drawings and paintings of patients depicted their experiences as they communicated with themselves or their doctors and guards about their perceptions, hallucinations, dreams, or feelings, just as some still speak out today (Fortier 2011). Still, too often we are unable to hear or understand their language from self-created images.

In Africa, as elsewhere in the Global South, colonial and contemporary "lunatics" seem voiceless, and this may be due not only to their clinical diagnoses, but because these colonial and postcolonial situations made them ill before carceral dimensions of their care worked to silence them. There is vital scholarship on psychiatric institutions located in Latin America, India, Southeast Asia, and Africa (for example, Vaughan 1983, 1991; Sadowsky 1999; Keller 2007; Ablard 2009; Jackson 2018; Edington 2019, 2021).

When we grapple with the history of mental illness and insanity, the experiences and perceptions of those directly affected should be central, as this volume underlines in new ways, and as Roy Porter long ago pointed out in his groundbreaking studies (Porter 1985, 1987; Micale and Porter 1994). Historical analysis is crucial for investigating colonial and postcolonial societies and their processes of inclusion and exclusion, and also for understanding the perspectives of those separated out as insane, "primitive," or "Other," those too often locked away for life. All these aspects have for some time been basic to histories of psychiatry and madness. The authors in this volume vitally refine approaches to reading archival traces, milieus, and situations to address the perceptions, experiences, and agency of those deemed insane, as in Büschel's analysis of Tanka's autobiographical writing about his experiences and "voices" heard (chapter 3); Quarshie's careful attention to one patient's petition and hallucinations (chapter 1); or Heaton's interpretation of questionnaire replies written down by Nigerian students regarding their concentration problems and the "fag" felt in their brains (chapter 6). The examples could go on in relation to the subtleties and novelties here.

All Those Involved

This book also suggests new and flexible interpretive edges for the concept of the *vernacular*, in keeping with Nancy Rose Hunt, who writes of "registers and amalgams of practice" and "residual traces, even if these are sometimes denigrated or romanticized" (chapter 10). The *vernacular* may stand for a wide residue of experiences, perceptions, and rituals, implying long streams of history and practice sometimes still residing unevenly in contemporary Africa and circling around mental illness, madness, psychiatry, and witchcraft—sometimes visible to colonial and European eyes yet open to being traced in African perspectives, practices, or objects.

The vernacular may signal those Africans or their practices, which participate in an "involvement cycle"—to use Erving Goffman's (1961, 79) term—that labels people or places through vernacular idioms suggesting *fou*, "deranged," or "bewitched," and even affected or altered by such attributions. We may know more about African healing and harming practices through drumming, cursing, and trance, and it is important to situate not only patients and kin, but also the positions and agendas of "witchdoctors," healers, and priests (Geschiere 1997; Hunt 2013).

The history of psychiatry in colonial contexts has often been conceptualized as one of opposition and conflict between Western or colonial and the indigenous or traditional (McCulloch 1995; Heaton 2013). This volume reminds us that such polarities cannot be sustained, and indeed often distort, in seeking the residual and the emergent in relation to an entire stream of facts: madness, psychiatric clinics, commercialized shrines, and spirit possession. The entwinements, exchanges, and translations of actors, spaces, and concepts involved a vast multiplicity of figures, tensions, interests, and power in a wide set of theaters that included anthropologists, psychologists, Guinea surgeons, and psychiatrists, whether punitive, conventional, or transgressive.

Governmentality

Let us return to Michel Foucault, that European master of theories of madness and psychiatric asylums. Yet let us recall less his familiar work on the history of psychiatry and the "totality" of psychiatric assessment, exclusion, and surveillance (Foucault 2006a, 2006b) and instead his studies on "governmentality" (Foucault 1991). From the context of this volume, the "governmentality" of psychiatric illness or madness might be inverted to suggest the vernacular practices of living with and also suffering from "madness," whether through cursing and "bewitchment," conjuring or disenchantment rituals, or with the expressions or other traces of the "mad" found in patient case files or the texts, art, or objects they created in these settings. The suffering might emanate from human subjects, the psychiatric institutions, or the expulsive, harming practices of healers, often called "witchdoctors," to invoke this vexed and enduring colonial cliché. Often enough, we can surmise, the suffering did not come from feelings of having lost one's kin or social scaffolding, thus control of one's rank or life. Rather, it came from something like a constant whispering with voices issuing orders, nightmares, or dark fantasies. So, deep sadness would begin.

Indeed, in the immense wake of Goffman and Foucault, as well as Robert Castel's *Order of Psychiatry* (*L'ordre psychiatrique*, 1976), the history of madness has often been described by historians and sociologists as tied up with social conflict or as a form of violence against members of a family or community (see Tiquet, chapter 9). Such perspectives remain justified. Still, as we have seen, the complexities of grasping the history of the insane cannot be left here alone.

The Vernacular and Suffering

I read this volume's call for studying psychopathology, carceral practices, and madness in relation to *vernacular* dimensions as also a plea for deeper histories of suffering. Utterly germane are phenomena and expressions of "madness"—the voices, deliria, agitations, pains, and feelings, which historians of psychiatry and madness too often have passed over. Yet Quarshie, Büschel, and Hunt (chapters 1, 3, and 10) are among those who render their import with nuance here. This disregard, largely surmounted here, may create the impression that psychiatric and psychological suffering is constructed out of the social and thus, as it were, that madness is fictive. This assumption is simply wrong. Wherever psychiatric suffering surfaces, it can be found or sensed through the voices that people hear, seemingly out of nowhere and sometimes linked to sensing angry ancestral spirits, and sometimes these sounds lead them to kill or to no longer be able to lead their lives with ease and harmony, since feelings of deep despair or misery overflow, assailing those who cower or weep.

Psychiatry and psychiatrists have made wrong and harmful decisions when they worked for colonial regimes, used primitivist language, and designed brainwashing programs, as was the case for John Carothers in Kenya when facing the Mau Mau (Carothers 1954; McCulloch 1995). Some administered medication, when conversations, sympathy, and friendship would have perhaps made a difference, though Wulf Sachs' experience in South Africa tells that suggestions of friendship could yield ambivalence (Sachs [1937] 1996). Still, many psychiatrists in colonial and all kinds of worlds have made false diagnoses and locked people up for weeks or decades in institutions resembling prisons. The colonial record surely suggests that few psychiatrists fought sufficiently against their own social coldness, isolation, ignorance, and racism (for important exceptions, see Keller and Mahone, chapters 7 and 8). Often enough, however, they reached certain limits that perhaps had them standing aside in inaction before faces and sounds of human—and colonial or postcolonial—suffering. Such scenarios were surely the case in colonial times, and they may still be part of Africa's mental health scenes today.

There are many psychiatric diagnoses to be found in the colonial archive, though some still remain unexplored in all their complexity by historians. The same is true with the suffering of those who lived with such maladies or diagnostic processes. It seems that historians should take such matters more seriously, and this volume shows ways to do so. The lack of historical and psychiatric research on diagnostic matters sometimes means not attending to destroyed lives or the violent ways that some were brought into asylums. The suffering of the untreated may lead to suicide, or not (Vaughan 2010, 2012). In historical and ethnological studies of depression in Europe, where doctors found widespread sadness, numbness, and emotional paralysis, or what Emil Kraepelin and Sigmund Freud (Lewis 1934) called "melancholia," a disorder not established with a separate diagnosis until the 1950s (Philipp, Maier, and Delmo 1991; Sadowsky 2021). Suffering from "depression" has rarely been studied by historians or anthropologists, although it was widespread in worlds with colonial and postcolonial entanglements, including in Africa (Field 1960; Vaughan 2010, 2012; Sadowsky 2021 and chapter 5 in this volume).

I would like to advocate something along these lines: in the future, historians would do well to set aside their reluctance before "recognizing" psychiatric illness as actuality (as we see in chapters 5 and 7–10), in order to get closer to both psychiatric practice and experiments, and also patient experiences and expressions of mental suffering in the past and the present. This volume moves in these directions, of course (see chapters 4 and 6–10) and manages to defy easy European–African or doctor–patient polarities (see chapters 1–4), signaling other veins to pursue in future work.

Usually, histories of suffering only glimpse catastrophe or difficult events and their psychological effects in the lives of individuals, friends, and families. In all historical studies of psychiatry, psychology, and madness, suffering is worth pursuing, along with the environments and the experiences of those afflicted. So it should be, even if the sources about such suffering are often rare or difficult to interpret. With greater attention to archival traces and the themes of anguish and affliction, we will better enter into what has been an understated concern in histories of madness and psychiatry, namely how societies dealt not only with Otherness or coloniality, with danger or dissent, but also with sheer pain and seams of suffering.

The history of madness in Africa, of course, can only ever be partly about "total institutions" or colonial mental institutions, as scholars have shown (Vaughan 1983, 1991; Sadowsky 1999; Keller 2007; Jackson 2018), while acknowledging that the topic and the archives could be mighty thin (Vaughan 1983). In the future, when investigating madness in coercive regimes or their postcolonial durations or effects, it would be wise to ask more about the expressions and actions of all those involved in labeling, navigating, and experiencing madness, in the manner often found here with richness and complexity. In other words, we need to investigate those who had to live with the label of "mad" and who may have suffered terribly from their dreams, voices, or visions (see chapters 1, 3, and 10). It is important to include families and friends of internees or patients (see chapter 9) and the intentions and practices of "witchdoctors" and healers, as well as medical doctors, psychiatrists, nurses, and guards in colonial and postcolonial settings. Vernacular healing like psychiatric experiments were experienced by people who, most of the time, suffered. Suffering was a fundamental aspect alongside psychiatric practices and diagnoses, and I believe it should be emphasized more as the crux or a pivotal facet in histories of psychiatry and madness.

Let us return to where I began: the visual or material remains of patient art. Such paintings and the like remind us how difficult it can be to read suffering into or out of a pictorial archive, created in this case by interned patients in colonial Nigeria. These images are wonderful and suggestive, but they often seem more light than dark. A perceptive analysis might pursue this tonality in relation to the total context, the colonial situation, or particular biographies (see chapter 2). Let me conclude with a question that ventures forth from the possible futures for such archival and painterly expressive traces. Along an extensive archival spectrum, what kinds of evidence enable a stronger turn to matters of suffering and the experiences and deliria of the mad? And how will visual—or textual or sensory—sources, whether patient-made drawings, scribbles, art, writing, texts, or even the results of cameras aimed at the unwell, enable new reflections on suffering? We know that cameras entered asylums, perhaps prisons and shrines too, and that the gaze and ambivalence (Hayes and Minkley 2019) found in such sources leave behind a rich litany of riddles about subjectivities seen, read, or interpreted (Du Plessis 2022). In sum, if historians of Africa are only beginning with such visual, aesthetic, and patient-created turns, suffering still needs to be central, complicating all queries in thorny, edifying, and mediated ways.

Sources

Archival Material

Collection Ulli Beier, Iwalea House, Bayreuth, Germany.

Literature

Ablard, Jonathan D. 2009. *Madness in Buenos Aires: Patients, Psychiatrists, and the Argentinian State, 1880–1983*. Calgary: University of Calgary Press.

Beier, Ulli. 1982. *Glücklose Köpfe: Malerei von Ver-rückten aus Nigeria*. Bremen: Edition Con.

Carothers, John Colin. 1954. *The Psychology of Mau Mau*. Nairobi: Government Printer.

Castel, Robert. 1976. *L'ordre psychiatrique: L'âge d'or d'alienisme*. Paris: Minuit.

Du Plessis, Rory. 2022. "A Haptic and Humanising Reading of the Subjects of Studio Portraits and Asylum Photography in Colonial South Africa." In *Embodiment and the Arts: Views from South Africa*, edited by Jenni Lauwrens, 155–80. Pretoria: Pretoria University Law Press.

Edington, Claire. 2019. *Beyond the Asylum: Mental Illness in French Colonial Vietnam*. Ithaca, NY: Cornell University Press.

Edington, Claire. 2021. "The Most Social of Maladies: Re-Thinking the History of Psychiatry from the Edges of Empire." *Culture, Medicine, and Psychiatry* 45:343–58.

Field, Margaret Joyce. 1960. *Search for Security: An Ethno-Psychiatric Study of Rural Ghana*. Evanston, IL: Northwestern University Press.

Fortier, Amanda, 2011. "Art Therapy Helps Mentally Ill Patients in Dakar." Voice of America, December 28, 2011. https://www.voanews.com/a/art-therapy-helps -mentally-ill-patients-in-dakar-136400123/159387.html.

Foucault, Michel. 1991. "Governmentality." In *The Foucault Effect: Studies in Governmentality*, edited by Graham Burchell, Colin Gordon, and Peter Miller, 87–104. Chicago: University of Chicago Press.

Foucault, Michel. 2006a. *Madness and Civilization: A History of Insanity in the Age of Reason*. New York: Taylor and Francis.

Foucault, Michel. 2006b. *Psychiatric Power: Lectures at the Collège du France 1973–74*. New York: Palgrave Macmillan.

Geschiere, Peter. 1997. *The Modernity of Witchcraft: Politics and the Occult in Postcolonial Africa*. Charlottesville: University Press of Virginia.

Goffman, Erving. 1961. *Asylums: Essays on the Social Situation of Mental Patients and Other Inmates*. London: Anchor.

Hayes, Patricia, and Gary Minkley. 2019. *Ambivalent: Photography and Visibility in African History*. Athens: Ohio State University Press.

Heaton, Matthew M. 2013. *Black Skin, White Coats: Nigerian Psychiatrists, Decolonization, and the Globalization of Psychiatry*. Athens: Ohio University Press.

Hunt, Nancy Rose. 2013. "Health and Healing." In *The Oxford Handbook of Modern African History*, edited by John Parker and Richard Reid, 378–95. Oxford: Oxford University Press.

Jackson, Lynette. 2018. *Surfacing Up: Psychiatry and Social Order in Colonial Zimbabwe, 1908–1968*. Ithaca, NY: Cornell University Press.

Keller, Richard C. 2007. *Colonial Madness: Psychiatry in French North Africa*. Chicago: University of Chicago Press.

Lewis, Arthur. 1934. "Melancholia: A Historical Review." *Journal of Mental Science* 80, no. 328: 1–42.

McCulloch, Jock. 1995. *Colonial Psychiatry and "the African Mind."* Cambridge: Cambridge University Press.

Micale, Mark Stephen, and Roy Porter. 1994. "Introduction: Reflections on Psychiatry and Its Histories." In *Discovering the History of Psychiatry*, edited by Mark Stephen Micale and Roy Porter, 3–36. New York: Oxford University Press.

Philipp, Michael, Wolfgang Maier, and Cynthia Delmo. 1991. "The Concept of Major Depression. I. Descriptive Comparison of Six Competing Operational Definitions Including ICD-10 and DSM-III-R." *European Archives of Psychiatry and Clinical Neuroscience* 240, no. 4–5: 258–65.

Porter, Roy. 1985. "The Patient's View: Doing Medical History from Below." *Theory and Society* 14, no. 2: 175–98.

Porter, Roy. 1987. *A Social History of Madness: Stories of the Insane*. London: Weidenfeld and Nicolson.

Prinzhorn, Hans. 1922. *Bildnerei der Geisteskranken: Ein Beitrag zur Psychologie und Psychopathologie der Gestaltung*. Berlin: Julius Springer.

Sachs, Wulf. (1937) 1996. *Black Hamlet*. Baltimore, MD: Johns Hopkins University Press.

Sadowsky, Jonathan. 1999. *Imperial Bedlam: Institutions of Madness in Colonial Southwest Nigeria*. Berkeley: University of California Press.

Sadowsky, Jonathan. 2021. *The Empire of Depression: A New History*. Cambridge, UK: Polity.

Vaughan, Megan. 1983. "Idioms of Madness: Zomba Lunatic Asylum, Nyasaland, in the Colonial Period." *Journal of Southern African Studies* 9, no. 2: 218–38.

Vaughan, Megan. 1991. *Curing Their Ills: Colonial Power and African Illness*. Cambridge, UK: Polity.

Vaughan, Megan. 2010. "Suicide in Late Colonial Africa: The Evidence of Inquests from Nyasaland." *American Historical Review* 115, no. 2: 385–404.

Vaughan, Megan. 2012. "The Discovery of Suicide in Eastern and Southeastern Africa." *African Studies* 81, no. 2: 234–50.

Von Beyme, Ingrid, and Sabine Hohnholz. 2018. *Vergißmeinnicht—Psychiatrieleben und Anstaltsleben um 1900: Aus Werken der Sammlung Prinzhorn*. Berlin: Springer.

Hubertus Büschel is a global historian of development and psychiatry, known for his postcolonial history of "help for self-help" development, *Hilfe zur Selbsthilfe: Deutsche Entwicklungsarbeit in Afrika 1960–1975* (2014) and his global history of the Rorschach test, *Der Rorschach-Test reist um die Welt: Globalgeschichten aus der Ethnopsychoanalyse* (2021). Professor of modern and contemporary history at the University of Kassel since 2019, he previously held posts in contemporary history at Groningen and in cultural history at GCSC JLU Giessen. His 2012 habilitation critiqued German forms of development cooperation in Tanzania, Togo, and Cameroon. In 2018, with his Heisenberg fellowship, he organized at Groningen the international conference "Global Histories of Psychiatry," a kick-off event for this anthology.

Raphaël Gallien is a doctoral student in history at Université Paris Cité, as well as the Center for Social Sciences Studies on African, American and Asian Worlds. He is also a research engineer at the CNRS. His work focuses on the history of psychological sciences (especially psychiatry and psychoanalysis) in colonial and postcolonial contexts. His dissertation focuses on madness in Madagascar. He recently edited a special issue on links between history and psychoanalysis (*L'autre*, 2023), and participated in several special issue projects in three academic journals: *History, Medicine and Health*, *Politique africaine*, and *La Revue d'histoire contemporaine de l'Afrique*.

Matthew M. Heaton is associate professor of history at Virginia Tech. His research concerns the history of health and illness, migration, and globalization in Africa, with an emphasis on Nigeria. He is the author of *Black Skin, White Coats: Nigerian Psychiatrists, Decolonization, and the Globalization of Psychiatry* (2013) and *Decolonising the Hajj: The Pilgrimage from Nigeria to Mecca under Empire and Independence* (2023). He is also coeditor with Toyin Falola of *The Oxford Handbook of Nigerian History* (2022).

Richard Hölzl is a provenance researcher at the Museum Fünf Kontinente (The Five Continents Museum) in Munich. He previously taught at the Universities of Göttingen, Kassel, and Erfurt, as well as the New School of Social Research in New York. His scholarly interests embrace the history of missions, colonialism, environmental history, and the history of health. His published monographs focus on scientific forestry in Germany (*Umkämpfte Wälder*, 2010) and colonial Catholic missions in East Africa (*Gläubige Imperialisten*, 2021), and his coedited volumes cover European forestry in comparison (*Managing Northern Europe's Forests*, 2018) and Christian missions in global contexts (*Mission Global*, 2014).

Nancy Rose Hunt, an anthropological historian of medicine and madness, has conducted fieldwork in ex-Belgian Africa since 1985. Her book *A Nervous State* (Duke University Press, 2016; Martin A. Klein Prize in African History) is about to appear in French (Editions de l'EHESS, 2024). Her ethnographic history of reproductive objects, *A Colonial Lexicon* (1999), received the coveted Herskovits Prize. She also received a Guggenheim and a year-long fellowship at Berlin's Wissenschaftskolleg. In 2016, when accepting a professorship in history at the University of Florida, Hunt became professor emerita of history (and of obstetrics/gynecology) at the University of Michigan, where she taught in the Joint PhD Anthropology & History program for nineteen years. With Achille Mbembe, she spearheaded Duke's book series, Theory in Forms.

Richard C. Keller is Robert Turell Professor of Medical History and Population Health and chair of the Department of Medical History and Bioethics at the University of Wisconsin School of Medicine and Public Health. He is the author of *Colonial Madness: Psychiatry in French North Africa* (2007) and *Fatal Isolation: The Devastating Paris Heat Wave of 2003* (2015), and the editor (with Warwick Anderson and Deborah Jenson) of *Unconscious Dominions: Psychoanalysis, Colonial Trauma, and Global Sovereignties* (2011). His work has been funded by the National Science Foundation, the

Andrew W. Mellon Foundation, and the Visiting Scholars program of the City of Paris.

Sloan Mahone specializes in the history of psychiatry and neurology, especially in Africa. Associate professor in the history of medicine at Oxford University, she has written about psychiatry, empire, the use of photography and visual sources in the history of psychiatry, and modern-day trepanation in East Africa. She is currently directing several interdisciplinary oral history projects on lived experiences of epilepsy in Africa, India, and Brazil. Known for her pioneering volume coedited with Megan Vaughan, *Psychiatry and Empire* (2007), her publications include "Colonial and Transcultural Psychiatries: What We Learn from History," in *The Palgrave Handbook of the History of Human Sciences* (2022) and a contribution to *Decolonizing the English Literary Curriculum* (2023).

Nana Osei Quarshie is assistant professor of history of science and medicine at Yale University, where he is affiliated with the Yale School of Medicine. A historian and anthropologist by training, Quarshie examines relationships among mental healing, immigration, and urban belonging in West Africa since the seventeenth century. His research has been funded by the Chateaubriand Fellowship, the Social Science Research Council's International Dissertation Research Fellowship, the University of Michigan, and Yale University. Quarshie's articles and essays have appeared in *Bulletin of the History of Medicine*, *Politique Africaine*, *Psychopathologie Africaine*, and *Somatosphere*.

Jonathan Sadowsky is a historian with degrees from Wesleyan, Stanford, and Johns Hopkins Universities; he also studied psychiatric epidemiology at Columbia University. As Theodore J. Castele Professor in History of Medicine at Case Western Reserve University, Sadowsky is also chair of history and associate director of the Medicine and Society Program in the Bioethics Department. He is the author of *Imperial Bedlam: Institutions of Madness and Colonialism in Southwest Nigeria* (1999), *Electroconvulsive Therapy in America* (2016), and *The Empire of Depression: A New History* (2020). His articles have appeared in *Culture, Medicine, and Psychiatry*, *Journal of the History of Medicine and Allied Sciences*, *Bulletin of the History of Medicine*, and *History of Psychiatry*. He is coediting *Cultural History of Madness*, a six-volume work (forthcoming).

Romain Tiquet is a researcher based at the Centre Marc Bloch, Berlin, and IMAF, Aix-en-Provence. Trained in history and political science, he has researched the history of police forces, forced labor, prisons, and the repression of urban marginality in Senegal and Burkina Faso. As principal investigator of a European Research Council–funded project, he directs collaborative work focusing on the social history of madness and decolonization in West Africa. He is the author of *Travail forcé et mobilisation de la main-d'oeuvre au Sénégal (années 1930–1960)* (2019); coeditor of a special issue on "ordinary" madness in *Politique Africaine*, vol. 157 (2020) with Gina Aït Mehdi; and author of an essay on colonial prisoners and their use of letters in prisons in 1930s Senegal in Marcis, Morelle, and Hornberger, eds., *Confinement, Punishment and Prisons in Africa* (2021).

Benedictine missions: racial divide in, 75–76; in Tanzania, 69, 71, 74–76, 80–81, 83

Benedict XV (pope), 77

Benjamin, Walter, techniques of nearness, 10, 291

Bewitching the Development (Smith), 213–14

binary colonial juxtapositions, 13

Biobaku, Saburi, 198–99

biomedicine, 21, 187, 191

biopolitical space of exception, 3

biopolitics: Foucault on, 105–6; in psychiatry in Africa, 3, 16, 106–7

Birnbaum, Karl, 99

Black populations, in United States: depression among, 166; madness and, 100–101

Black Skin, White Masks (Fanon), 247

Bleuler, Eugen, 103–4

Bonhomme, Julien, 7–8, 46

Bontemps, Alex, 293

Boroffka, Alexander: Freud as influence on, 97–98; Lambo and, 111–12; Tanka as patient of, 93–94, 97, 116, 118–19, 121–22; WHO and, 94

Bostock, Peter Geoffrey, 219

Botsio, Kojo, 57

Bowen, Elenore Smith, 164

Brahim, Rachida, 250–51

brain fag syndrome: for African students, 200–201; economic class markers for, 182; as form of madness, 189; Lambo and, 182; Last on, 180–81, 190; medicalized narratives of, 181; methodological approach to, 181–94; nervousness and, 194–200; in Nigeria, 179–200; Nigerian personality and, 182; Prince and, 179–86, 197–98, 200–

201, 202n1; questionnaires on, 181–86, 191, 193, 195, 197, 201, 202n1; schizophrenia and, 112; student responses in study, 186–94; suicidal ideation and, 187–88; symptoms of, 180, 182, 192–93, 202n1; vernacular healing and, 187; Yoruba culture and, 189–90

Braverman, Bill, 213

Brierre de Boismont, Alexandre, 239–41

British Togoland, 49, 63n35

Brown, R. Cunyngham, 167

Burkina Faso, 43

Burton, Robert, 298

Busia, Kofi Abrefa, 57, 59

Byung-Chul Han, 17

Cameroon, 94; healing rituals in, 96; as independent nation, 115; lunatic asylums in, 110; Menka society in, 117; Roman Catholic Christianity in, 95; schizophrenia in, 118; witchcraft in, 96. *See also* Tanka, Benedict Nta

Canguilhem, Georges, 11, 282–83

capaciousness, madness and, 17, 26

Cape Verde Peninsula, 257

Caribbean region, French colonialism in, 243

Carothers, John Colin, 24, 285, 319; on depression, 170; in Kenya, 11–13; on Mau Mau rebellion, 167; racism of, 11–12

Castel, Robert, 318

Casting out Anger (G. Harris), 214, 229

category work, for psychiatry, 9, 12–13; epistemic objects and, 11; errors in, 10; reshaping of, 11; Williams on, 20

Catholicism: in Cameroon, 95; Holy See, 77, 89n26; Second Vatican Council, 82

Catholic missions, 74; Africanization of, 71–72; docile bodies in, 76, 86; for Taita people, 215

Chale, Sebastian, 74

Chavafambira, John, 6–7

children, global mental health for, 8–9

China, 109

Christianity, for Taita people, 219–20

Christian missionaries, 72

citizenship: in Algeria, 243–44; in France, 236–37; under Jonnart Law, 243–44; passive, 244

civilization: diseases of, 158; madness as result of, 158

Claxton, Ercroide, 298–99

Cohen, David William, 46

Cold War, historiography of, 7

Collomb, Henri, 258–59, 265, 270

Colombia, 109

colonial Africa: Madagascar, 147–50; mental asylums in, 2, 6; mental illness in, 158–59

colonial Algeria, 234–36, 238–51; psychiatrists in, 237

colonialism: binary juxtapositions and, 13; dominant, 6; emergent, 6; ethnopsychiatry and, 7; Fanon on, 135; madness and, 14–15, 87n1, 149–50; particular and, 237; psychopathology and, 3, 69; racial inferiority/superiority as element of, 137; racialization as element of, 3; residual, 6; subjectivity and, 135

Colonial Madness (Keller), 234, 246

Congo: healing methods in, 5; psychiatric hospitals in, 9–10; suicides in, 4–5

Congo Free State, 304n3

COVID-19 pandemic, in France, 235

Crémieux Decree of 1870, 241, 243

crisis of presence, 282

critical race theory, 251

cults, women and, 228

cultural relativism, 251

culture, cultural capacity and: of depression, 160, 162–63; guilt as symptom of, 169–71; madness and, 151

Czechoslovakia, 109

Dakar, Senegal, 22; under colonial decrees, 260; historiography of, 261; kinship letters, 259–73; psychiatric clinics in, 258–59; psychiatric internment in, 257–73; societal changes in, 264

dance and gesture, on slave ships, 298–301

Danzer, Beda, 88n12

Daston, Lorraine, 101–2

Declaration of the Rights of Man and Citizen, 239

decolonization, of Africa, 2; missionary decolonization, 72, 85; psychopolitics of, 5, 23, 41; racial classifications after, 137; social pathology of, 11

dejection, suicide and, 293–94

Deleuze, Gilles, 4, 28

delirium: in Anjanamasina, Madagascar, 142, 145; geographical content for, 28; political content for, 28; prophetic, 7–9; racial content for, 28; in Senegal, 266

delusion, in Anjanamasina, Madagascar, 143

dementia praecox: schizophrenia and, 98, 103, 115; Schreber and, 98, 115

Denmark, 109

dependence, Fanon on, 151

depression, in Africa: at Aro Mental Hospital, 160; biological basis

Freud, Sigmund, 6, 123n1; Boroffka influenced by, 97–98; on depression, 169; on melancholia, 319–20; Schreber analysis by, 97–99
Front National Party (France), 234

Gabon, 5, 8; schizophrenia in, 7
genetics, schizophrenia and, 105
genocide, in Rwanda, 27
German East Africa, 304n3
German Empire, 71
gesture and dance, on slave ships, 298–301
Ghana: Accra Psychiatric Hospital, 23, 47–48, 50–51, 53–54, 61n1, 63n35; Aliens Compliance Order, 59; Fourth Anglo-Asante War, 54; herbal healing techniques, 54; lorry dreams in, 304n4; mental illness in, 265; money-doubling spirits in, 53–54; National Liberation Council in, 51, 59; Nkrumah and, 49–51, 56–57; period of crisis in, 50–51; postcolonial era in, 61; private medicine men in, 53–54; refugees from, 59; schizophrenia in, 107; Second Republic in, 59; in United Nations, 49; worldmaking in, 23
Ghana Mental Health Authority, 61
global mental health: African context for, 7–9; for children, 8–9; emergence of concept, 8–9; psychotherapeutic turn and, 8; war zones and, 8–9
Global North, schizophrenia in, 104
Global South: madness in, 2; "Medicine in Developing Countries" in, 94; schizophrenia in, 109
glocalizations, 101
Goffman, Erving, 99, 317

Gold Coast: colonial administration in, 49–50; Field in, 13, 27–28; lorry dreams on, 289–90; madness in, 283–84; schizophrenia in, 107–8
Good, Byron, 164
Good, Mary-Jo DelVecchio, 164
GOOD GOLDMANGOD, in "Akla-Osu" case study, 52–56
governmentality, 17, 273, 318
Greenlee, T. Duncan, 167
Guattari, Félix, 28
Guba, David, 240
Guha, Ranajit, 69–70
guilt: depression and, 169–71; melancholia and, 169; in Nigeria, 169; as symptom of cultural capacity, 169–71
guilt cultures, 169

Hacking, Ian, 10; ecological niches for, 282; on schizophrenia, 102
Haiti, depression in, 163
Harrer, Heinrich, 222
Harris, Alfred, 211, 218
Harris, Grace, 211, 229; on anger among Taita people, 212–15; diagnosis of women, 227; on pepo as illness, 223; on possession hysteria, 223–34; Taita people and, 211–15
Head, Bessie, 14
Heaton, Matthew, 102
Heckel, Benno, 70–71
Hegba, Meinrad, 84–85
Henckes, Nicholas, 28n2
Hinsley, Arthur, 77
Histoire de la folie à l'âge classique (Foucault), 150
Hobley, Charles William, 219
Hofbauer, Father Severin, 72–73, 78, 87n5
Holola, Pauli, 87n9

Holy See, 77, 89n26
Horace, 88n16
Hunt, Nancy Rose, 196, 317
Huxley, Aldous, 222
hysteria, among Taita people, 217–18

"Idioms of Madness" (Vaughan), 5
Ike, Chukwuemeka, 198
illness narratives, 25
Imperial Bedlam (Sadowsky), 101,
    171–72, 260
India, 109, 120
Indochina, 136
Indonesia, 11
Inner World of Mental Illness, The
    (Kaplan), 99
insanity cases: in French Empire,
    238; legal supervision of, 152n1;
    in Madagascar, 136; among Taita
    people, 209, 215, 217
insecurity, missionary anxiety and,
    70–71, 87n2
*International Statistical Classifi-
    cation of Diseases and Related
    Health Problems*, 108
intersectionality, 251
Islam: in France, 236; in North Africa,
    235, 242; as pathogenic force, 235
Islamic medicine, 21

Jackson, Lynette, 45
Jadhay, Sushrut, 160, 172
Jahoda, Gustav, 53, 55
Janet, Pierre, 169
Janzen, John, 299
Japan, shame culture in, 169
Journal of African History, 20

Kaplan, Bert, 99
Keller, Richard, 234, 246
Kennedy, Dane, on psychopathology
    of colonialism, 69

Kenya: Carothers in, 11–13; Catholic
    missions in, 215; depression in,
    163–64; Mathari Mental Hospital,
    211, 215; Mau Mau in, 11–13, 210,
    319; *Psychiatric Disorder among
    the Yoruba*, 165; Taita people in,
    209–31
Khalfa, Jean, 170–71
KidaBida philosophy, among Taita
    people, 210, 213
Kimani, Njambe, 173n1
Kimbangu, Simon, 4, 17
kinship letters in psychiatric clinics,
    in Senegal, 259–60, 272–73; al-
    coholism, 262; before entrance in
    clinic, 261–65; family care forms
    in, 263, 265–71; language use in,
    264; mental illness in, 261–62;
    precarity and, 269–71; public
    orders and, 265–69
Kirmayer, Laurence, 202n1
Knox, John, 291
Kocher, Adolphe, 242
Komba, James, 86
Kraepelin, Emil, 103, 169, 319–20
Krahl, Wolfgang, 121
Kramer, Fritz, 220
kutasa ritual, 213, 215

Lacan, Jacques, 18
La Folie Colonisée (Storper-Perez),
    265
Lambo, Thomas Adeoye: at Aro
    Mental Hospital, 95; Boroffka
    and, 111–12; brain fag syndrome
    and, 182; depression and, 165–66;
    *Psychiatric Disorder among the
    Yoruba* and, 165; psychiatrist
    training for, 94; reshaping of co-
    lonial psychiatric categories, 11
land use system, for Taita people,
    216–17

Lange-Eichbaum, Wilhelm, 99

Lantoro Mental Asylum, 312–16

Lantum, Dan N., 94

Last, Murray, 21–22; on brain fag syndrome, 180–81, 190

Leopold II (king), 4–5

Lerner, Paul Frederick, 83

letters, as archival material, 47

Lewis, I. M., 228

Lewy body dementia, 173n1

Lindblom, Gerhard, 226–27

lorry dreams, 284; depression diagnosis and, 287; ethnographic cases, 285–87; Field and, 285–89; in Ghana, 304n4; in Gold Coast, 289–90; translation of, 287–89; velocity in, 287–89; among women, 286–87

Luongo, Katherine, 226

Mabanckou, Alain, 14

Macron, Emmanuel, 233, 236

Madagascar: *Assistance médicale indigène*, 152n2; automobile in, 144; colonial model in, 147–50; in French colonial empire, 136; insane asylum in Anjanamasina, 136–46; insane populations in, 136; legal supervision of insane in, 152n1; madness in, 135–52; medical model in, 152n2; psychiatric hospitals in, 136; School of Medicine in, 146; Sikidy practices in, 146

"Madman, The" (Achebe), 14

madness: in Africa, 3–4, 159–60, 320–21; in Algeria, 136; Black populations and, 100–101; brain fag syndrome as form of, 189; capaciousness and, 17, 26; civilization as influence on, 158; collective form of, 11; colonial processes

and, 14–15, 87n1, 149–50; as concept, 14–17; crisis of presence and, 282; cultural factors for, 152; definition of, 1; diagnosis of, 15; as disorder, 149; as expression of wishes, 149; Fanon on, 135–36; Foucault on, 1–2, 15; in Global South, 2; in Gold Coast, 283–84; historiography of, 159–60, 320–21; history of race and, 14–15; individual factors for, 152; individualization of, 11; as language, 147–50; in Madagascar, 135–52; mobilization of history and, 143; multiple connotations of, 303n1; Muslims and, 246; periodization of, 1; political borders and, 148–49; in precolonial Africa, 21; psychiatry and, 1; psychopolitics and, 18; racial inferiority/superiority and, 136–37; as refractory domain, 26; as reinvention of reason, 150–52; relation to the future, 148–49; in Senegal, 273; on slave ships, 292–93, 302, 303n1; social borders and, 148–49; textuality of, 141; vernacular dimension of, 5, 15; vivacity and, 15–16; in West Africa, 273

Madness Is Better Than Defeat (Beauman), 72

Mad Travelers (Hacking), 10

magic, as subaltern technique, 12

Mahone, Sloane, 77–78

Mair, Lucy, 214–15

Maji Maji War, 71

Makanjuola, Roger, 189

Making Ethnic Ways (Braverman), 213

Malanda, Ted, 157–58, 172

Mannoni, Octave, 151

Margetts, Edward, 211–12, 217–20, 226, 230

Marie, Auguste, 242

Marks, Shula, 5–6

Martino, Ernesto de, 12, 21, 282

masked depression, 159, 173n7

mass hysteria, in Uganda, 11

Mathari Mental Hospital, 211, 215, 217

matrilineal societies, in Tanzania, 79

Mau Mau: Carothers assessment of, 167; in Kenya, 11–13, 210, 319; Taita people and, 210

Mayer, Doris Y., 106

Mba, André Ondo, 7, 46

Mbembe, Achille, 18, 141

M'Bengue, Pape Malick, 257

McCaskie, Tom, 57

McKnight, Robert, 222–23

Mead, Margaret, 105

medical systems: biomedicine, 21, 187, 191; Islamic, 21

medicine, history of, 100

"Medicine in Developing Countries," 94

medicine men, in Ghana, 53–54

megalomania, 83, 147–48

Meilhon, Abel-Joseph, 242

melancholia: definition of, 170; Fanon on, 170; Field on, 302; Freud on, 319–20; guilt and, 169; medicalization of, 172; on slave ships, 297–99, 302

mental illness: in Egypt, 239–40; financial costs of, 269; in Ghana, 265; in kinship letters, 261–62; moral costs of, 269; Muslims on, 248–49; in North Africa, 246; rehabilitation vocabulary for, 270; in Senegal, 263, 267; social abandonment as result of, 258–59; stigmatization of, 268–69; suppression of, 268–69; violence and, 266

Mestri, Archbishop Guido del, 80

Middle Passage: as milieu, 291–301; space and, 295–96; suicides during, 283; as temporal distortion, 284; tonality and, 295–96. *See also* slave ships

milieu, 3, 11; Canguilhem on, 282–83; lorry dreams and, 284–89; Middle Passage as, 291–301; shrines and, 284–89; slave ships as, 291–301

Millar, George, 300

missionaries, missions and: in Africa, 4; Africanization of, 71–72, 83–84; Benedictine missions, 69, 71, 74–76, 80–81, 83; Catholic, 71–72, 74, 76, 215; Christian, 72; as cultural brokers, 68; exploitation of, 88n11; isolation from African population, 72; moral panic among, 84; nationalism among, 84–85; on neurasthenia, 5; racial discrimination in, 82–83; syphilis in, 77–78; transition to secular career, 73–74; violence against African priests in, 85–86; white superiority and, 82–83, 86–87

missionary anxiety: cultural associations and, 79; definition of, 70; failure as part of, 70–71; insecurity as part of, 70–71, 87n2; megalomania, 83; as nervous state, 87n2; process of, 72; psychoneurosis diagnosis, 83; as source of conflict, 85

Mitchell, William John Thomas, 11

Mkinga, Laurenti, 86

mobility themes, 25

modernity, Foucault on, 283

Mofolo, Thomas, 4

Momah, Chike, 198–99

money-doubling spirits: "Akla-Osu" case study and, 52–56; magical, 55; technological, 55

Moradi, Robert, 164
Moreau de Tours, Jacques-Joseph, 240–41
Moya, Lily, 6
Mudimbe, Valentin-Yves, 45–46, 76
Muslims: as behaviorally distinct from Europeans, 235, 242, 249; Fanon on, 248–49; in French colonial culture, 243; under Jonnart Law, 243–44; madness and, 246; on mental illness, 248–49; in North Africa, 250; in postcolonial Africa, 250; in Tanzania, 88n22; tropes about, 245
Mwageni, Father Gregory, 86
Mwariri, Henry, 218

National Archives (Ghana), 47
nationalism, among missionaries, 84–85
National Liberation Council, in Ghana, 51
Native Council, in Nigeria, 311–12
naturalized citizens, in Anjanamasina, Madagascar, 144
nearness, techniques of, 10
necropolitics, 283
neoliberalism, 27; in Africa, 9
nervousness, brain fag syndrome and, 194–200
neurasthenia: depression and, 165, 173n5; missionaries on, 5
Ngala, Ronald, 217
Ngoni clan, in Tanzania, 73
NGOs. See nongovernmental organizations
Nicaragua, depression in, 173n8
niches, of psychiatry, 9, 12–13; definition of, 10–11; ecological, 10, 282
Nietzsche, Friedrich, 11, 18
Nigeria: Aro Mental Hospital, 95, 160, 179–80; brain fag syndrome in,

179–201; British colonial government in, 311–12; depression in, 165–66; economic development in, 181; epidemic of psychiatric disorders in, 179–80; false prophets in, 45; guilt in, 169; Lambo and, 94; Lantoro Mental Asylum, 312–16; Native Council in, 311–12; schizophrenia in, 107–9, 120; spirit possession in, 21–22; University College Hospital in Ibadan, 95, 97, 111–13, 196; Yaba Lunatic Asylum, 6; Yoruba culture in, 165–66, 189–90
N'Koi, Maria, 4–5
Nkrumah, Kwame, 49–50, 56–57; National Liberation Council and, 51, 59; overthrow of, 51; political downfall of, 59
Nkwenke, Nontetha, 17
Noble, Clement, 292, 295, 299–300
No Longer at Ease (Achebe), 196, 200–201
nongovernmental organization (NGOs), 9–10, 105
North Africa: Crémieux Decree of 1870, 241, 243; French colonialism in, 234, 240; Islam as pathogenic force in, 235; Jonnart Law in, 243–44; mental illness in, 246; Muslims in, 250; primitivism and, 245; Taïeb in, 245–47; tropes about, 245
Nyame, Solomon, 265
Nyere, Julius K., 82, 87n7; Catholic Church and, 88n22; uhuru campaign for, 84

object use, for Taita people, 220, 226, 228
Odhiambo, E. S. Atieno, 46
Okigbo, Christopher, 198

Okonkwo, Obi, 200
oral traditions, in precolonial Africa, 4
Orders of Psychiatry (Castel), 318
Oughourlian, Jean-Michel, 17
Oxford English Dictionary, 1

paganism, syphilis and, 80
paranoid imperialist formations, 4
Parin, Paul, 7
particular, the: colonialism and, 237; race and, 250; universalism and, 237
pepo, as illness, 221, 223
pepo dance rituals, 218–20; pepo as illness distinct from, 221; photography of, 221–23
Pinel, Philippe, 237; theory of mind for, 238–39
Pius XI (pope), 77
Plessis, Rory du, 45
popular, vernacular and, 282
Porot, Antoine, 242–43
Porter, Roy, 100, 316
possession hysteria: G. Harris on, 223–34; among Taita people, 212, 223–31; women as susceptible to, 223–31
postcolonial Africa, 2; anthropologists in, 46; Muslims in, 250
precarity, kinship letters and, 269–71
precolonial Africa: Fabian study on, 4; madness in, 21; nineteenth-century explorers in, 4; oral traditions in, 4
"primitive" societies, schizophrenia in, 105, 123n1
primitivism, 123n1, 245
Prince, Raymond, 24, 158–59. *See also* brain fag syndrome
Pringle, Yolanda, 11
Prins, A. H. J., 219

Prinzhorn, Hans, 315–16
prophetic deliria, 7–9
psychiatric clinics: Fann clinic, 258–59; kinship letters and, 259–73; in Senegal, 258–59
Psychiatric Disorder among the Yoruba, 165
psychiatrists: in colonial Algeria, 237; in Senegal, 266; for Taita people, 217–20
psychiatry: from below, 101; in history of medicine, 100; vernacular history of, 98–103
psychiatry, in Africa, 2–6; anthropological approaches to, 25; from below, 98–100; biopolitical initiatives in, 106–7; category work for, 9–13; connection in, 13; data sources for, 210; decentering of, 13; depression disorders, 157–72; diagnostic languages in, 12; episodic data on, 7; ethics in, 27; ethnographic perplexities in, 12; Eurocentric influences on, 21; global mental health context for, 7–9; historical analysis of, 316–18; historiography of, 140–41, 159, 273; illness narratives, 25; madness in, 1; methodological approach to, 23–26; mobility themes for, 25; in neoliberal Africa, 9; niches of, 9–13; prophetic deliria and, 7–9; provincializiation of, 13; racial inferiority/superiority in, 136–37; schizophrenia and, 7; sensibilities for, 13–14; sensing in, 13–14; techniques of nearness, 10; therapeutic insurgencies for, 12; *tradi-practiciens* of, 9, 27; transcultural psychiatry, 22–23; trauma zones, 27; Vaughan on, 102; vernacular practices, 10

psychoneurosis, missionary anxiety and, 83

psychopathology: Agamben on, 3; as biopolitical space of exception, 3; of colonialism, 69; colonialism and, 3; difference and, 4; origins of, 3

psychopolitics, 26; of false prophets, 45; geography of patient gnosis, 45; madness and, 18; politicization of mental illness, 17; scope of, 17; subalterns, 17–18

psychosis: systematized, 145, 150; among Taita people, 218

psychosocial, 29n5

psychotic depression, 169

public orders, in Senegal, 265–69

race and racism: of Carothers, 11–12; after decolonization of Africa, 137; delirium and, 28; discrimination and, 82–83; Fanon on, 18; in French colonial empire, 235, 250; in French Empire, 235; madness and, 14–15; particularization and, 250; universalism and, 250

racecraft, 166

racialization, colonialism and, 3

radical antipsychiatrists, 17

Rakotomalala, Malajaona, 142

Ranger, Terence, 73

reactive suicides, 5

Read, Ursula M., 102, 265

reason, madness as reinvention of, 150–52

republicanism, 237

residual: colonialism, 6; in vernacular, 20

Return to Laughter (Bowen), 164

Rheinberger, Hans-Jörg, 102

riots, 3

Robertson, Roland, 101

Rousseau, Jean-Jacques, 238–39

Rugambwe, Cardinal Laurean, 80–82

Rwanda, genocide in, 27

Sachs, Wulf, 6–7, 285; in South Africa, 13

Sadowsky, Jonathan, 45, 101, 171–73, 260

Saint Alban hospital, 247–48

Saka Complex, 223–27; individual expression and, 228; psychological interpretation of, 229

Sankara, Thomas, 43, 48, 61

Sarkozy, Nicolas, 235

Saro-Wiwa, Ken, 198

Satires (Horace), 88n16

Sayad, Abdelmalek, 250

schizophrenia: affect and, 103; ambivalence and, 103; association of ideas and, 103; autism and, 103; Bleuler and, 103–4; brain fag syndrome and, 112; in Cameroon, 118; colonial studies on, 105; control of, 105; core causes of, 117; dementia praecox and, 98, 103, 115; in developing countries, 120; diagnosis of, 102–3; economic damage of, 104–5; epistemic cultures and, 108–10; in Gabon, 7; genetic definitions of, 105; Ghana in, 107; in Global North, 104; in Global South, 109; in Gold Coast, 107–8; Hacking on, 102; historical approach to, 103–4; as in-between state, 117–18; modernization as influence on, 106, 112; myths about geographical prevalence, 104; in Nigeria, 107–9, 120; primary symptoms, 104; in "primitive" societies, 105, 123n1; psychiatry context for, 7; secondary symptoms, 104; as

Middle Passage, 283; reactive, 5; on slave ships, 293–96; Vaughan study on, 160

SUPERLANDLORD, in "Akla-Osu" case study, 49, 56–60

superstitions, in Africa, 4

Swartz, Sally, 181

syphilis: among missionaries, 77–78; paganism and, 80; social context for, 78, 80; social Darwinism and, 78

systematized psychosis, 145, 150

Taïeb, Suzanne, 245, 249; Jewish identity for, 246–47

Taita people, in Kenya, 231n1; acts of violence among, 216; alcoholism in, 216; anger among, 212–15; Catholic mission and, 215; Christianization of, 219–20; A. Harris and, 211; G. Harris and, 211–15; hysteria cases among, 217–18; incarceration of, 210–11; insanity cases among, 209, 215, 217; KidaBida philosophy among, 210, 213; *kutasa* ritual, 213, 215; land use system for, 216–17; Margetts and, 211–12, 217–20, 226, 230; Mathari Mental Hospital and, 211, 215; Mau Mau rebellion and, 210; object use for, 220, 226, 228; observation of, 215–17; pepo as illness for, 221, 223; pepo dance rituals, 218–23; political aspirations for, 216; possession hysteria among, 212, 223–31; psychiatrists for, 217–20; psychosis diagnosis for, 218; source material on, 211–15; stress for, 209; witchcraft and, 211, 216, 219, 230

Tanganyika African National Union (TANU), 74

Tanka, Benedict Nta: Boroffka and, 93–94, 97, 116, 118–19, 121–22; cosmology for, 94–95; dream protocols for, 97; ego-documents and, 98–103; "Medicine in Developing Countries," 94; schizophrenia diagnosis for, 95, 111–12, 114–18, 121; self-construction as patient, 118–20; self-empowerment for, 110–11; self-expression for, 120–21; vernacular history of psychiatry for, 98–103; voices in head, 93–95; writings of, 96–98, 110–11, 119

Tansi, Sony Labou, 14

TANU. *See* Tanganyika African National Union

Tanzania: Benedictine missions in, 69, 71, 74–76, 80–81, 83; colonial secondary school system in, 73; East African School of Psychiatry, 77–78, 88n15; German Empire in, 71; Maji Maji War, 71; matrilineal societies in, 79; missions in, 69, 71; Muslim population in, 88n22; Ngoni clan in, 73; TANU, 74; uhuru campaign in, 84; witchcraft in, 230

techniques of nearness, 10

theory of mind, 238–39

therapeutic pluralism, 22

Thomas, Lynn, 29n3

Thumiger, Chiara, 164

Tilley, Helen, 123n1

tonality, slave ships and, 295–96

Tooth, Geoffrey, 106, 167

Towne, James, 291, 298

tradi-practiciens, 9, 27

transcultural psychiatry, 22–23

trauma zones, 27

Trotter, Thomas, 291, 293, 295, 300

Trump, Donald, affective temporality under, 11
Truth and Reconciliation Commission, in South Africa, 27
Tunisia, 241–42
twin studies, for schizophrenia, 123n2

Uganda: mass hysteria in, 11; psychic epidemic in, 11
uhuru campaign, in Tanzania, 84
UN. *See* United Nations
United Kingdom, 109
United Nations (UN), 49
United States (US), 109; depression rates in, 166; as guilt culture, 169; madness in, 100–101
universalism: Fanon on, 247; French colonial discourse on, 237, 247; particular and, 237; race and, 250
University College Hospital in Ibadan (Nigeria), 95, 97, 111–13, 196
US. *See* United States

Vaughan, Megan, 5, 303n1; on mental asylums in colonial Africa, 2, 15–16; on psychiatry in Africa, 102; on psychopathology of colonialism, 69; on suicide in Africa, 160
vernacular, 23; antivernacular, 300; authenticity movement and, 21; dominant in, 20; ego-documents and, 22, 282; emergent in, 20; etymology for, 19; Fabian on, 19; in history of psychiatry, 98–103; interpretive analysis of, 317; for madness, 5, 15; popular as distinct from, 19; for psychiatry in Africa, 10; registers of practice and, 282; residual in, 20; for slave ships, 298–301; as social category, 3; spatiality of, 3; suffering and,

318–21; tonality of, 3; traditional senses of, 281; as unresolved term, 20; Raymond Williams on, 20
vernacular healing, brain fag syndrome and, 187
vernacular resistance, in Algeria, 234–51
violence: against African priests, 85–86; in Algeria, 242; mental illness and, 266; by Taita people, 216
Virilio, Paul, 289, 301
vivacity, 15–16, 18, 295
voice, for patients, structural silencing of, 100
voices in head, for Tanka, 93–95

Walsh, Father Richard, 87n7
war zones, global mental health and, 8–9
Weidner, Tobias, 84
West Africa, madness in, 273
West African Pilot, 198
White, Luise, 46, 153n20
white superiority, white supremacy and, among missionaries, 82–83, 86–87
WHO. *See* World Health Organization
Wilkinson, R. A., 215
Wilks, Ivor, 304n5
Williams, Raymond, 3; on categories, 20; on vernacular, 20; versatile language for, 6
Williams, Robin, 157
Wilson, Isaac, 293–98
witchcraft: in Cameroon, 96; deadly forms of, 230; depression and, 157; Taita people and, 211, 216, 219, 230; in Tanzania, 230
witch doctors, 318
women, mental illness and: in Anjanamasina, Madagascar, 141–46; cult activities among, 228; de-

pression among, 168–69; G. Harris, diagnosis of, 227; hysterical label for, 144–45; lorry dreams and, 286–87; on slave ships, 26; stereotyping of, 227–28

World Congress of Psychiatry, 223

World Federation for Mental Health, 105

World Health Organization (WHO), 94; depression estimates, 160–61; health policies of, 17; *International Statistical Classification of Diseases and Related Health Problems*, 108; pharmaceutical guidelines, 9; pilot study, 111–12, 114–18; schizophrenia and, 105, 108–12, 114–18

worldmaking, in Ghana, 23

Wretched of the Earth, The (Fanon), 99, 170

Yaba Lunatic Asylum, 6

Yoruba culture: brain fag syndrome and, 189–90; depression and, 165–66

Zanzibar, 81

zar practices, 303–4n2

Zimbabwe, false prophets and delusional speech in, 45

Zulu people, 229